BEYOND GLASSES!

BEYOND GLASSES!

THE CONSUMER'S GUIDE TO LASER VISION CORRECTION

by

FRANETTE ARMSTRONG

with an introduction by

JAMES J. SALZ, MD

LIC
BOOKS

BEYOND GLASSES!
The Consumer's Guide to Laser Vision Correction
by Franette Armstrong

Published by:
UC Books
43 Danville Square, Box 1036
Danville CA 94526

UC Books publications are available at special discounts for bulk purchase. Special editions or excerpts can be created to specification. For details contact the Vice President of Marketing, UC Books: 510-820-3710 Fax 510-820-3711 email ucbooks@aol.com

UC Books is a subsidiary of Uncommon Communications Inc.
LaserVision® is a registered service mark of LaserVision Centers Inc.

Printed in the United States of America   10 9 8 7 6 5 4 3 2 1
Copyright © 1997 by Uncommon Communications Inc.

ISBN: 0-9656505-0-2

Publisher's Cataloging-in-Publication Data
Armstrong, Franette
        Beyond glasses! : the consumer's guide to laser vision correction /
by Franette Armstrong ; with an introduction by James J. Salz,
        p. cm.
        Includes bibliographical references and index.
        ISBN 0-9656505-0-2
        1. Cornea—Laser surgery—Popular works. 2. Lasers in surgery. I. Title.

RE86.A76 1997   617.7'19

In remembrance of my brother,

DANIEL LEE ARMSTRONG

May 9, 1951 — April 17, 1996

"He had the sort of eye that can open an oyster at 60 paces."

—P.G. Wodehouse

Acknowledgements

I am grateful for this chance to thank, publicly, the doctors and inventors whose intuition and perseverance made my new natural vision possible: Drs. Steven Trokel, Marguerite McDonald and Francis L'Esperance, Charles Munnerlyn, Ph.D, and Terrance Clapham.

This book was made possible by the help of all the ophthalmologists and optometrists listed in Chapter 4, who demonstrated their commitment to patient education in the hours they spent with me in interviews and reviewing manuscript pages. I especially want to acknowledge the work of five of these physicians who made personal projects out of helping me understand the concepts, treatments and patient issues discussed in the book: Drs. Roger Steinert, James Salz, Steven Schallhorn, Robert Maloney and Christopher Blanton. Thank you very much.

An additional thanks goes to Charles Munnerlyn for all the time he spent with me on optics and lasers and reviewing chapters; to the laser manufacturers: VISX, especially Lola Wood and Shareef Mahdavi, and Summit Technology; to the U.S. Navy, and Pat Kelly in particular; to Dr. Carl Hirsch; to Rick Sutter at Frame by Frame Digital; and to Dana Donahue and the Beacon Eye Institute for all their help with graphics and other information. To all the executive assistants and nurses who coordinated patient interviews, I send my hopes that someone as organized as they are will help them with a project some day. Especially helpful were Sandi Chamberlain, Eileen Russell, Melissa Richardson, Andrea Dent, Bridget Van Dyke, Jan Ashton, Karen Gimbel, Barbara Carrington and Sandy Richards.

My brother, John Armstrong, gave the manuscript a careful, perceptive reading from his "Every Myope" point of view and made numerous improvements. To him and everyone else involved I offer a deep bow and the consolation that, no matter how hard all of you tried to prevent it, I am bound to have made a few mistakes. For those I accept full credit.

Finally, first and last, there was my agent, Joe Regal, who shared my vision for this project from the first day and was responsible for its seeing the light of day. Thanks, Joe.

Table of Contents

PART THREE

LOOKING AT YOUR OPTIONS

Introduction

When I was a first-year ophthalmology resident at the University of Southern California, I learned about a doctor in Bogota, Colombia who was helping patients see without glasses by removing and freezing their corneas, reshaping them so they would bend light differently, and then sewing them back on the patients' eyes. That was in 1966 and the work that Dr. José Barraquer was doing then laid the foundation for the laser vision correction procedures that were developed 20 years later.

In the mid-1980's Dr. Barraquer's formulas for reshaping the front of the human eye were refined and computerized, and it was no longer necessary to remove the cornea, because a new type of laser could reshape the eye in seconds. As a result, most of the risk and unpredictability of refractive (vision correction) surgery disappeared. In the ten years since laser vision correction was developed, hundreds of thousands of patients all over the world have been treated with the new procedures and nearly all achieved good, functional vision without vision aids.

Laser vision correction has survived rigorous medical scrutiny and has evolved to the point where nearly any qualified ophthalmologist with adequate training can achieve an excellent result. Best of all, the side effects and potential risks are well known and minimal. The FDA has approved laser vision correction because it has been found to be both safe and effective for solving certain vision problems.

If you purchased this book, chances are you are wondering what life would be like without glasses or contact lenses. Glasses, especially strong ones, can limit vision, be a nuisance, and are useless in many situations. Contact lenses are hard to keep clean, difficult to wear in certain environments and uncomfortable for many people. With either alternative there can be optical problems and for both the cost is continually increasing.

Why Vision Correction is *Not* Cosmetic Surgery!

In my practice, I find that patients don't opt for vision-correction surgery to look better: they want good natural vision so that they can *function* better. Even though most people look better without glasses than with them, laser vision correction is not cosmetic surgery! It is not performed to make the eye *look* better, it is performed to improve the function of the eye—to make the eye *see* better.

If you were hard of hearing, you might be given two choices. You could be fitted with a low-cost hearing aid which would be safe and relatively inexpensive, but you would be dependent on that hearing aid whenever you wanted to hear well. The other option might be to have your hearing permanently corrected with an operation. The surgery would have some potential risks, and might be more expensive than the hearing aid, but it would more than likely cure your hearing problem. Your decision between these two options would take into consideration how well the hearing aid would fit into your lifestyle, whether it would work adequately, what the benefits, side effects and risks of surgery would be, and whether you could afford the more expensive option. Laser vision correction requires the same analysis.

How This Book Can Help You

It has only been since the 1980s that people with poor vision had the option of a safe, effective and permanent cure for their vision problems. With the new options, however, come a confusing array of choices. Laser vision correction is not for everyone. In order to find out if it is right for you, you need to understand the procedures so you can make a truly informed decision. This book was written to help you sort out the possibilities for your own eyesight, choose an appropriate treatment facility, and, with an experienced doctor, make the right decision.

There have been many textbooks written about the various techniques of vision-correction surgery, and I have contributed a few of them myself. Unfortunately, they all have one flaw in common: They were written by ophthalmologists for ophthalmologists—so anyone outside the field would have difficulty comprehending the jargon. By contrast, *Beyond Glasses!* was written by a professional writer—not a doctor—and, even better, one who was formerly nearsighted and has experienced what it is like to go through the laser vision-correction experience.

As a result, you will be able to understand this book. It is extremely accurate and written in a clear and comprehensible manner. It is based upon information gathered by an extensive reading of the research in the field of refractive surgery and interviews with many of the leading refractive surgeons in the world. The human impact of vision-correction has been as carefully researched—Ms. Armstrong has followed the experiences of a wide variety of patients as they progressed through the process. By understanding your options, and the risks and benefits of various procedures, you will be prepared to ask the right questions. I am confident *Beyond Glasses!* will prove to be an invaluable source of information that will help you make the right decisions.

James J. Salz, MD

CLINICAL PROFESSOR OF OPHTHALMOLOGY
UNIVERSITY OF SOUTHERN CALIFORNIA

When "What if?" Isn't Enough

What if you could open your eyes tomorrow morning and see the picture on the wall across the room?

What if you could just throw on your sweats and go for your morning run without stopping to put in your contacts?

What if you could walk in the rain without windshield wipers for your glasses?

And what if you could look at your loved ones without a barrier of plastic between your eyes and theirs?

These and a million other "what ifs" are propelling people like you into doctors' offices all over the country. They want to know: Can the new laser treatments help *me* live without glasses or contacts?

Laser vision correction (also known as PRK) promises to become one of the most-performed surgeries in North America. Why? Because there are at least 75 million people who can benefit from it *and* because it is safe, fast, easy, and amazingly effective in solving common vision problems. Ten minutes in a doctor's office can change your life. It changed mine, and that's why I wrote this book.

WHAT IS PRK? PRK is an acronym for Photorefractive Keratectomy—using laser light to reshape the cornea of the eye to change the way it "sees." This process is described in detail in Chapter 6.

My Journey into PRK

At the time I "got my eyes fixed," PRK was still being investigated in the U.S. I had heard about the coming laser technology for several years, but my local eye doctor, who wanted me to have RK (a surgical procedure involving a knife), told me the laser treatment was years away from becoming practical.

In October of 1994, though, I turned on *CBS This Morning* and Paula Zahn was conducting an interview with a doctor in New Jersey *while* he was performing the laser treatment on a patient! The entire procedure took less than a minute—a perfect primetime subject. The news was that the FDA had issued the first "pre-market approval" for PRK. Final approval was expected to take about a year.

The rest of that day I was on the phone—calling every teaching hospital I could think of to try to find a way into the FDA clinical trials. Unfortunately, there were no open trial sites in my area and all the others required patients to live within a certain radius of their clinics. In desperation I called VISX, the company whose laser was used in the CBS segment, and asked for their sales manager.

"Tell me where you've sold lasers in Canada!" I demanded, almost without preamble. Fortunately, the sales manager, Phil Davis, had a sense of humor as well as compassion, and told me how I could go about getting my 20/500 nearsightedness cured.

I had to wait six weeks for an appointment at a local hospital for pretesting and another six weeks for the treatment. But finally, on a rainy Monday in January of 1995, I flew up to the doctor in Canada. I had both eyes treated a day apart, flew back to California on Wednesday, and drove home from the airport without glasses!

No one ever has accused me of being shy, but I was so afraid that I would be turned down at every step in the process, that I couldn't bring myself to ask any questions other than *"to whom do I make out the check?"* As a result, there was much I didn't know going into the procedure and many things I could have done to make my recovery easier.

Even so, I wouldn't trade my new eyes for six months on a beach in Tahiti. I paid $3000 per eye (including aftercare at the local hospital) and I would pay double that now, if I could afford it. Do I care whether I could have saved $2000 by waiting a year? Honestly, no—and I am, by nature, a tightwad. For me, having a year of good natural vision for the first time in my life made that just about the best money I ever spent.

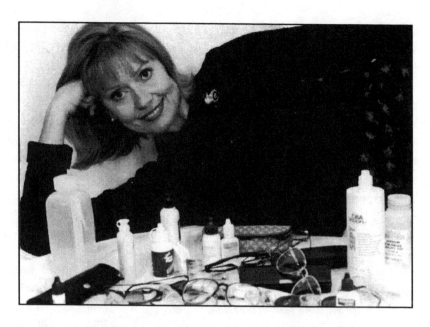

This was my vision "wardrobe" on the day I left for Canada. Now I need only a pair of drug-store reading glasses, for reading in dim light, and non-prescription sunglasses.

Why a Book on PRK?

I decided to write this book three weeks after my eyes were done. I was euphoric and couldn't understand why my nearsighted friends said things like, "Well, it sounds great, but I'd need to read a book on it." I finally realized most people want to look before they leap—even if they need glasses or contacts to do it.

Now PRK is available throughout the U.S. and Canada through all kinds of organizations with all kinds of treatment options. There are doctors who have performed thousands of procedures, and doctors who are just getting trained. There are FDA-approved lasers, lasers that have been used all over the world *except* in the U.S., brand-new lasers just entering trials, and even lasers that are being jury-rigged in doctors' back offices.

In other words, PRK is not something you go into a store and buy. Your results will be determined by the skills of your doctor, the idiosyncrasies of your own vision, and the type of treatment you receive. There are options you should understand before you show up on a doctor's doorstep.

This book will give you the information you need to find a good doctor, ask the right questions, make the right decision, and get the best possible vision for your uniquely beautiful, but currently dysfunctional, eyes.

You Should Be Glad I'm Not a Doctor...

...not because I would make a bad doctor (who knows?), but because I came to this book only with a background in writing about technology and my own enthusiasm about laser vision correction. After doing some intensive research through the medical and government databases and contacting equipment manufacturers, I networked from one doctor to the next throughout the U.S. and Canada. If I had been a doctor, you would have heard only from me.

Doctors being accomplished as they are, are also confident and self-assured in their opinions. As a result, after each of my early interviews I was left with the feeling that I had the whole story—no need to go further. I soon learned, however, that many of the issues at the outer limits of laser vision correction are far from resolved and hotly debated. Whenever I sniffed a little controversy I would research further and interview more doctors until I felt I had heard from representatives of all the viewpoints.

This doesn't mean I talked to every doctor in North America, but I did interview—intensively in many cases—nearly two dozen of the leading eye surgeons who have shaped PRK into the procedure it is today (their careers are briefly summarized in Chapter 4). Many of these physicians spent hours reviewing manuscript pages and chapters to help me get the facts straight.

To learn about the laser and the mechanics of reshaping the cornea, I spoke with all the inventors of PRK as well as executives of the two manufacturers whose lasers are approved by the FDA. To learn about how the eye functions I spent hours with optometrists and an optometry professor.

Finally, to find out how other people have fared with laser vision correction, I interviewed 18 patients—many of whom were just recovering from various procedures. All their stories are told as they related them to me.

So, while I have my own experience and my own bias, I have tried to go beyond all that to bring to you the informed opinions of some of the best doctors in the world, a comprehensible summary of research where it is relevant, and some real-life experiences to give you a sense of how vision-correction procedures affect the people who have them. Your own experiences will be different and, if you feel they'll help readers of the next edition of *Beyond Glasses,* I hope you'll share them (please see the Afterword).

The Quick Tour

If you're in a hurry, read Chapter 4, then skip to Part Two, skim the first chapter so you understand what kind of vision problems you have, read the chapters about getting ready, the procedure, and the side effects, and then take the time to read about alternative treatments for your vision problem in Part Three. Whatever you decide, you'll make better choices for having taken the time. When you're ready to choose a doctor, there's a list of expert resources in Chapter 7.

Here's looking at *you*, kid!

Franette Armstrong
20/25 in California

Is Laser Vision Correction (PRK) For You?

"I have such poor vision, I can date anybody."

—GARRY SHANDLING

24

1

PRK Q & A

Since 1988 laser vision correction (PRK) has been used to cure nearsightedness, astigmatism and, in fewer cases, farsightedness, in over half a million eyes in 40 countries around the world.

In all those cases, and unlike other surgical alternatives, no one has ever been blinded by PRK. It is considered safe and effective by the U.S. Federal Drug Administration (FDA) for treatment of nearsightedness, and U.S. eye surgeons who want to do the procedure must first go through a training program.

By contrast, the FDA has never evaluated any of the alternatives to PRK, such as radial keratotomy (RK), LASIK, or ALK. These procedures are dependent on an individual surgeon's skills, but there is no standard training for doctors who perform them: Anyone with a medical degree and the right instrument can offer them.

As a vision correction alternative, PRK represents a major leap forward in safety, predictability and effectiveness, but it's not for everyone and it doesn't solve every visual problem. Below are short answers to the most frequently asked questions about PRK. The chapters that follow examine these, and many other important issues, in more detail.

What Is PRK?

PRK stands for **p**hoto**r**efractive **k**eratectomy, a procedure that uses a cool-light laser to vaporize a thin layer of tissue from the front of the eye. Because the light is cool, rather than hot like other lasers, only the exact tissue targeted is affected by the treatment and there's no residual burning or damage. Each pulse of light is exactly the same and removes exactly the same amount

of tissue. The number of pulses and their placement determines how much
your vision is changed.

How much does it cost?

As of this writing the cost is about $1500-$2200 per eye plus some prescription medications, and most insurance plans will not cover it unless you can prove a medical or vocational necessity. See Chapter 12 for more information on how to get the best price, and how you might be able to obtain help from your insurance company and the Internal Revenue Service.

How is PRK performed?

The PRK laser is remarkably precise: a doctor enters the desired amount of vision correction into the laser's computer and the computer determines exactly how many pulses of light are needed and exactly where they should go. Chapter 6 explains in detail how PRK works.

How do I know it's safe?

The safety and effectiveness of PRK was proven on hundreds of animal eyes and ten patients with nonfunctioning eyes before the first human sighted eyes were treated in 1987. After that, several thousand patients had PRK as part of the FDA trials. The FDA trials are fully described in Chapter 13.

How is PRK different from RK?

RK (Radial Keratotomy) is performed by an eye surgeon who uses a scalpel to cut incisions directly into the surface of the eye to cause the eye to change shape and become less nearsighted. The depth, number and placement of the incisions control the amount of correction and the type of correction, but the results can be unpredictable—especially for moderate to high nearsightedness—and "tune-up surgeries" are frequently needed. RK is not an effective treatment for farsightedness.

PRK involves only a laser beam which is controlled by a computer, not a surgeon's hand, and the results are more predictable than with RK. In the nearly two decades RK has been in use in Canada and the U.S., a significant number of serious vision-threatening incidents have been reported, in addition to common problems such as starburst effects at night and vision that continues to change years after the surgery. We have not seen these problems with PRK, although long-term follow-up studies are still in progress, and PRK has its own side effects. Chapter 14 discusses the RK option in detail.

How long does PRK take?
A typical procedure takes about 30-40 seconds of actual laser time, but you'll probably be in the doctor's office for about an hour, start to finish, for each eye treated.

What will I feel during the procedure?
Absolutely nothing in the treated eye because your doctor will place anesthetizing eye drops in it ahead of time, which take an hour to wear off. You might feel nervous (everyone does), but the procedure goes so quickly, it will be over before you have a chance to work up a real worry. Chapter 9 describes the PRK procedure.

Will I be conscious while it's being done?
Yes. In fact, your role will be to keep your eye still during the procedure. This is something people worry about, but it's not hard.

Can I have both eyes done at once?
In Canada and other parts of the world this is routine. In the U.S. the FDA currently recommends (but doesn't require) waiting three months between eyes unless there is a "compelling" reason to do otherwise. There's more about this option in Chapters 8 and 11.

How long does it take to heal?
The outer layer of the eye heals in 1-5 days, in most cases. This is the period in which discomfort, if there is any, occurs, but many people leave the doctor's office and go straight back to work without skipping a beat. Chances are good that your eye will be 20/40 or better by the end of the first week or so. After this period, it takes 3-6 months, on average, for the eye to reach its final visual result. Chapter 10 gives you information you need to speed your recovery after PRK.

I've heard PRK is painful and recovery is slow...
This was true several years ago, but not today. Patients having PRK now have a much happier experience than those who were part of the FDA trials, which did not allow doctors to use medications and other methods to increase patient comfort. But even during the trials, most patients felt little sensation after the first day. So if you hear rumors about pain, long recovery periods and other scary drawbacks, try to put them out of your mind until you read Chapter 11 and what real PRK patients have to say throughout this book.

Like every medical procedure, PRK is right for some people and not for others, and there is a wide range of responses. In addition, there are rare complications that need to be understood before you make a decision that can affect your vision or way of life. The purpose of this book is to give you the fullest possible understanding of what is *usual* and what is *possible* with PRK as well as the other vision-correction alternatives. Only then can you make the best decision for your own eyesight.

Can my doctor guarantee a result?

No, unfortunately, because different eyes—even in the same head—heal at different rates, in different ways. However, in thousands of PRK cases it's been shown that about 95-98% obtain enough improvement to be able to drive without lenses. If you end up with less correction than you hoped for, chances are your eye can be retreated simply and effectively with PRK to take it the rest of the way. Chapter 11 tells you more about the risks and rewards.

Is there anyone who can't have PRK?

Yes, several factors could prevent you from being a candidate either temporarily or permanently. See Chapter 3 for more details.

Can I go to any eye doctor for PRK?

Not if you care about your outcome. Chapter 7 will tell you what kind of doctor to look for and how to find out whether she or he is qualified to perform the PRK procedure. It also contains a resource list of the some of most experienced PRK surgeons in the U.S. and Canada. Don't make a decision without reading this chapter!

Why do some people from the U.S. go to Canada for PRK?

Until quite recently PRK was still investigational in the U.S., so Americans who couldn't get into the clinical trials (like me), had to go North for any version of the treatment, and even Canadians had to flock to a few major cities. Now, most people can find an eye surgeon with enough PRK experience much closer to home.

In addition to PRK for low-to-moderate nearsightedness, there are PRK treatments for high nearsightedness and farsightedness which are available only in Canada or through clinical trials sites in the U.S. Other types of treatments now being studied in both the U.S. and Canada. To know what's best for you, you need to read about all the options discussed in Part Three.

I'm farsighted, not nearsighted. What can PRK do for me?

PRK for farsightedness still is considered investigational in Canada, but being performed frequently. In the U.S. clinical trials are well underway, but it is not yet approved by the FDA. In addition another type of laser procedure is being tested for farsightedness. To find out more, read Chapter 18.

I need bifocals or reading glasses with my contacts. Will PRK solve both my distance and reading vision problems?

It depends. PRK does not make reading vision worse. In about 25% of cases, it improves it. Some people who could read by removing their distance glasses find themselves needing reading glasses after PRK. Reading vision can be taken into account during the PRK procedure to reduce or eliminate the need for reading glasses. There also are new treatments designed especially to solve reading vision problems. All these possibilities and more are discussed in Chapter 17.

What if my Doctor says I should have RK, or another procedure, instead?

In addition to personal qualifications, not all eye surgeons have access to the laser needed for PRK—it costs about $500,000 plus $50,000-100,000 *a year* to maintain, and that requires a very large or a combined practice to justify it.

Some doctors might make a case that other, incisional surgeries (such as RK) are better than PRK or that they are the only options available for your case— and they might be. But before you make a decision, you need to understand what kinds of treatments and results are being obtained in all of North America, not just in the States or in your doctor's office.

Part Three presents and compares all the alternatives and offers the views of leading surgeons and researchers. Chapter 7 will help you find a second opinion.

I work outside and wear sunglasses all the time anyway, so how can PRK benefit me?

You won't have to carry two pairs of glasses and switch between them during the day. If you wear photosensitive lenses, you don't have this problem, but your eyes might be increasingly less able to adapt to changes in light levels.

After PRK you'll most likely need only nonprescription sunglasses—which can be less expensive so you won't worry as much about losing or breaking them, and they are lighter in weight so they won't irritate the nose and ears as much. Most important, indoors and at night you probably won't need any lenses at all, so you can see your clock when you wake up at night and find the soap in the shower before you step on it.

What's the big deal? I can see fine with my glasses and contacts!

If that's how you feel, you're one of the lucky ones whose lifestyle and personality are a perfect fit with the lowest-cost, easiest, most predictable way of solving vision problems. You're who the FDA had in mind when they took the PRK lasers through the most rigorous testing and trial process ever before required of a medical device. With glasses and contacts such a readily available, affordable, effective alternative, they asked, why risk causing even a single vision problem?

But even if you feel this way now, your attitude might change when you start to need reading glasses, or if your vision, your job or your lifestyle changes. This book will help you understand the technologies that are available now, and the ones that are coming, so that if you ever need a solution, you'll know where to look for it.

2

What is "Perfect" Vision
and Who Needs It?

What would it be like to have the best vision on the planet? To find out, I talked with Dr. Steven Schallhorn,* a former Navy F-14 pilot, instructor at the "Top Gun" Navy fighter Weapons School and now a Navy ophthalmologist.* "The average Top Gun students are experienced, hand-selected fleet pilots in their late twenties," Dr. Schallhorn said, "and their vision *has* to be good."

What is "Perfect" Natural Vision?
A naval aviator has to pass vision tests most of us never even take. They include measures of reaction time, high- and low-contrast vision, spot detection, far-to-near and near-to-far shift of focus, and night vision. In addition, color perception is critical because of the need to differentiate the colors of instrument lights and landing signals. In a study that compared Navy jet pilots to college students, the pilots out-performed college students on all but one of the vision tests: the ability to shift focus from distance to reading.[1]

This isn't surprising given the job Navy pilots do. "A pilot's eyes are constantly searching, scanning and transmitting sensory information to the brain. Vision is a pilot's most important input—being able to look out and know if the aircraft next to them is their wingman or the enemy, or see the tanker they're supposed to find when it's just a dot on the horizon," Dr. Schallhorn said. "At night, visual acuity is even more important—a carrier looks tiny when you're approaching it, and the pilot has to be able to detect small changes in the angles between the lights that guide his landing. The difficult task of inte-

---

Throughout this book Dr. Schallhorn is presenting his own views, which do not necessarily represent the views of the U.S. Navy.

grating all of this information and coming up with an instant response—like move the stick, or give it a little more power—is where the training comes in."

According to Dr. Schallhorn, distance vision plays a crucial role in tactical flying. Most Navy pilots have better than 20/20 vision, typically 20/15 or even 20/10, and some are slightly farsighted. But even these "perfect" eyes have their limitations: "At night, vision degrades as the pupil widens to take in more light, so some pilots wear "cheaters," glasses that compensate for a little latent myopia or astigmatism," Dr. Schallhorn said. "When lives depend on it, you wear glasses when you need them!"

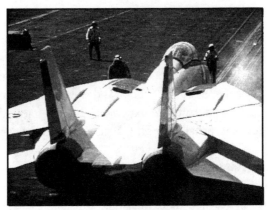

PHOTO BY CDR STEVEN SCHALLHORN, MD. NOT AN OFFICIAL NAVY PHOTO.

An F-14 moments after its landing on a carrier.

Forget Perfect—What's Good Enough?

Most of us don't have to find a runway on a bucking carrier in the middle of the night, but our careers might require special visual skills. Truck drivers, photographers, rescue workers and surgeons all need highly developed visual systems, but their needs are very different. Computer programmers and editors who read all day can get along fine at work without being able to see clearly beyond the end of their arms.

The bottom line is, you need the vision *you* need—not what someone else requires. This is important to remember when you evaluate the pros and cons of PRK or any vision correction procedure: It is possible to get an "imperfect" result, and still come out with vision that is good enough to change your life, eliminate glasses and contacts, and make you happy you went to the expense and bother.

VIEW FROM THE COCKPIT OF AN F-14

Before Dr. Steven Schallhorn became a Navy ophthalmologist, he flew F-14s as part of a fighter squadron, trained at the prestigious Navy Fighter Weapons School (Top Gun) and then went on to become a Top Gun Instructor.

"I have to admit, real life pales by comparison. The flying that men and women do in the Navy is the best in the world, with the best training you can possibly imagine. Nothing can come close to hurling a 30-ton plane at an aircraft carrier and landing it.

"You fight the way you train. At Top Gun the training is as close as it can get to the stress of air combat. This builds in the reflexes that will automatically take over when people start shooting at you and your mind goes to Jell-O.

"There is nothing better at keeping skills razor sharp than landing on aircraft carriers, especially at night. Navy pilots have to do that time after time—the entire battle group depends on it. When you're out on a mission you're flying at 500-1000 mph, but the sensation at altitude is about the same as looking out the windows of a commercial aircraft. It's when you're down low that there's the incredible sensation of speed.

"A typical landing on a carrier at night involves precision-instrument flying until you're about three quarters of a mile from the carrier. At that time you transition to a visual approach. You radio the Landing Signals Officer and say '*Tomcat Ball,*' meaning you're in an F-14 and you can see the gyroscopic Fresnel lens that projects a colored glide slope behind the ship. This changes from orange to red if you're dangerously below the glide slope. From there on in, that's what you're flying: the Ball and the drop lights that give you a 3-D representation of the carrier deck. You fly the lights right or left of center, you fly up or down the glide slope, you fly airspeed based on the angle of attack—and you go as slow as you can while remaining powered up enough to take off instantly if something goes wrong.

"There were times I landed at night in zero visibility and the only way I could tell I had touched down was by the tug on my shoulder straps. You train and train to be able to do night landings and finally qualify, but that qualification ends seven days after your last night landing. After that, you have to requalify. The Navy doesn't take chances with its pilots or planes."

Dr. Schallhorn has been researching PRK for the Navy as part of the FDA trials. "Doing laser surgery is fairly straightforward. It's not like landing on an aircraft carrier, I can tell you that!"

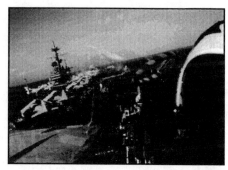

This pilot is making a visual sighting just prior to landing on a carrier.

You Probably Have More Vision Than You Think

Nearsightedness, farsightedness and astigmatism only affect one of your visual skills: visual acuity. Laser vision correction can solve visual acuity problems and help compensate for focus problems. In addition, lasers often can correct defects in the eye when they interfere with visual skills such as night vision and contrast sensitivity.

To see well, however, you need a variety of other skills, all working together to give you an accurate picture of what's going on around you.

OUR VISUAL SKILLS AND WHAT THEY OFFER

Visual acuity
Fine central vision allows distant objects out in front of us to appear sharp and clear.

Peripheral vision
When we look straight ahead we can see about 180 degrees to the left and right. Images aren't in sharp focus, but we can tell they are there. This skill is critical for everyday functioning.

Depth perception
We can perceive the relationships between us and the objects we view, even in unfamiliar environments or when we and they are moving.

Stereoscopic vision
Both eyes work together to create 3-dimensional vision in the mid- to near distance. This is part of depth perception and is required for Navy and commercial pilots, but not for others: You could get a noncommercial pilot's license with only one functioning eye.

Contrast sensitivity
We are able to perceive stationary, low-contrast images (a white rabbit in the snow, a boat on a sun-dappled sea), especially in low light or at night.

Night vision
Dimly lit objects can be perceived and lighted objects can be seen clearly against a dark background without flaring or glare.

Dynamic visual acuity
We are able to detect that an object is moving. This was a survival skill eons ago.

Visual tracking
Our eyes can smoothly pursue an object as it moves across our field of vision.

Focus
Our eyes automatically change focus from distance to near without causing blurring or eyestrain. This skill usually diminishes with age.

Are You a Candidate
for PRK?

Ask any ten people who had PRK why they did it and I'll bet eight will mention water sports. One after another, patients told me they couldn't wear glasses and water ski, they got lost at sea when their windsurfer deep-sixed them and their contacts, or they had a hard time seeing while scuba diving. Some just wanted to be able to swim in the neighborhood pool and know if it was their kid who was falling in at the other end.

Along with the frustrated flippers there are those who wanted freedom from burning, tearing eyes, or a better appearance. Or they wanted time to do something besides deal with contact lenses morning and night.

Still others talked about needing three pairs of glasses (for reading, computer screens and distance) because they were unable to tolerate bi- and trifocals. I heard from a golfer who said every time he looked down at the ball, his glasses slipped off his nose. A runway model said her career was limited because she could no longer tolerate contacts. A would-be cop ended up in the reserves. The head of a major corporation told me every time he traveled he had to pack a separate duffel bag for all his glasses and contact lens supplies.

A suddenly single 44-year old man felt that relearning the dating game was going to be hard enough without thick glasses getting in the way. A flight

"His eyes are so bad he has to wear contacts to see his glasses."
—Unfunny Joke

attendant gave up international routes because of chronic dry eyes from wearing contacts on long flights, an attorney said she suddenly realized during the Los Angeles earthquake that she wouldn't have been able to help her family to safety had she lost her glasses.

I had many of these feelings as well. I also got tired of trying to find my eyes behind glasses that demagnified them more every year, but my eyes were too dry for even the softest contact lenses. I hated the irritation of glasses bouncing on my nose and ears, the lenses continually popping out of the frames and screws falling out of the nosepads and arms. The day I tried progressive lenses was the day I knew I had to find another way to see.

Whether your motivation is athletics, appearance, convenience, comfort or career, you've got company.

THE BENEFITS OF GOOD NATURAL VISION

Even if your glasses or contacts give you 20/20 vision, you probably don't realize that your vision isn't all it could be. If you're nearsighted, the objects you view are demagnified and your eyes look smaller through your glasses than they actually are. If you're farsighted, it's the reverse. With glasses your peripheral vision can be distorted and backlighting and glare can make it hard to see at night. You might find it hard to use binoculars, cameras and telescopes.

Contacts solve many of these problems but with them can come infections, eye fatigue, irritation, dry eyes and difficulties during allergy season. Long-term use can cause irregular astigmatism, scarring or problems from depriving the eye of oxygen. Toric lenses to correct astigmatism can make clear vision a sometime thing. And cleaning solutions or disposable lenses are expensive.

With good natural vision, nearly everyone comments that they never knew what they were missing; they feel much more alert and alive when they have the full use of their eyes. Like Barry Manilow, when they look up, suddenly they can see the stars.

Too Good to Be True?

As varied the reasons people have for going into the experience, the comments afterward all sound the same, and all the sentences end in exclamation points:

"It was a miracle. I was almost blind, and now I can see!"

"It was the best thing I ever did for myself!"

"I wish I could have done it 20 years ago!"
"It was so easy. I'd do it again if I had to!"
"It has changed my life in ways I never expected!"
"I feel so much better about myself!"
"Amazing!"

I know. It's difficult to relate until you've been there. In fact, the co-developer of the first laser system for PRK, Terrance Clapham, didn't have his own treatment until late '95. "As close as I was to all of this, I really didn't understand the magic until it happened to me," he said.

Beyond these reactions, nearly all patients mentioned something that surprised them after they had PRK:

"Strangers treat me better now that I don't wear glasses. It's like being able to see my eyes makes them realize I'm human, too."
"I can't believe how little time it takes to get ready in the morning."
"I can see better now than I ever did with my glasses."
"I love being able to buy inexpensive sunglasses just to go with an outfit."
"Colors seem so much brighter now."
"I can see my feet in the shower!"

Joyce Puckett has been a reserve police officer for over 15 years and before that was in the National Guard—not jobs for the meek and mild (her story is in Chapter 11). Nonetheless, because she was teased constantly about her glasses, she grew up feeling ugly and different. "Even as an adult, subconsciously my bad vision always made me feel inferior, even when I wore contacts. Since PRK I have much more self confidence. I feel I'm just like everyone else."

When I was a kid (back in the early days of television) Clairol ran a commercial with the tagline *"You only have one life. Wouldn't you rather live it as a blonde?"* Except for a brief period in high school, I've never wanted to be a blonde, but I have *always* wanted to be able to see. PRK was the ticket to that life, and it almost *is* too good to be true.

"Many complain of their looks, but no one complains of his brains."
—Hasidic saying

EVERYTHING IS COPASETIC!

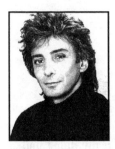

Name
Barry Manilow,
California

Occupation
Entertainer, Songwriter

Pre-Op Vision
-3.5 (nearsighted)
with slight astigmatism

Procedure
PRK with no
astigmatism treatment

Surgeon
Robert Maloney, MD

I contacted Mr. Manilow about three weeks after his PRK experience, just as he was leaving to begin a tour in England. He kindly faxed this reply to my questions.

Dear Ms. Armstrong:
Happy to be of any help. My eye is still healing but there's been an incredible improvement. I haven't worn my glasses since the procedure. Amazing.

Before the surgery, I couldn't see very far. I needed glasses for TV and movies. Onstage I suffered with contact lenses—which I'd rip out as soon as I exited.

I'd read about the PRK procedure for years and since I'm fearless(!) decided to check it out. I was referred to Dr. Maloney and felt confident that it was the right thing for me.

I was nervous before the procedure. I don't need my second eye done, but if I did, I wouldn't be nervous again. It was quick, painless and simple. The staff made me feel totally at ease. The recovery wasn't too bad. Just some annoying soreness.

A few hours after the procedure I had a costume fitting and two meetings with musicians. On the following two days I had two photo sessions. PRK never even slowed me down! I can wholeheartedly recommend this procedure for anyone who wants to throw away their glasses or contact lenses.

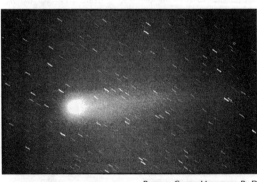

PHOTO BY CHARLES MUNNERLYN, PH.D.

Dr. Charles Munnerlyn, co-developer of the PRK laser, used a telescope he constructed to take this photo of Comet Hyakutake, which Barry Manilow saw in March of 1996.

When I returned for my checkup the next day, I actually saw a woman in tears because she could see so clearly after having blurry vision all her life. And last night, I looked up into the sky without my glasses and saw the comet! Yipes! It's a miracle!

Very clearly yours,

Barry Manilow

IS PRK FOR YOU?

Analysts who claim to know the market for vision-correction surgery expect that in the next five years 5-8 million eyes will be treated with PRK in the U.S. alone. At this writing it is estimated that over 600,000 people worldwide have had PRK. Chances are, someone you know has had it, or is about to have it. Is it for you?

Realistic Expectations

If your experience is "typical" of at least 95% of the people who have had PRK, this is what you realistically can expect:

- 20/40 eyesight or better. This is good enough to drive without glasses or contacts.
- 1-4 days of mild "something's in my eye" discomfort.
- Temporary difficulty reading or doing close-in work if you have both eyes done at about the same time.
- Temporary glare, haloing and/or flaring of lights at night which disappears in 2-3 months.
- A number of visits to your doctor: the day after, three-four days after, two weeks after and once a month for several months after the procedure.
- A regimen of using prescription eyedrops that will start out several times a day and gradually diminish over 3-4 months.

Finally, you probably will have to pay for all or part of the procedure yourself, as most health and vision insurance plans do not cover "elective" procedures such as PRK. There's more on this in Chapter 12.

Chapter 11 talks about exceptions to these "average" experiences and Chapters 14-18 describe alternatives.

A Compatibility Test

Here's a simple true/false quiz to help you decide if you really are ready to change the way you see.

T F   Contacts or glasses allow me to do the things I like to do.

T F   I need glasses only for reading.*

T F   I am happy with the way I look most of the time.

*PRK is not designed to correct presbyopia (the inability to read without glasses that begins at about age 40), so if you need glasses only for reading, skip to Chapter 17 and 18 to see what might be available to help you. Chapter 5 contains some background information on what's behind this normal phenomenon.

T F   I don't have any comfort problems with glasses or contacts.

T F   My contacts work fine in just about all situations.

T F   I can't tolerate even a few days of vision "downtime."

T F   I lead a fairly inactive life.

T F   Reading is much more important than distance vision to me.

T F   I don't mind change, as long as it doesn't upset my routine.

T F   Seeing perfectly is more important than seeing without help.

T F   I don't worry about needing to see in an emergency.

T F   I am planning a career in the U.S. military.

T F   Getting rid of glasses or contacts probably wouldn't change my life much.

T F   Getting rid of glasses or contacts might change my life *too* much!

T F   PRK is too expensive! I don't have money to spend on nonessentials.

T F   I have a strong dislike of doctors, medicines and feeling uncomfortable.

T F   I'm a busy person and I don't like inconvenience.

T F   I'm happy with my vision exactly the way it is.

T F   I'm not that vain!

T F   "Don't fix what ain't broke," I always say.

If you answered "T" to most of the above, it is *unlikely* you would be a good candidate for *any* vision-correction procedure. Save the money and take a vacation instead.

Another Kind of Attitude

Let's look at the statements of people who *are* good candidates:

"I'd rather have good vision without glasses or contacts than 'perfect' vision with them."

"I can't wear contacts comfortably for more than a few hours."

"Every year my activities seem to be more restricted by my need for glasses."

"I'm usually grouchy at the end of the day because of irritation from my contacts or glasses."

"I feel handicapped because of my vision."

"A few days of downtime would give me a good chance to relax."

"I would enjoy sports and exercise so much more without glasses slipping off my face."

"I think I would look much better without glasses or red, irritated eyes from contacts."

"I have allergies that affect my ability to wear contacts."

"I won't mind my vision being in transition for a few weeks to several months."

"I have faith in technology and medical science."

"Getting good natural vision would be worth putting off buying other things."
"I am prepared for the possibility that I might have to have a "tune up" proce-dure after six months or so."
"I wouldn't care if being able to see into the distance without glasses caused me to need reading glasses sooner."
"I welcome change and adventure. 'Nothing ventured, nothing gained, I al-ways say.'"

If you see yourself in most of these statements, chances are you'll be happy with your outcome if you have PRK.

GIRLS ALWAYS MAKE PASSES AT...?

When Steve Floyd showed up in my figure skating class suddenly wear-ing glasses I couldn't resist skating right over for an impromptu interview. "What's with the glasses?"

"I needed a new valance," he replied, deftly executing a hockey stop.

"A *what?*"

"A new valance. You know, a new front. These are just plain plastic—to give me a new look."

"Oh." I hesitated, but then had to ask, "What for?"

"I figured I'd meet a different kind of young lady wearing these."

By this time we were skating back crossovers in unison so I felt com-pletely comfortable intruding still further. "What kind of young lady is that?"

"The more serious type," he said. "More studious." I asked if the glasses had worked yet. "Not so far, but it's only been a week," he said, gliding away.

The following Tuesday Steve showed up, but the glasses didn't. "Ex-periment over?" I asked. He gave me a sly grin. Then I noticed he wasn't skating alone.

Which Front Worked?
Steve Floyd, 35, with and without his new "valance."

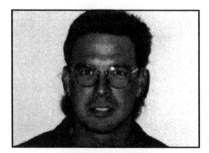 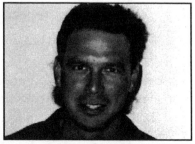

PHOTOS BY FRANETTE ARMSTRONG

SOME PEOPLE MIGHT NEED TO WAIT

Before having PRK, or any vision-correction procedure, your vision prescription should be stable for about two years. There are some exceptions to this rule, such as for those who need good natural vision in order to get or keep a job, but if your vision is still changing, the results might not be permanent and you might need a "touch up" procedure later on.

If you've added a reading prescription in the last two years, or if your reading glasses have needed strengthening, don't worry. This factor alone won't exclude you from having PRK.

There are physical conditions (such as pregnancy) and certain medications which can cause short-term vision fluctuations. Be sure to mention any medications you are taking to your doctor. In order to achieve accurate results with PRK, your doctor has to be certain she can obtain an accurate measure of your vision.

Physical and Lifestyle Barriers

If you have any one of the following conditions, you probably are *not* a candidate for PRK. However, the only way you can know for sure is to schedule an evaluation with a cornea specialist who has a strong background in PRK as well as other refractive procedures. See Chapter 7 for help finding a doctor with these qualifications.

Physical Conditions That Can or Will Prohibit PRK
- Autoimmune diseases which create healing problems, such as lupus or rheumatoid arthritis
- Cataracts or diabetic retinopathy with loss of vision
- Uncontrolled glaucoma
- Keloid scars after surgery
- Severely dry eyes (keratitis sicca)
- Keratoconus (thinning and steepening of the cornea)
- Amblyopia (wandering eye)
- Unusually large pupils
- Age under 18 years
- Still progressing nearsightedness
- Current use of Accutane or Cordarone.
- Chronic eye infections or irritations (must be fully healed before PRK)
- Pregnancy (can cause short-term vision changes)
- Inability to lie still and to focus during treatment (mental or physical handicaps)

Consult Your Doctor If You Have Had
- Herpes Simplex or Zoster virus
- Previous Radial Keratotomy (RK)

Lifestyle Conditions That Would Prohibit PRK
- You need 20/20 vision for your job and can't tolerate less than perfect vision—even for a short period.
- You can't accept a final result of less than 20/20 in both eyes.
- Perfect night vision is crucial to you.
- You are unwilling/unable to commit to a series of follow-up visits.
- You have difficulty taking prescribed medications on a schedule.

While FDA approvals limit PRK to people over age 18, studies are being conducted using PRK to treat children and teenagers—especially for conditions that cannot be corrected with ordinary glasses or contacts, such as "wandering eye." The results appear to be about the same as for adults, but since children's eyes are still changing, the patients might find themselves needing retreatment when they are older.[1]

PRK ON THE JOB

There is a wide variety of careers in which people have to perform in conditions that can cause glasses to break or fall off or make contact lenses impractical or dangerous—law enforcement, firefighting, and rescue work, to name a few. Others require near-perfect vision but allow glasses or contacts as long as the worker isn't too nearsighted without them. Many have no restrictions on PRK or other vision-correction procedures.

If you are considering PRK for career reasons, be sure to check with your future employer before making a decision and read Chapter 12 to find out how your health insurance might cover the cost.

Vision Correction and the Military
If you are thinking about a career in the U.S. military, Pat Kelly, Public Affairs Officer for the Naval Medical Center of Sand Diego, offers this caution: "Don't have any vision-correction procedure performed before you enlist. With current regulations, refractive [vision correcting] surgery will prohibit acceptance into the U.S. Armed Forces. If you have surgery after you are in the service, it could limit your career potential in areas such as aviation and diving."

Admission doctors might not be able to tell if you've had PRK, however. Unlike incisional procedures (such as RK) which leave scars, after most cases of PRK the eye heals so completely that another ophthalmologist might not be able to tell that you had the procedure. In a few cases there is residual cloudiness in the cornea, however, so if you are serious about a military career, wait until you're fully enlisted before proceeding with PRK. Waiting could have another advantage: you might get the procedure done for free as part of your service..

Will Military Restrictions Change?

Will the military change its regulations now that PRK is approved in the U.S.? Because more than 20% of Navy personnel is nearsighted, according to Dr. Steven Schallhorn, the Navy has been investigating all vision-correction techniques very carefully and there currently are joint Navy/Army trials of PRK.

Eyesight is a functional issue during times of war or crisis. A recent Navy study on PRK said that glasses and contacts are often inadequate. Navy SEALs (SEa/Air/Land commandos) operate in such a wide variety of environments, that no one solution is perfect: glasses don't fit under masks and become dirty and scratched in sandy, marshy terrain. Contacts, while compatible with face masks and goggles, are impossible to keep clean on a long field mission. The study concluded that a safe, effective cure for nearsightedness would be of "profound benefit" to the Navy.[2]

VISION IN WARTIME "Contact lenses were a major problem in the Gulf War, where blowing sand, heat and humidity combined to cause injury and infection. Gas masks cannot be worn over eyeglasses which present severe operational problems in the event of chemical warfare."

—Pat Kelly, Public Affairs Officer
U.S. Naval Medical Center, San Diego

PRK for Pilots?

The U.S. military regulations against vision-correction surgery were put in place when radial keratotomy (RK) was first being performed because the incisions in the eye weaken it structurally and make it more susceptible to infection. PRK, which doesn't affect the stability of the eye at all, might someday soon be acceptable by the military, even for pilots. A1993 Navy newsletter speculated that "approval of [PRK] would clear the way. It is expected that most aviation, diving and special warfare careers would be open to personnel who had their eyesight corrected by [PRK]." [3]

As of this writing, however, a waiver to become a pilot has never been granted for anyone who has had vision-correction surgery. "What it comes down to is whether there is a manpower need for more pilots," Dr. Schallhorn said. "If they have more applicants than they can accept, the armed forces probably won't change their rules."

How to Get the Most
from This Book

To figure out what vision correction options are available to you, you need to know your vision prescription. 20/200 or 20/800 tells you something, but not quite enough to judge whether certain treatments might be right for you. If you carry your glasses/contacts prescription in your wallet (which you should until you get your eyes fixed!) take it out and look at it. Table 4.1 shows my prescription *before* PRK:

AUTHOR'S PRESCRIPTION BEFORE PRK			Table 4.1
	Sphere	Cylinder	Axis
O.D. (right eye)	-5.50	1.50	080°
O.S. (left eye)	-4.50	1.00	080°
Type Bifocal			
O.D. (right eye)	+1.50		
O.S. (left eye)	+1.50		

The "-" sign next to the "Sphere" number (-5.50) shows that I was nearsighted—I couldn't see the big E on the eyechart, in fact. A "+" sign before this number (such as +5.50) would mean that I was farsighted.

The next two numbers indicate that I had astigmatism. If the "Cylinder" and "Axis" columns are blank on yours, it means you don't have astigmatism.

"Bifocal" is the reading lens strength, if glasses are needed for reading. If your prescription is formatted differently, be sure you understand which number is "Sphere," which is "Cylinder" and which is reading glass strength. Your doctor's assistant should be able to answer any questions.

What PRK Can Do

This is my prescription today, about 18 months *after* PRK. It hasn't changed in at least six months:

AUTHOR'S PRESCRIPTION AFTER PRK			Table 4.2
	Sphere	**Cylinder**	**Axis**
O.D. (right eye)	0.0	0.50	020°
O.S. (left eye)	-0.25	0.50	035°
Type Bifocal			
O.D. (right eye)	+0.75		
O.S. (left eye)	+0.75		

This prescription shows that I now have no nearsightedness in my left eye and only a tiny amount in my right (which was intentional—see Chapter 17). My astigmatism has been greatly improved.

This prescription indicates that I need reading glasses—although only half the strength of the ones before PRK—but in actuality, I can read nearly anything without glasses in good light—and I'm 49. I test my reading vision once a week at Sunday Brunch by reading the smallest type on the sugar substitute packets. Because of my residual astigmatism, in dim light I need weak reading glasses to read paperbacks or the stock reports—anything with low contrast or fuzzy type.

In the next Chapter we'll get into the different kinds of vision problems and what causes them, but for now, just make sure you have your vision prescription. If you don't, call the last optometrist, optician or ophthalmologist you visited and ask someone to dictate it to you over the phone. They should be happy to give you this information. If it is more than two years old, you probably have a sense of whether your vision has improved or worsened and can use your prescription as a rough guide.

Keeping The Vision You Have...Or Will Have

100% of people in a dozen different surveys rate vision as their single most valued physical attribute. You probably feel the same, so whatever your decision turns out to be about PRK and other vision correction procedures, you should visit an optometrist or ophthalmologist at least once a year after age 40, and immediately at any age if you notice changes in your vision. This simple, painless, relatively inexpensive step can help make sure the vision you have, or will have, stays with you for life!

GUIDE TO THE DOCTORS IN THIS BOOK

In the coming chapters you will hear from a great many of the doctors who have shaped PRK and other vision-correction procedures into the safe, effective treatments they are today. To avoid having to repeat each doctor's background every time I quote one of them, below is a one-stop reference to who they are and how they gained their expertise.

Beyond their contributions to PRK, these doctors gave generously and patiently of their time to teach me about the human eye, the way it sees, and the way surgeons are helping eyes see better. They helped review manuscript pages and offered suggestions to improve the contents and scope of this book. For some, this meant a contribution of many hours.

Chapter 7 contains a complete list of their addresses and telephone numbers along with those of other doctors who participated in the FDA trials for PRK and PTK.

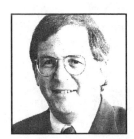

Richard L. Abbott, MD

Dr. Abbott is one of the four voting members of the FDA's Ophthalmic Devices Panel—the committee which made the recommendation for PRK approval. He currently is conducting PRK trials for a new laser and for the intrastromal corneal ring segments described in Chapter 14. Dr. Abbott received his medical degree from George Washington University, completed his residency at Pacific Presbyterian Medical Center in San Francisco, and held a corneal fellowship at the Bascom Palmer Eye Institute, Miami. Dr. Abbott is professor of ophthalmology at the University of California at San Francisco, co-director of corneal and refractive surgery of UCSF's Beckman Vision Center, and a research ophthalmologist with the Francis I. Proctor Foundation.

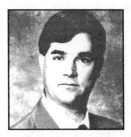

Christopher L. Blanton, MD

Dr. Blanton was one of the Navy ophthalmologists who participated in the Navy's segment of the FDA clinical trials for PRK and has been part of a multicenter trial investigating the effects of steroids and analgesics after PRK. Dr. Blanton received his medical degree from the Medical College of Ohio, completed his residency at the National Naval Medical Center, and held a fellowship in cornea at Wills Eye Hospital in Philadelphia. At the time he was interviewed for this book, Dr.

Blanton was director of cornea service at the Naval Medical Center of San Diego and assistant clinical professor with the Uniformed Services of the Health Sciences. He has since entered a civilian private practice in ophthalmology in Colton, California.

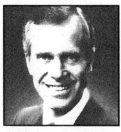

Howard Gimbel, MD

Dr. Gimbel's was the first clinic in Canada to use the Summit laser for PRK and he has been a primary evaluator of four other excimer lasers. Dr. Gimbel has performed over 10,000 PRK and astigmatic PRK procedures, is currently conducting a randomized study comparing LASIK to PRK, investigating hyperopic LASIK, and studying the effects of anti-inflammatory drugs on healing. Dr. Gimbel received his medical degree from Loma Linda University in California and completed his residency at the White Memorial Medical Center in Los Angeles. He holds clinical professorships with the University of Calgary, Loma Linda University and the University of California, San Francisco. Dr. Gimbel is an ophthalmologist in private practice in Calgary.

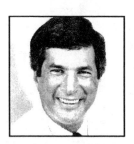

Michael Gordon, MD

Dr. Gordon was the first doctor in the U.S. to use the Summit laser for PRK. In 1989 he conducted the Blind Eye Study, treated the first human sighted eyes with PRK and then participated in all phases of the PRK and PTK trials. He currently is investigating mutizone PRK, astigmatic PRK, hyperopic PRK, and LASIK. Dr. Gordon received his medical degree from State University of New York, Buffalo, completed his residency at the University of Colorado Medical Center and held a fellowship in cornea and external disease of the eye at the University of California, San Diego. He is an ophthalmologist in private practice in San Diego.

Lewis R. Grodin, MD

Dr. Grodin served as a principal investigator in the U.S. FDA trials for PRK and PTK. He received his medical degree from SUNY-Buffalo School of Medicine, completed his residency at Eye and Ear Hospital at the University of Pittsburg, Pennsylvania, and held a cornea fellowship at Wills Eye Hospital. He is associate professor and director of refractive surgery at the Albert Einstein College of Medicine and medical director of the 20/20 Laser Center in White Plains, New York.

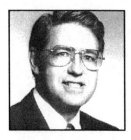

W. Bruce Jackson, MD

Dr. Jackson manages one of Canada's three academic research centers for PRK and conducted the first clinical tests on the VISX laser as well as the first 25 hyperopic PRK cases for that laser. He currently is investigating multizone and hyperopic PRK. Dr. Jackson received his medical degree from the University of Western Ontario, completed an ophthalmic residency at McGill University, Montréal, and held a cornea fellowship with the Francis I. Proctor Foundation for Research in Ophthalmology at the University of California, San Francisco. He is now department chair and professor of ophthalmology at the University of Ottawa and director general of the University of Ottawa Eye Institute, Ottawa General Hospital.

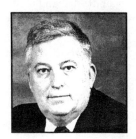

Donald G. Johnson, MD

Dr. Johnson has performed over 8,500 PRK procedures in Canada since 1989, and since 1991, two thirds have included laser treatment for astigmatism. He has pioneered multizone PRK techniques and conducts ongoing investigations into new lasers for the treatment of nearsightedness and farsightedness. Dr. Johnson received his medical degree from the University of Western Ontario and completed an ophthalmology residency at the University of British Columbia. He is an ophthalmologist in private practice in Vancouver.

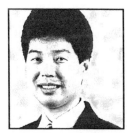

David Tat-chi Lin, MD

Dr. Lin has been involved with PRK since 1988 and has since performed over 4,000 PRK procedures and several hundred LASIK treatments. Dr. Lin received his medical degree from McGill University in Québec and completed his residency at the University of British Columbia. Dr. Lin held cornea fellowships at Louisiana State Medical Center and Pacific Presbyterian Medical Center, San Francisco. He currently is clinical assistant professor of ophthalmology at Stanford University and the University of British Columbia and an ophthalmologist in private practice in Vancouver.

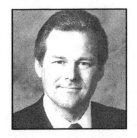

Richard L. Lindstrom, MD

Since 1988 Dr. Lindstrom has performed over 1000 PRK and several hundred LASIK procedures in private practice and as a clinical investigator of PRK and PTK for the U.S. FDA trials. Dr. Lindstrom was one of the nine surgeons involved in the National Institutes of Health ten-year study of the effects of radial keratotomy (PERK Study) and he developed the "mini-RK" procedure which is in wide use today. He currently is clinical investigator for the intrastromal corneal ring segments. Dr. Lindstrom received his medical degree from the University of Minnesota, was a research fellow in ophthalmology with the National Institutes of Health and held fellowships with University Hospitals in Minnesota, Mary Shiels Hospital in Texas and the University of Utah. Dr. Lindstrom is clinical professor of ophthalmology at the University of Minnesota Medical School, a member of the board of directors of the American Board of Eye Surgery, and an ophthalmologist in private practice in Minneapolis.

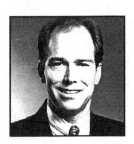

Robert K. Maloney, MD

Dr. Maloney's experience with PRK began in 1989 as an investigator in the FDA clinical trials. He conducted the first LASIK trial in the U.S., has investigated astigmatic PRK, and currently is conducting a trial comparing multizone PRK to LASIK for high levels of nearsightedness. Dr. Maloney graduated summa cum laude from Harvard University, was a Rhodes Scholar at Oxford University, and received his medical degree from the University of California, San Francisco. He completed his residency at Johns Hopkins Hospital and held a cornea fellowship at Emory University, Georgia. Dr. Maloney is assistant professor of ophthalmology at UCLA and director of refractive surgery for the UCLA Laser Refractive Center in Los Angeles.

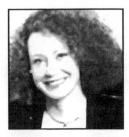

Marguerite B. McDonald, MD

Dr. McDonald treated the very first human eyes with PRK in June of 1987 as the principal investigator in the VISX FDA Phase I clinical trials and she participated in the Phase I trials for hyperopic PRK. She currently is conducting trials for new types of ophthalmic lasers. Dr. McDonald received her medical degree from Columbia University, completed her residency at Manhattan Eye, Ear and Throat Hospital, and a cornea fellowship at Louisiana State University Medical Center. She is clinical professor of ophthalmology at Tulane University in New Orleans and director of the Refractive Surgery Center of the South at the Eye, Ear, Nose and Throat Hospital of New Orleans.

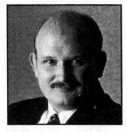

Mihai Pop, MD

In June of 1990 Dr. Pop was the first surgeon in Canada to perform PRK. Since then he has performed over 6,000 PRK procedures at his clinics in Québec. He currently performs multizone PRK for low to very high levels of nearsightedness, astigmatic PRK, and hyperopic PRK. Dr. Pop received his medical degree from, and completed his residency at, the University of Sherbrooke, Québec and completed an additional surgical residency in ophthalmology at Hôpital Notre-Dame at the University of Montréal. He is head of the ophthalmology department of Centre Hospitalier Regional de L'Outouais in Hull, Québec, and an ophthalmologist in private practice in Montréal.

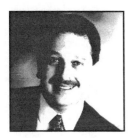

Jeffrey Robin, MD

Dr. Robin conducted Phase III clinical trials of PRK for the FDA study and is currently investigating PRK and LASIK. He received his medical degree from Jefferson Medical College in Philadelphia, completed his residency at Georgetown University, Washington D.C., and held fellowships at Estelle Doheny Eye Foundation, and Louisiana State University. Dr. Robin currently is president of the International Society of Refractive Surgery and is medical director of the NuVista refractive surgery and laser centers.

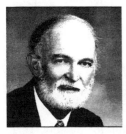

James J. Salz, MD

Dr. Salz was a principal investigator for the VISX FDA trials of PRK and was one of the nine surgeons who participated in the National Institutes of Health study of the effects of radial keratotomy (PERK Study). He currently is conducting FDA trials for hyperopic PRK and independent studies of Clear Lens Extraction for Hyperopia. Dr. Salz received his medical degree from Duke University and completed his residency through the University of Southern California at the LA County Medical Center. One of the few surgeons in the U.S. who has performed every type of vision-correction procedure, Dr. Salz is clinical professor of ophthalmology at USC, has been a volunteer surgeon on Project Orbis (the "flying eye hospital") in Yugoslavia, India and Cuba, and is an ophthalmologist in private practice in Los Angeles.

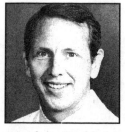

Steven C. Schallhorn, MD, CDR USN

Dr. Schallhorn* was a principal investigator in the Navy/FDA clinical trials of PRK. He currently is conducting a broad-based Army/Navy study of PRK and astigmatic PRK to determine how these procedures affect visual performance. Dr. Schallhorn received his medical degree from the Uniformed Services University of the Health Sciences in Bethesda, Maryland, completed his residency at the Naval Medical Center in San Diego, California and held a cornea fellowship at USC's Doheny Eye Institute. He was a Navy F-14 fighter pilot and instructor at the "Topgun" Navy Fighter Weapons School. Dr. Schallhorn directed the Navy's "visibility of air-to-air missiles" project through the Naval Aerospace Medical Research Laboratory. He is director of cornea service at the Naval Medical Center in San Diego.

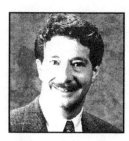

Raymond M. Stein, MD

Dr. Stein has performed well over 3500 PRK procedures. Co-author of *The Excimer, Fundamentals and Clinical Use* (Slack, 1995), Dr. Stein received his medical degree from the University of Toronto, completed an ophthalmology residency at the Mayo clinic and was a corneal fellow at the Wills Eye Hospital in Philadelphia. He is chief of ophthalmology at Scarborough General Hospital in Toronto, teaches ophthalmology at the University of Toronto Medical School, is medical consultant for the Beacon Eye Institute in Toronto and is an ophthalmologist in private practice in Toronto.

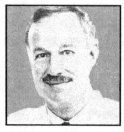

Roger F. Steinert, MD

Dr. Steinert began experimenting with excimer lasers at the Massachusetts Institute of Technology in 1983 and has authored two textbooks on ophthalmic lasers. He was a principal investigator for Summit Technology's FDA clinical trials for PRK and currently is investigating astigmatic and hyperopic PRK. Dr. Steinert graduated from Harvard College summa cum laude and Harvard Medical School. He completed his ophthalmic residency and advanced cornea training at Massachusetts Eye and Ear Infirmary. In addition to his position as assistant clinical professor of ophthalmology at Harvard Medical School, Dr. Steinert has held visiting professorships at numerous institutions including Yale University, USC and Georgetown University. Dr. Steinert is a consulting ophthalmologist in private practice in Boston.

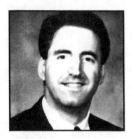

Vance M. Thompson, MD

Dr. Thompson was a clinical investigator in the U.S. FDA trials for PRK and was national medical monitor for all of Summit Technology's PTK clinical trials. He currently is national medical monitor for holmium laser trials treating hyperopia and astigmatism and a principal investigator for PRK treatments of high near-sightedness, astigmatism, and hyperopia. Dr. Thompson received his medical degree from the University of South Dakota, completed his residency at the University of Missouri, Columbia, and held a fellowship in refractive and corneal surgery at the Hunkeler Eye Clinic in Kansas City, Missouri. He is assistant clinical professor of ophthalmology at the University of South Dakota, director of refractive surgery at Sioux Valley Hospital, medical director of the excimer laser center at St. Luke's Hospital in Sioux City, Iowa, and is a regional medical director for Summit's excimer laser centers as well as an ophthalmologist in private practice in South Dakota.

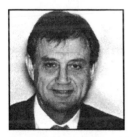

Stephen L. Trokel, MD

Dr. Trokel was the inventor of PRK and the first to use the excimer laser to change the way the eye sees. He currently is training surgeons in the use of the VISX laser and working with VISX to refine treatments for nearsightedness and to develop techniques for using PRK to treat farsightedness. Dr. Trokel graduated from Cornell University with a degree in physics and obtained a master's degree in radiation biology and then a medical degree from the University of Rochester, New York. He completed a residency in ophthalmology at Presbyterian Hospital, held a fellowship with Columbia University and was a Special Fellow with the National Institutes of Health. He currently is professor of clinical ophthalmology at Columbia University College of Physicians and Surgeons.

---

*Throughout this book Dr. Schallhorn is presenting his own views, which do not necessarily represent those of the U.S. Navy.

The Optometrists in this Book

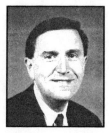

Louis Catania, OD

Dr. Catania, whose eyes were treated with PRK by Dr. Michael Gordon (see biography above), provides optometrist training for Global Vision, Inc., an international laser management company which operates laser vision correction centers in the U.S. Dr. Catania completed a two-year residency in primary eye care and corneal disease in Rochester, New York where he also taught primary care optometric and medical interns and residents in the University of Rochester School of Medicine's Associate Hospital Residency Program. Dr. Catania currently is a clinical optometrist and an associate professor at the Pennsylvania College of Optometry, as well as vice president of professional services and optometric director for Global Vision in Jacksonville, Florida.

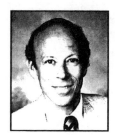

Carl Hirsch, OD

Dr. Hirsch had his own eyes treated with PRK by Dr. David Lin (see biography above) and provides pretesting and follow-up for PRK patients. Dr. Hirsch received a degree in electrical engineering from the University of Vermont, a degree in optometry from the New England College of Optometry, and completed a vision therapy residency at SUNY in New York City. He is an optometrist in private practice in Walnut Creek, California.

Getting It Done

"We can be absolutely certain
only about things we do not understand."

—ERIC HOFFER

5

If You're Not Seeing Clearly, Here's Why

To understand how PRK and other vision-correction procedures work, you need to know a little about how the eye sees, what causes it to see poorly, and how vision problems are measured

THE MIND'S EYE: HOW LIGHT IS TRANSFORMED INTO PICTURES

We see when objects out in the world reflect light. Our eyes detect that light and transmit it to the brain in the form of electrical energy. Then our brain has to interpret the signals and transform them into images, literally, in our mind's eye. All the way along this pathway there is the opportunity for a bad connection, so it's amazing most of us see as well as we do.

There are only three parts of the eye you need to know about to understand how laser vision correction works:

The Cornea

This is the most important part of the eye to a laser surgeon, because it is the part that can be reshaped easily to compensate for vision problems. The cornea is a thin, clear dome that perches on the front of the eyeball like a cover. Because it protects the inner eye from injury, it has more nerve endings than just

---

"The eye sees only what the mind is prepared to comprehend."

—Henri Bergson

about any other part of the body. It also contains a UV filter to help protect the eye from sun damage.

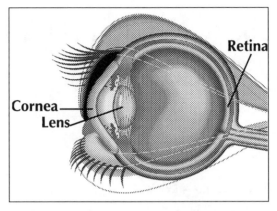

FIGURE 5.1   Diagram of the eye.

The cornea holds up the **tear film**: a water, oil and protein layer that makes the surface of the eye completely smooth, like a highly polished lens. Less than a third the thickness of a single blood cell, the tear film is crucial to vision because it picks up light waves and bends them so they enter the cornea at an angle. Have you ever had the experience of staring at something for too long, and finding your vision becoming blurred? This was because the tear film dried out. A blink restores it. One of the reasons people with dry eyes have trouble with contact lenses is because the lens either absorbs the tear film or becomes embedded in it, instead of floating on top of it.

Just below the tear film is the **epithelium**, a thin layer of cells which protects the cornea from injury. Like enamel on a tooth, the epithelium covers the nerve endings in the cornea so you and your eye can hang out in the sun, wind and cold.

The inner cornea is made up mostly of collagen fibers. By making tiny changes to the shape of the cornea, surgeons can change the way light is transmitted by the tear film, improving the way you see.

Behind the cornea is the **pupil** which opens and closes to control the amount of light that enters the eye. The **iris** is the ring around the pupil that gives us our eye color.

The Lens

About the size of a thumbtack, the lens picks up light as it comes through the cornea and finetunes the angle it takes as it continues through the eye.

Focusing muscles surround the lens to bring images into focus—just like the lens of a camera does when you twist it. When near images need to be seen, the focusing muscles contract to make the lens thick in the center, like a magnifying glass. When distant objects need to be seen, the muscles relax and the lens becomes thinner in the center, like glasses for distance. This function is automatic but diminishes with age.

If the lens becomes cloudy, as with cataracts, the image doesn't transmit clearly, if at all.

The Retina

The retina, at the very back of the eyeball, is like film in a camera. As light passes through the lens and comes to rest at the retina, the retina records it, converts it into an electrical signal, and then relays it to the optic nerve which takes it to the brain. What we see is a direct result of how focused the light is when it reaches the retina.

The retina is made up of ten layers, one of which contains cones for differentiating colors and all the cones and rods for seeing in bright as well as dim light. Like camera film, the retina can become damaged from overexposure to sunlight. This is why we should all wear UV-filtered sunglasses when we're outside on bright days and *never* look directly at the sun.

WHAT IS GOOD NATURAL VISION?

Good natural vision occurs when light comes through the cornea and focuses at a single point right at the retina. When you want to shift from distance to near vision, or from near to far, the eye muscles automatically accomodate to make the lens bend light a little more or less. For good natural vision, all parts of the visual system have to work together: from the tear film to the brain (Figure 5.2).

WHAT IS BLINDNESS?

There are two types of blindness. The first is "total" blindness, where no image is perceived. This usually is caused by damage to the back of the retina, injury to the optical nerve, or trauma to the visual center of the of the brain.

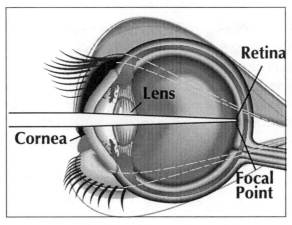

COURTESY OF BEACON EYE INSTITUTE

FIGURE 5.2   An eye with perfect visual acuity. Light is refracted by the tear film and then the lens to come to focus at a single point exactly at the back of the retina.

In rare cases psychological trauma can result in "hysterical blindness," which is quite real even though the causes aren't physical. A case of hysterical blindness is described in Chaper 13.

The second type of blindness is partial, or "legal," blindness—which is defined as best-corrected vision of 20/200 or worse. In other words, *with* glasses or contacts, the *best* the person can see from 20 feet is what a person with 20/20 vision can see from 200 feet.

The causes of partial blindness can be the same as those which cause total blindness plus clouding or scarring of the cornea, cataracts on the lens, and other eye diseases. For some of these conditions, treatments such as PTK and other types of laser surgeries, lens implants or cornea transplants can offer dramatic improvement. Chapter 19 describes some of the therapeutic treatments of the cornea now being performed with the laser used for PRK.

VISION ALERT!   Good visual acuity is possible only when light waves come together at a tiny spot on the retina—called the *macula lutea* that is about 1/20 of an inch in diameter. Macular degeneration erodes the macula and can result in the loss of all but peripheral (side) vision. It is the major cause of blindness in people over 60 but its most destructive form, if caught soon enough, can be treated with a laser—another good reason to have your eyes checked every year.

Understanding Visual Acuity

Everyone has seen the Snellen Chart: letters or numbers that you read with each eye covered, then with both eyes together. The Snellen Chart tests *visual acuity*, or sharpness of distance vision.

Having 20/20 eyesight simply is the ability to see the 20/20 line from a distance of 20 feet (see Figure 5.3). Does this mean perfect vision? Actually, it is possible to have a vision problem and still read the 20/20 line. And, as we saw in Chapter 2, visual acuity is only one of many important visual skills.

Only about four out of ten of us have natural visual acuity of 20/20 or better. The rest of us either are nearsighted (myopic) or farsighted (hyperopic). With either of these conditions we can have astigmatism or we can have astigmatism alone.

If you have 20/200 vision, you have to be at 20 feet to see something a person with 20/20 vision can see from 200 feet. In other words, you have to stand *nearer* the object to see it.If your vision is 20/10 you can see at 20 feet what someone with 20/20 vision can only see from 10 feet.

Best Corrected Vision versus *Uncorrected Vision*

If you wear glasses or contacts, your best-corrected acuity is the line you can see on the Snellen Chart with your glasses or contacts *on*. Your *uncorrected* acuity is what you can see with them off.

The goal of PRK and all other vision-correction procedures is to improve your uncorrected acuity enough so you won't need glasses or contacts for most of your daily activities.

How Vision Problems Are Measured

Leaving the extremes of perfect acuity and blindness, we come to ordinary vision problems that can be corrected with glasses and contacts. To be accurate and less confusing later on, we'll call these "refractive" problems because they all are caused when the light entering the eye is bent (refracted) too little or too much to allow sharp vision.

I suggested in Chapter 4 that you obtain a copy of your vision prescription. To determine that prescription, your doctor used set of trial lenses to see how much power needed to be added to, or subtracted from, your eye in order for you to see the eye chart clearly. The lens power he ended up with was the one that would best move the point where light naturally focuses in your eye to the back of the retina when you view the chart from 20 feet. The distance between the natural place light comes to focus in your eye and the retina is called called

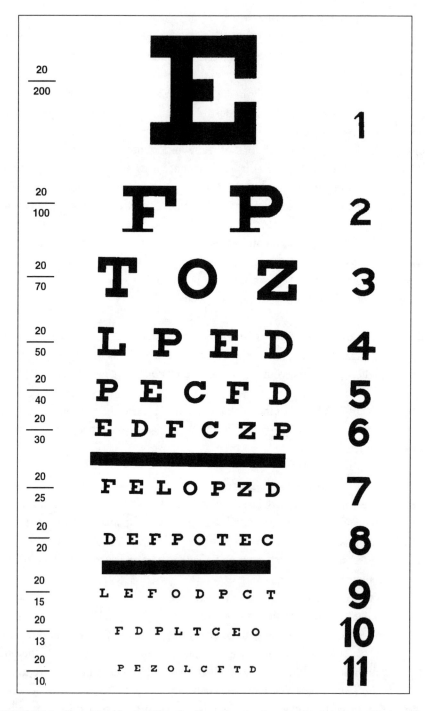

FIGURE 5.3 The original Snellen Chart for measuring visual acuity, shown here, was designed in the late 1800s by Hermann Snellen. Later versions display non-Western alphabets, numbers, or are language-free (use shapes instead of letters).

your *refractive error.* If there is no error (light comes to a focus right at your retina), your "sphere" reading will be 0.0, or "plano." If there is any error, it is expressed in terms of "diopters." So with this prescription:

Sphere
_____
O.D. -5.50 D   O.S. -4.50 D

I had 5½ diopters of nearsightedness in the right eye and 4½ diopters in the left eye. With both eyes together my uncorrected acuity was about 20/400. After PRK it was 20/25 and 20/20.

Refractive error is important, because that's what tells your doctor how much correction you need to achieve good functional vision: Acuity is the measure of your functional distance vision.

Let's see how all this works with the three types of refractive vision problems: nearsightedness, farsightedness and astigmatism.

NEARSIGHTEDNESS (MYOPIA)

The nearsighted person (myope) can't see images clearly at a distance: They look fuzzy or blurred. This is because the myopic eye cannot refract light all the way back to the retina. It comes to a focus before it gets there and then fans out again. By the time it reaches the retina it is out of focus. I think the English have it right: they call nearsightedness "shortsightedness" because the focal point falls *short* of the retina (Figure 5.4).

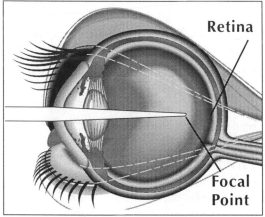

COURTESY OF BEACON EYE INSTITUTE

FIGURE 5.4   Nearsighted eyes are too long so light comes to a focus before it arrives at the retina.

WHO IS NEARSIGHTED?   Nearsightedness, while it affects over 25% of the population, is not an equal-opportunity disability. If you're nearsighted you are more likely to be:
- Older rather than younger
- Female rather than male
- Wealthier rather than poorer
- More educated rather than less
- More likely Caucasian than Black
- More likely Asian than any other group.[1,2]

How Nearsightedness Affects Vision

A nearsighted prescription always has a minus sign in front of it because the prescribed lens *subtracts* refractive power from the eye to bring light to a focus farther back. These lenses are thinner in the center than they are at the sides and they demagnify the appearance of the eye as well as everything the eye sees.

One diopter of nearsightedness is equal to about one meter of focusing power. If your vision was -3.0 D, your eye would naturally be focused about ⅓ meter (13") out in front of you—perfect for reading. Anything farther out would become blurry unless you were wearing lenses to correct for this refractive error.

If you had -3.0 D, the smallest line you could read on the Snellen Chart from 20 feet probably would be the 20/200 line, although this would depend on the size of your pupils and the amount of ambient light.

Table 5.2 shows the approximate conversion of diopters to visual acuity as measured on the Snellen Chart—with a hypothetical extension beyond the chart's upper limit of 20/200.

A "high myope" has a focal point that falls quite short of the retina, and a refraction over -7.0 diopters. A "low myope" has a focal point almost to the retina and has a refraction below -3.50.

Very sharp visual acuity—better than 20/20—is possible if the optical system (cornea, lens and retina) is better than average. For the same reason, some people with any given refractive error might have better than expected visual acuity.

A Little Myopia Can Go a Long Way

With slight nearsightedness (20/40) you can drive in most states. Most myopes don't feel they a visual problem until they are worse than this.

About 95-98% of nearsighted patients who have PRK achieve uncorrected acuity of 20/40 or better, and most of them are improved all the way to 20/20.

HOW REFRACTION RELATES TO ACUITY			Table 5.2
	Refraction		**Acuity**
No refractive error	0.0 D	=	20/20 +
	-0.5 D	=	20/30
	-1.0 D	=	20/50
Low myopia	-1.5 D	=	20/80
	-2.0 D	=	20/100
	-2.5 D	=	20/150
	-3.0 D	=	20/200
	-3.5 D	=	20/300
	-4.0 D	=	20/400
Moderate myopia	-5.0 D	=	20/500
	-5.5 D	=	20/550
	-6.0 D	=	20/600
	-7.0 D	=	20/700
High myopia	-8.0 D	=	20/800
	...and higher		

The Permanent Cure for Nearsightedness

Doctors have known for over a century that myopia could be cured by reducing the distance between the front of the cornea and the back of the retina, and that the easiest way to do this is to flatten the center of the cornea. But it has taken most of that time and some amazing technology before doctors had a way to do this safely and predictably.

PRK, and related procedures, have been used to treat nearsightedness all the way up to -30. Treatment options for high myopia are described in Chapter 15.

HOW NEARSIGHTED ARE WE?   Of the 75 million myopes in North America, 80% have less than 6.0 diopters of nearsightedness. Right eyes tend to be more nearsighted than left eyes.[3]

WHAT CAUSES·MYOPIA?

We know why nearsighted eyes have trouble seeing, but there appears to be more than one cause of the problem. Some children are nearsighted from birth, which fits neatly with the explanation that the eye is too long. Others become progressively nearsighted throughout childhood, but is this because the eye is changing shape, or because the child is using her eyes differently? Nearsighted parents tend to have nearsighted children, but how do you separate genetics from environment? And some people don't become nearsighted until long after their eyes have stopped growing. How is this possible?

To learn more about the different theories of myopia, I talked with Dr. Martin Banks, professor of optometry and psychology at the University of California at Berkeley, and Dr. Carl Hirsch, an optometrist in Walnut Creek, California.

The Self-Regulating Eye and Progressive Myopia

"Some believe that the eye has a self-regulating mechanism which assures it will grow to the right length," said Dr. Banks. "If the eyes start out farsighted, as most kids' do, the child finds he has to pull his focus in to see clearly. This might exert a force on the eye and make it longer. Thus the child becomes myopic."

Why are so many schoolkids just fine until about third grade and then they suddenly start squinting? "That's about the time they start reading," Dr. Banks said. "Their doctors prescribe distance glasses and guess what? They need stronger glasses next year. This happens because the child, whose natural focal point might be one foot, suddenly has to focus as if it were 20 feet when he wants to read. 'Progressive myopia' is actually the result of mismanaging the problem."

Dr. Hirsch agrees. "I wish kids who need distance glasses would wear bifocals with no prescription in the bottom half, but many parents won't permit it. At the very least children should take their distance glasses off to read."

Dr. Roger Steinert cautions, however, "this theory hasn't yet been proven and is the subject of much debate."

Nature *vs* Nurture

The "environmental" explanation is that our eyes were designed to gaze out on fields, not stare at computer screens or do crossword puzzles. "Nearsightedness is increasing all over the world," said Dr. Banks, "and it's probably because more people are spending more time doing close-in work. Studies show that Eskimos who never went to formal school are not nearsighted, but their grandchildren who sit in classrooms all day, are. It's no secret that people with formal education are much more likely to be nearsighted."

Myopic Bookworms?
Some people get all the way through college with no vision problems and find themselves needing distance glasses in graduate school. What's going on? "For the focusing muscles in a normal eye, spending hours reading is like carrying a heavy suitcase five blocks," Dr. Hirsch said. "When you stop, your muscles remain tight and it takes awhile for them to loosen their grip.

"If a 22-year old isn't susceptible to this kind of stress, she can spend six hours reading, then look up and her eyes will relax automatically to allow her to see into the distance," Dr. Hirsch explains, "then they refocus when she looks back down at her book. Others have a visual system that no longer can deliver both near and far vision equally well. Their eye muscles go into permanent spasm and they can only focus images that are close. So they get glasses for distance, wear them to read, the eye muscles cramp even more, and they need even stronger glasses to see into the distance.

"This phenomenon leads to the belief that wearing glasses will weaken the eyes and make them dependent on glasses. The right glasses worn in the wrong way can!"

FARSIGHTEDNESS (HYPEROPIA)

I'll give you a clue to what causes this: The English call it "longsightedness." That's because the eyeball either is too short, or the refractive powers of the cornea and lens are too weak, so the light enters the eye and goes all the way to the retina without ever coming to a single point. The place at which light waves would come to focus is *longer* than the eyeball. (Figure 5.5)

It's a common misconception that farsighted people (hyperopes) can see much farther than myopes. If that were true, however, an extremely farsighted person could see ants on a mountaintop from the valley below, and an extremely nearsighted person could see the cells in a fingernail. Obviously, nobody has telescopic or microscopic vision—and it would be impractical if they did!

In actuality, moderate to severe farsightedness can be an even bigger handicap than nearsightedness because both near and distant images are blurred. Hyperopes can need reading glasses much sooner than anyone else.

How Farsightedness Affects Vision
A farsighted prescription always has a plus sign in front of it because corrective lenses have to *add* refractive power to bring the light to a point at the retina. These lenses are thicker in the middle than at the edges and magnify the eyes as well as everything the eye sees.

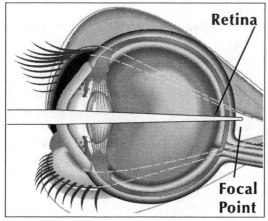

Figure 5.5 Farsighted eyes are too short, or the refractive power of the cornea and lens is too weak, so light waves aren't fully focused when they reach the back of the retina.

Young people can be quite farsighted without experiencing any vision problems. In fact, Navy pilots are allowed up to 3.0 diopters of farsightedness. As hyperopes get into their thirties, though, they begin to have trouble focusing on objects close to them: Someone who is farsighted has no natural focal point. Without focusing capabilities, everything far *and* near is out of focus. In order to see, their eye's focusing muscles have to "tune in" the light waves, and the closer the object, the more tuning power is needed.

Once the eye is fully grown (in the mid-teen years, usually) farsightedness doesn't increase. However, as hyperopes get older, their focusing ability diminishes, and they need glasses or contacts to see distant images, and reading glasses to read.

Farsightedness is harder to live with than nearsightedness because the focusing muscles have to work in both directions: for near and distance viewing. This can cause headaches and eyestrain which are easily solved with glasses or contacts.

The Permanent Cure for Farsightedness

To cure hyperopia, we have to increase the distance from the front of the cornea to the back of the retina. This is a tougher problem than correcting myopia, because no one has figured out a way to make the eyeball physically longer. Instead, research has focused on steepening the curve of the cornea to change the way the tear film refracts light.

PRK for hyperopia (HPRK) is considered investigational in Canada and is in FDA clinical trials in the U.S. In addition, another type of laser is being tested for the treatment of very mild (up to +2.0) hyperopia. See Chapter 18.

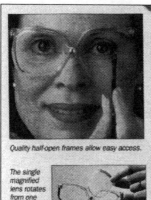

COURTESY OF SELFCARE CATALOG

As this catalog ad illustrates, even the moderately farsighted have trouble seeing both near and far. Without glasses or contacts, tasks like applying makeup can be as difficult as throwing darts.

GLASSES ON CHICKENS?

Chickens have quirky eyes. Apparently you can put lenses of any prescription on a hen and her eyes will adjust and become the opposite of the prescription in the lenses. For example, put a farsighted contact on one of a chicken's eyes, and the eye will become physically longer until five days later it's nearsighted. Put nearsighted lenses on, and the opposite happens. Even odder, the eye without the lens changes, too. I won't tell you what they did to prove that all the physical changes were controlled by the chicken's brain—but researchers showed that the changes weren't caused by a reaction of the eye to the contact lens.[4]

Doesn't it make you wonder why anyone thought to try this in the first place? If human eyes could be made this reactive, we might someday be back to glasses and contacts as the permanent solution to our vision problems.

ASTIGMATISM

Astigmatism is caused by an irregularly shaped cornea that projects light waves at two points inside the eye rather than one. The difference between the two points causes the brain to "see" a blurred image. It is possible to have astigmatism with nearsightedness—the two points fall short of the retina—or with farsightedness, when the points never come to a focus inside the eye. It is also possible to have astigmatism by itself with no other refractive error: two points of light come to focus right on the retina.

The two focal points are created when the eye is steeper in one dimension and flatter in another—like an egg rather than a golfball. Light waves enter the cornea and are bent one amount by the steeper side and another amount by the flatter side, so they go in slightly different directions and never meet up, as shown in Figure 5.6

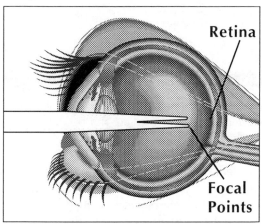

COURTESY OF BEACON EYE INSTITUTE

FIGURE 5.6   Astigmatism causes light to enter the eye unevenly, so it comes to two focal points rather than one. About a third of all of us have some astigmatism, but over two thirds of myopes have it. This illustration shows a nearsighted eye with astigmatism.

How Astigmatism Affects Vision

A prescription for astigmatism has two parts: the amount (cylinder) and the orientation (axis). Depending on the amount of space between the two focal points and where the astigmatism occurs on the cornea, symptoms can range from eye strain to blurring. Some astigmatism only shows up during reading, when characters might appear doubled or blurred.

Astigmatism can be corrected easily with glasses or, with more difficulty, by "toric" contacts which are weighted to keep the lens correctly positioned on the cornea. It has been estimated that there are more than 60,000 different toric lens shapes available—which gives you some idea of the number of ways the cornea can be shaped. Anyone who has worn toric lenses knows that keeping them correctly positioned on the eye is crucial to seeing a clear image.

The Permanent Cure for Astigmatism

To cure astigmatism, the steeper and flatter dimensions of the cornea need to be equalized so light is refracted into a single point. PRK can smooth out the longer or steeper areas to remove most or all astigmatism at the same time nearsightedness is being corrected. This procedure is called Astigmatic PRK (APRK).

Outside the U.S. APRK usually is done at the same time nearsightedness is treated—it's just another step with the laser and I had it as part of my own PRK. In the U.S. APRK is just completing FDA clinical trials for the VISX laser, and another procedure, Astigmatic Keratotomy (AK) has been used in the U.S. instead. You'll learn more about these treatments in Chapter 16.

PRESBYOPIA:
LOOKING OUT OF THE EYES OF TIME

As most of us settle into our forties, we begin to lose our ability to bring near images into focus. For myopes, this begins with having to take distance glasses off to read, and then needing bifocals and sometimes even trifocals for mid-range viewing of things like computer screens. Hyperopes might find themselves in bifocals. And those who never had a single vision problem could be trying on reading glasses in the drugstore.

The problem is called "presbyopia" and no one really knows what causes it. We do know that it is not a *refractive* error: people with perfect refraction can become presbyopic just like the rest of us. You can need reading glasses with myopia, hyperopia or no refractive error at all. And you can have astigmatism with all of these conditions. Whatever vision problem you have going into middle age, you most likely will continue to have it *plus* the problem of presbyopia— unless you do something about it.

Presbyopia and Refractive Vision Problems

Most of us are born with 20 diopters of focusing power—babies can see their
own noses—but we lose half of it by the time we're in our early twenties. That
still leaves plenty to spare, however. "No refractive error and 10 diopters of
focusing power would give you the visual acuity of a Navy pilot," said Dr. Richard Lindstrom.

By the time we're 40, the steady loss of focusing power becomes more noticeable. To bring a distant image into the range of about 40" (1 meter), requires 1
diopter of focusing power. To take it from there to 20" requires another diopter.
And to take it to reading distance requires one more diopter: 3 diopters in total.

So someone who has no refractive vision problem will need 3 diopters of
focusing power to read. If his focusing power has diminished to less than 3
diopters, he'll need reading glasses to make up the difference.

A nearsighted person, on the other hand, has eyes that are naturally focused
at reading distance or closer without glasses *or* the need to focus her eyes. But
when she puts her distance glasses on, suddenly she is exactly like people who
have no refractive problem: She has to be able to focus 3 diopters to read or she
must wear reading glasses.

A farsighted person, say +4.0, would need 4 diopters of focusing power to see
fairly large objects clearly and 3 diopters to be able to bring small print into
focus. So he would need 7 diopters (+4 +3) of focusing power in order to read
the same material that a nearsighted person would be able to read without glasses.
That's why farsighted people need reading glasses sooner than nearsighted—
they are starting from a longer focal point and so they require more focusing power
to read.

The reason some myopes need reading glasses after PRK when they didn't
before is because having their vision corrected is the equivalent of installing
permanent distance lenses: their eyes are now focused at the distance. If they

don't have 2 or 3 diopters of focusing power left, they might need reading glasses to bring near images into focus. (See Chapter 17 for ways around this problem.)

A Word About Reading with Glasses

Nearly every ophthalmologist and optometrist I spoke with had the same advice: The longer you can stand to put off wearing reading glasses, the longer you'll be able to read without them. I heard about one doctor who is 59 and still not wearing glasses to read. Not wearing reading glasses when they are necessary, however, can cause severe headaches and eyestrain.

As mentioned above, younger people might be able to keep their nearsightedness from getting worse by taking off their distance glasses when they are going to read for any length of time.

But when it's time to go, it's time to go. The question is, where? A person with good distance vision whose eyes function identically can buy inexpensive "readers" at the drugstore and stash them all over the house. For the rest of us, it's not that simple: If we have astigmatism, or if each eye needs a different correction, we're going to have to go to an optomestrist and plunk down money year after year for prescription readers, bifocals or trifocals.

HOW LOW WILL YOU GO?   From about age 40 to 66 most of us can expect our focusing ability to weaken until we can't focus up close at all without help. In fact, optometrists say they can guess your age fairly accurately just by checking your reading vision. Here's the additional magnification usually needed to read newsprint at 13″ by people with 20/20 vision. Very detailed work, like embroidery or watch repair, might require even stronger magnification.   Nearsighted people tend to need less magnification, as explained above, while farsighted people need more.

Age	Added Lens Power Needed
40	+0.50
45	+0.75
50	+1.00
55	+1.50
60	+2.00
65	+2.50

Will PRK Make Me Need Reading Glasses?

As mentioned above, PRK and other surgical techniques for correcting vision don't cause prebyopia—because the cornea isn't a factor in creating the problem. However, if you're nearsighted now, you might begin to need reading glasses if you are corrected to 20/25 or better, because your eye will no longer be focused naturally at the near point. Conversely, if you end up slightly undercorrected after laser surgery (20/30 for example) in one or both eyes, you might not need reading glasses until you're a senior citizen! We will look at this in more detail in Chapters 17 and 18.

What Causes Presbyopia?

No one is sure why presbyopia occurs, but there are three plausible theories:
1) The eye's focusing muscle tires out from years of overuse and loses its ability to thicken the lens.
2) The lens of the eye becomes fibrous and rigid, making it harder for the muscles to thicken it.
3) The ligaments which hold the lens become rigid, perhaps because the white part of the eye hardens as we age.[6]

No matter the cause, for most of us there'll come a day when we try to shift focus from watching the birdfeeder to looking at the weather map in the paper. Our eye muscles will stay relaxed, the lens will remain thinned out for distance viewing, and we won't be able to read the small print. The only benefit of being nearsighted is that it might postpone this fate by a few years.

Is there a Cure for Presbyopia?

Some optometrists recommend eye exercises that are time-consuming enough to rule out most busy people. Doctors suggest that you can delay presbyopia by forcing your eyes to focus instead of relying on reading glasses, but many of us can't take the eyestrain or headaches and give up. Dr. Hirsch tried biofeedback in his optometry practice to help patients re-teach their eyes how to focus. "It worked for a few patients, but they had to come in twice a week and most didn't have the time."

As Baby Boomers enter the "reading glasses" years, there will be huge profits for anyone who can solve the presbyopia problem permanently, safely and predictably.

Myopes frequently have PRK performed to optimize one eye for distance and one eye for reading, or to undercorrect both eyes just slightly but this doesn't work for everyone (see Chapter 17). PRK has also been used to sculpt a "bifocal" right onto the surface of rabbit corneas (so now they can read *Peter Rabbit* to their grandkids).

Another method implants a microscopic magnifying lens into the cornea—giving the patient the same "built-in" bifocal effect. A third alternative involves surgery on the white part of the eye. In addition, treatments with lasers are being tested which, in effect, make a farsighted or 0.0 eye slightly nearsighted for reading, or make each eye capable of seeing both far and near (multi-focal). All of these procedures are still investigational and are described in Chapter 17.

Currently available are methods such as bifocal contact lenses—which have been met with limited success—and monovision contacts, where one eye is corrected for distance and the other either is left without a lens or is undercorrected so it can be used for reading.

The only alternatives which do not involve a tradeoff between fine distance vision and the ability to read are reading glasses, bifocals and trifocals. As we know, however, these require other compromises.

Life is Hard—See Well

Lots of people live with their glasses and contacts up until the point they can't see well near or far. Then they start carrying around prescription distance glasses for outside and inside, along with prescription reading glasses. Or they begin fussing with bifocals, progressive lenses or trifocals, and monovision or multivision contacts. Sometime around age 45, many of us just say "life is hard enough!" and start to look for a solution that will remove, at least, the worst of our vision problems.

If you're in this situation—or if you're ahead of your class and ready to give up your dependence on glasses and contact lenses even earlier—the time has never been better.

The following chapters will describe the risks and rewards of the new laser vision correction procedures and compare them to other approaches available today, or on the horizon.

VISION ALERT! Did you know that medications can cause blurred vision, dry eyes or trouble seeing at night? If you ever notice a sudden change in your vision you should see your optometrist or ophthalmologist. Be sure to speak up if you are taking any of the following types of medications:

Acne medications	Antihistamines/allergy medications
Anticonvulsants	Antidepressants
Appetite suppressants	High-potency vitamins
Corticosteroids	Muscle relaxants
Tranquilizers	

WHAT'S YOUR VISION ?

Vision	Refraction	Symptom
Good acuity	-0.5 to +0.5	You see distant images clearly
Myopic	-0.75 or greater	You see better near than far
Hyperopic	+0.5 or greater	You have trouble seeing far and near
Astigmatic	+.25 or greater	You see blurred or doubled images close in, far away, or both
Presbyopic	Begins about age 40	You can't focus on images that are closer than about 20"

6

How the New "Cool" Laser Solves Vision Problems

*I*n 1983 an eye surgeon discovered that an industrial laser, called the "excimer," could reshape the cornea without harming the underlying tissue. This news catapulted vision surgery into the world of high technology, spawned a half-dozen new companies, and generated over a hundred million dollars in investment capital.

"Until Dr. Trokel got his hands on the excimer laser, nobody was able to reshape the front of the eye directly," said Dr. Roger Steinert, who was experimenting with lasers at M.I.T. at that time.

All the other methods of correcting vision were indirect: Some used incisions to cause the cornea to bulge, or hot needles to shrink it into shape. Others required the surgeon to cut a "cap" off the cornea, reshape it or the underlying tissue, and put the cap back on. Donor corneas were turned on a lathe and sewn on patients' eyes to create "living contact lenses."

Compared to all these methods PRK requires much less surgical skill and involves much less risk to the patient. The laser simply "polishes off" just enough corneal tissue to make the eye see clearly.

Other forms of lasers are now used to solve vision problems—they are discussed in Chapters 18 and 19—but only the excimer is approved in the U.S. for vision correction.

"Everything must be made as simple as possible but not one bit simpler."
—Albert Einstein

High-Tech Buff 'n Polish

PRK, or Photorefractive Keratectomy, uses ultraviolet light to "dust off" excess tissue from the cornea—a fragment at a time. It's a computer-controlled buffing process so precise that the tissue removed is measured in quarters of microns. The name of the procedure is shorthand for the process: *Photo* (light) *refractive* (bending) *kera* (cornea) —*ectomy* (removal of tissue): Using *light* to change the *light-bending* power of the *cornea* by *removing tissue*.

For nearsighted people, the eye is microscopically flattened in the center, to reduce the angle that light is bent so that it can fall farther back in the eye. For farsighted people, the eye is steepened in the middle of the cornea, to increase the angle that light is bent, and make it focus closer to the retina.

Bloodless

The cornea does not contain blood vessels, so there's no bleeding during PRK. There is no knife used, so there's no potential for cutting into the eye. The risk of infection is remote.

Painless

The eye is anesthetized with drops during the procedure, so there's no sensation at all. For about a day or two afterward most patients feel only a sensation of irritation—similar to the feeling of a speck of dust in the eye or something under a contact lens.

Safe

The laser beam for PRK is made from very cool ultraviolet light waves, not the hot infrared light waves of most other lasers. It works by breaking apart the bonds that hold the collagen molecules of the cornea together, not by heating up the tissue. As a result, fragments of collagen can be removed without damaging the rest of the cornea. The epithelium, which is removed during treatment, grows back in less than a week. The patient has functional, unaided vision within the first day to two weeks which continues to improve over a period of several months.

Permanent

Once molecules are removed from the cornea, they are gone forever, so PRK is permanent. Because the eye isn't compromised with knife incisions, a second "tune-up" PRK can be performed without risk to the stability of the eye. This comes in handy if the patient needs a little more correction after the first procedure, or if the eye changes later, which might happen if the patient's nearsightedness is still progressing.

HOW SMALL IS A MICRON?   If you ever have to measure something in microns, you'll need a microscope to do it. A single micron is 1/1000 of a millimeter, or 1/25,000 of an inch. In normal room light the average person's pupil is about 3.5 millimeters (1/8 inch) wide: that's *3,500* microns. By contrast, the cornea is only about 500 microns thick—half a millimeter or 1/50 of an inch. Now you know what they mean by the term "microsurgery."

This circle is six millimeters, or about 6000 microns, in diameter: the size of the PRK treatment zone.

OH, WHAT THAT EXCIMER CAN DO!

Excimer lasers for PRK work when two gases—argon and flourine—which normally don't combine, are forced into combination. The molecules that are generated by this "shotgun" marriage stay together only a short time before breaking up. Their break-up produces extremely intense energy in the form of ultraviolet light—energy so intense that it can blast apart the carbon-to-carbon, carbon-to-nitrogen and carbon-to-hydrogen bonds of the molecules that make up the collagen in the cornea.

The Safety Zone
It turns out that the short wavelengths of the excimer cannot go through the cornea into the eye. This is because all the energy from the beam is entirely absorbed by about 1 micron of corneal tissue. As the energy is absorbed, fragments of the tissue disappear into dust.

A pulse of the excimer beam could be shot across a room or a football field—the distance wouldn't matter— right at a cornea, and when it got to the cornea it would remove 1/4 of a micron of tissue and stop. What remained would be a very smooth impression in the exact shape of the beam.

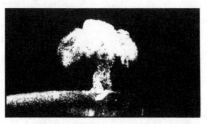

AN ATOMIC EXPLOSION AT THE MICROCOSMIC LEVEL Fragments of collagen literally turn into dust when a single pulse from the excimer reaches the surface of the cornea. Dust particles explode from the surface of the cornea at speeds of over a *mile a second*...while leaving the rest of the cornea undisturbed.

Wide-Area Ablation

In 1983 Dr. Stephen Trokel discovered that pulses from the excimer could remove tissue from the cornea without damaging what remained, but the question was, how should the laser be used? As the "Brief History" section below describes, doctors first attempted to use the beam as a knife, by performing RK-like incisions with it (RK is described in Chapter 14) but this didn't work because knives cut by separating tissue, not by removing it. When even a very fine laser beam is used as a knife, it creates a gap which doesn't easily refill because the molecules are no longer there to grow back together.

The key to PRK was the discovery by Dr. Trokel, Charles Munnerlyn, Ph.D., and others that a wide beam could be used to "ablate," or remove, tissue right from the front of the cornea. Since nearsightedness is caused by a too-steep cornea, this proved to be an ideal way to flatten it.

The process that evolved was called "wide-area ablation." To correct near-sightedness, the amount of tissue removed is greatest at the center of the eye and least at the edges of the ablation zone. This flattens the cornea, decreases its refractive power, and moves the focal point of the eye back to the retina where it belongs.

In the mid-'80s Charles Munnerlyn, an optical engineer devised the computer formulas for determining exactly how much tissue to remove for any given degree of nearsightedness—the procedure he named PRK. One of his great contributions was the concept that the surface of the patient's cornea was irrelevant. "A doctor doesn't have to measure your cornea to fit you with glasses," Dr. Munnerlyn explained, "so why would we measure it before we

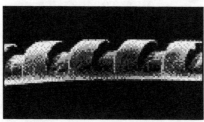

COURTESY OF VISX , INCORPORATED AND IBM CORPORATION

This early electron micrograph of a human hair demonstrates the effect of about 100 pulses from the excimer laser. A hair is about 50 microns wide. As you can see, the pulses created very well-defined trenches without damaging what remains of the hair. Most PRK treatments remove less than the width of a hair from the central cornea.

reshape it? If we know how nearsighted the eye is, we know how much to take off the cornea to correct it."

Working with Terrance Clapham, an electrical engineer, Dr. Munnerlyn developed the first complete ophthalmic excimer. As a result of their work, today's ophthalmologists simply enter the patient's desired correction into the PC that controls the laser, and the software automatically calculates the number of pulses and the diameter and depth of the ablation.

The depth of the ablation is determined by the diameter of the treatment zone. Through experimentation, doctors have learned that a 6-millimeter zone is optimal for most patients. To correct one diopter of nearsightedness with a 6-millimeter diameter, 12 microns of tissue must be removed. To correct -5.0 diopters of myopia, 60 microns would be removed. That would take precisely 240 pulses—about the thickness of a human hair. One pulse lasts only billionths of a second, and the laser emits the pulses in bursts of 5-10 per second. So 240 pulses would take 24-48 seconds.

Some of the earliest experiments involved finding ways to remove scars and infections which can result in the need for corneal transplants. This procedure, called Phototherapeutic Keratectomy (PTK), is described in Chapter 19.

HOW THE EXCIMER
SOLVES VISION PROBLEMS

The word "laser" is an acronym for "Light Amplification by Stimulated Emission of Radiation." All that is a very complicated process in its own right, but for PRK, the laser itself is just one box in the system.

What Happens During PRK

Your cornea is very, very thin: about 500 microns, or about the width of 10 human hairs stacked tightly together. PRK removes only 1/4 micron ($\frac{1}{2000}$ of the cornea) with each pulse.During PRK, the pulses begin with the aperture set to a fairly narrow circle—less than one millimeter wide—and then the aperture gradually widens to 6 millimeters. This produces a pattern that is deeper in the center than at the edges. Since the cornea is rounded, no indentation is made in the surface.

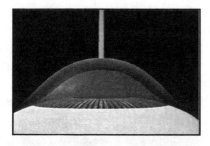

PRK begins with a narrow beam...

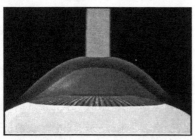

which gradually widens...

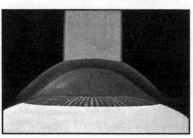

to about 6 millimeters in diameter.

ANIMATIONS COURTESY OF SUMMIT TECHNOLOGIES

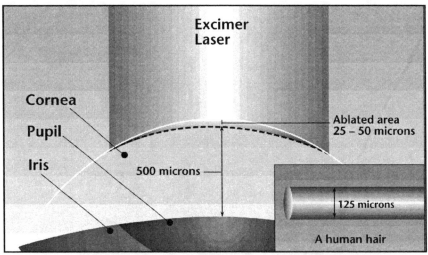

COURTESY OF VISX , INCORPORATED

This graphic illustrates that about 20-40% of the thickness of a human hair is removed from the cornea during a typical PRK.

Astigmatic PRK (APRK)

Astigmatism results from the eye being "out of round." One method of APRK corrects this with an aperture that opens in a gradually widening slit positioned to match the orientation of the astigmatism on the patient's eye. This produces an elliptical ablation. Nearsightedness and astigmatism can be treated simultaneously with two apertures, one round and one rectangular. Another method uses a mask applied to the lens to produce the elliptical ablation. These treatments are described more fully in Chapter 16.

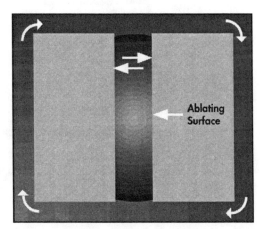

An elliptical ablation smooths out the irregularity which causes astigmatism.

COURTESY OF VISX, INCORPORATED

Hyperopic PRK (HPRK)

The excimer manufacturers are well into trials of the excimer to correct hyperopia—farsightedness. One method uses a technique which rotates an off-centered beam to create an ablation in a ring around the central visual area. Another method uses a mask in the lens of the laser to create the same effect. Both result in a cornea that is steeper in the center and flatter at the periphery, moving the focal point of the eye forward. Chapter 18 describes these and other treatments for hyperopia.

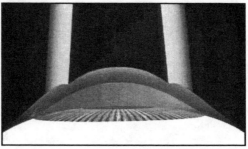

COURTESY OF SUMMIT TECHNOLOGY

HPRK for farsightedness removes corneal tissue in a ring to steepen the curve of the central cornea.

Phototherapeutic Keratectomy (PTK)

PTK has revolutionized treatment of corneal scars, dystrophies and other diseases that used to result in cornea transplants. During PTK the beam begins in the full-open position so that tissue is removed evenly with minimal change to the refractive power of the eye. This treatment is described in Chapter 19.

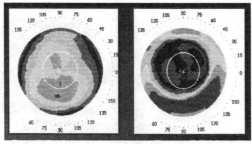

COURTESY OF VISX, INCORPORATED

The photo on the left shows a cornea with severe scars. After PTK, the haze is gone from the central visual area (circled), indicating the scar has been removed.

What Goes into the PRK System?

Like a shutter in a camera, the computer-controlled aperture of the PRK system controls the size and shape of the laser beam (Figure 6.1). The aperture controls the size and shape of the beam and directs it down to the surface of the eye where it vaporizes ¼ of a micron of tissue with each pulse.

The excimer laser is just the beginning. To use it as a predictable, safe vision-correction tool, developers had to integrate dozens of elements including:

- A cryopump
- A computer
- Programmed software
- A surgical microscope
- Optical lenses and mirrors
- Alignment and calibration instruments
- An aperture system
- Safety controls, and monitors

Not Just for Eyes

From computer chips to weapons to surgery, the cool excimer laser has left its mark in a number of fields. According to Michael Barra, vice president of marketing for Summit Technology, military excimers were first used in the Star Wars anti-missile technology of the 1980s. In addition to vision correction, they have been used in other forms of surgery.

Clinical trials are now in progress to investigate a procedure called Transmyocardial Revascularization (TMR) which might combat narrowing of coronary arteries in patients who can't have angioplasties or bypass surgery. Heart surgeons drill 20-30 channels through the heart wall to enable oxygen-rich blood to flow into the heart. Similarly, excimers are taking part in brain surgery to clear blockages in the carotid artery.

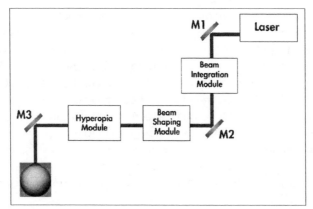

COURTESY OF VISX, INCORPORATED

FIGURE 6.1 Between the excimer laser and the eye, there are mirrors, beam rotators, integrators and a lens, in addition to all manner of safety systems and instruments.

A BRIEF HISTORY OF THE EXCIMER LASER

In a funny, touching essay I recently heard on public radio, a wedding photographer said the best part of his job was watching people dance at receptions. After describing a few couples, he made the general observation that, unlike lawyers who tend to dance in one spot, up and down like a pogo stick, doctors usually dance all over the place.

From what I've learned about how refractive surgery has developed in the last two decades, this description of doctors rings true. Not only are the leading surgeons trying many solutions at once (most of the FDA trial physicians who contributed to this book are running trials on more than one new procedure at this writing), but they converse across national and political borders, work on each other's problems, publish their results internationally and involve any and all manufacturers who are willing to listen. The result is worldwide cross-pollination of technology with technique at supercomputer speeds.

PRK evolved in just this fashion. While the excimer laser and the PRK procedure were indisputably invented in the U.S., the developers lost no time involving their counterparts in Germany and England, lighting a fuse that sizzled through 40 countries and ended in an explosion of innovation for reshaping the way people see. As the following story tells, these doctors truly were "dancing all over the place."

A NEW KIND OF MAGIC

Lasers have been used by ophthalmologists since the early '70s to treat problems like glaucoma and retinal bleeding, but they all worked by producing extreme heat. Then Dr. S.R. Srinivasan, a photochemist at IBM's Watson Research Center, discovered a way to use the excimer to etch and ablate organic polymers—so he could etch circuits in tiny microcomputer chips without melting the silicon sand from which they were made.

A couple of years later, Dr. Stephen Trokel, in his lab at Columbia-Presbyterian Medical Center, was reading about lasers in a book by a military physicist, John Taboda. Dr. Taboda had performed safety tests on the excimer which included seeing if the beam was harmful to animal eyes. It was.

"But one man's damage is another man's surgery," said Dr. Trokel. "When Taboda demonstrated that the excimer would make an impression on the surface of an animal cornea, I figured it could have the potential for refractive surgery."

Compared to that leap of imagination it was a short hike to Srinivasan's lab with a bucket of cow eyes. "Dr. Srinivasan was extremely gracious. He let me experiment with his laser just to see what kind of surgery it could do. That was in June of 1983 and we were all young, full of energy and looking for a new kind of magic."

On July Fourth, Dr. Trokel was out in Silicon Valley to test another kind of laser Dr. Munnerlyn and Mr. Terrance Clapham were developing. Afterward, he asked Dr. Munnerlyn, to give him a ride back to the airport. On the way he casually mentioned his excimer tests. "Look," he said, "I think this thing is going to work. It really does something neat on the surface of the cornea."

"I instantly knew what he had," said Dr. Munnerlyn. "It was a brand new way of dealing with the eye—a way to shave off a little cornea and change the refractive powers of the eye."

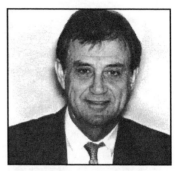

Stephen Trokel, MD

Dr. Trokel began his animal studies at Columbia-Presbyterian Medical Center in Fall of 1983. By day he'd operate on animal eyes. By night he'd pack up the eyes, catch the red-eye to London, and have the ocular pathologist, Dr. John Marshall, create electron micrographs so that he could prove that the laser worked without damaging the underlying tissue. Then he'd fly back to New York to perform more experiments.

During this period he made numerous sidetrips to Germany to share his results with doctors there and to try to convince companies—including ones who later developed their own excimers—that the laser was ideal for ophthalmic surgery, but they weren't interested. "It got to be fun watching customs agents when they went through my luggage and found the jars of eyeballs," Dr. Trokel recalls.

A few months later Dr. Trokel showed Dr. Munnerlyn some of the scanning electron microscope photos and Dr. Munnerlyn said, "Yep. That's it," and he and Mr. Clapham began working on the first ophthalmic excimer system for PRK.

Despite this early success, the PRK procedure had yet to be developed and proven. That began in earnest in fall of 1984, with financing out of Dr. Trokel's own pocket. He started performing the first wide-area ablations on monkey and rabbit corneas using a 3.5-millimeter treatment zone. His studies proved that the eyes would heal clearly, the corneas would flatten, and the optics of the eye would change. Along the way he intentionally induced infections and scars to prove the laser could remove them.

"I talked to anyone who would listen back then, but people were skeptical. But when I published my results in late '83, everyone became interested, patents started being filed by people faster on their toes than I was, companies were formed and suddenly the research turned into a race."

THE SHOT SEEN 'ROUND THE WORLD   This is one of Dr. Trokel's early electron micrographs that had the medical community on its feet. It shows a clearly etched indentation made by an excimer laser in a cow cornea with no damage to the surrounding tissue.

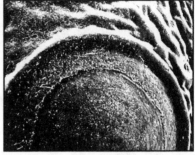

BY STEPHEN TROKEL, MD, COURTESY OF VISX, INCORPORATED

Knife or Polisher?

But a debate had begun: Use the laser as a knife, or as a polisher? In early '85 Dr. Theo Seiler in Berlin began working with Meditec's first prototype excimer. Using a 1-millimeter beam, Dr. Seiler did some incisions in non-functional eyes and some wide-area ablations by moving the beam back and forth. In 1986 he started treating astigmatism using the Meditec laser to make incisions. His results made it clear that the excimer was going to have a profound effect on vision surgery, but using the laser as a knife didn't work very well: the beam created a 1-millimeter-wide "trough" that wasn't as fine as doctors could obtain with a diamond-blade knife.

"At the beginning we were all chasing RK," Dr. Roger Steinert recalls. "We thought we were going to make slits with the laser. We even got the incision width down to just 40 microns. But we didn't realize the laser could do something even better—it could optically reshape the central cornea. A knife just can't do that because it causes scars."

Monkey Trials

Back in New York, Dr. Trokel was running out of money. He needed to do studies on monkeys with a machine that had a controlled ablation pattern but the animals and laser equipment were expensive. He solved one of his problems by getting Drs. Herbert Kauffman and Marguerite McDonald involved. As part of the faculty of Louisiana State University, Dr. McDonald had access to a primate facility in New Orleans, and she began working with Drs. Trokel and Munnerlyn to refine the ablation formulas on rabbit and monkey corneas and give them feedback on the laser design.

"It took a lot of dedication for Marguerite to keep going," Dr. Trokel said. "Back in '85-86 she was having trouble getting the rabbit studies to work and even her young research Fellows were bailing out on her. But she stuck with it."

Meanwhile, Dr. Trokel was working on ablation techniques using very simple, inexpensive equipment. "This turned out to be a blessing because other researchers were trying more complicated solutions without any success," Dr. Trokel remembers. "It turns out it works best when you keep it simple. One lens, a positioning device and a small circle for the aperture was all it took."

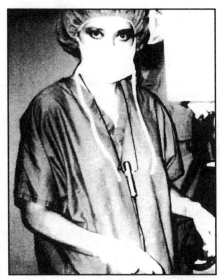

COURTESY OF LOUISIANA STATE UNIVERSITY

Dr. Marguerite McDonald in 1986 during experiments with the early excimer.

At Long Last, Real Patients

Finally, Dr. McDonald felt she had proved Dr. Munnerlyn's system on hundreds of rabbit and primate corneas and they were ready to move on to the FDA Phase I trials: live patients. In June of 1987, Dr. McDonald treated the first ten human blind eyes and the first human sighted eye with PRK. (See "The Amazing Double-Blind Study" in Chapter 13).

At the same time that Drs. Trokel and Munnerlyn were working on PRK, Dr. Francis L'Esperance, Dr. Roger Steinert and others were designing and conducting experiments with other excimer systems. In February of 1987, Dr. L'Esperance used an excimer laser to perform the first clinical treatments for removal of corneal scars on three blind patients, as a prelude to performing PRK on sighted eyes.

Dr. Munnerlyn's laser was the first complete excimer system designed for human clinical use. It had a 5-millimeter beam and was fully programmable using the algorithms he developed. He and Mr. Clapham formed VISX, Incorporated, which later merged with a company founded by Dr. L'Esperance. In parallel, Summit Technology was developing its own ophthalmic excimer and, by the late 1980s all three companies were traded on the U.S. public stock exchange.

And They're *Still* Going and Going and...

Dr. Trokel became a VISX founder and assigned his patent application to the company. He was their Medical Director during the FDA trials, trained all the clinical investigators at the trial sites and is currently working with investigators on new procedures for hyperopia and astigmatism. He and Dr. L'Esperance are professors of ophthalmology at Columbia-Presbyterian Medical Center.

Dr. Munnerlyn retired from his position as CEO of VISX two years ago but has continued to work with the company as a research consultant and to pursue his interest in telescopes. The VISX system received FDA approval on his 56th birthday.

Mr. Clapham is vice president of research and development for VISX

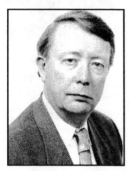

Terrance Clapham

and recently had his own -9.0 nearsightedness corrected by Dr. Bruce Jackson using the VISX Star laser he helped develop. "I waited until we had long-term results on treating high myopia and had the first eye undercorrected a little so I could read without glasses." At this writing, Mr. Clapham's treated eye had met its target and he was awaiting his second procedure.

Dr. McDonald has continued her research into new vision correction techniques and is conducting FDA trials for new types of lasers at Louisiana State University Medical Center in New Orleans. Her stories are in Chapters 13 and 15.

Dr. Seiler worked with Summit's initial prototype system. He continues his research into PRK techniques and is a professor of ophthalmology in Dresden.

Dr. Steinert became the principal investigator for Summit Technology's FDA clinical trials and currently is assistant clinical professor at Harvard Medical School and a consulting ophthalmologist in private practice. In May of 1996 he finally had his own vision treated with PRK. His story is in Chapter 9.

While it's fashionable to rail against the rising cost of new drugs and procedures, it's healthy to remember that many of the stunning advances in medical technology have come through the nearly superhuman efforts of a few dedicated scientists like the ones who developed PRK. Nearly any other enterprise they could have engaged in would have been more financially rewarding, faster, but few would have greater impact on as many lives.

"You can't depend on your eyes when your imagination isn't seeing clearly."
—Mark Twain

WHAT IF HIS GRANDMA HAD BEEN NEARSIGHTED?

Before becoming an inventor, Dr. Charles Munnerlyn worked on reconnaissance and tracking systems for the Air Force. "But ever since grade school, my primary interest was optics—telescopes and spectrascopes and other things you could look through." I asked how that interest began.

"When I was about 10 years old I was rummaging through a dresser drawer and found my grandmother's old round spectacles. I put one of the lenses in each end of a tube, looked out the window with it and said 'hey, the cow's upside down!'

"So that was my first telescope and after that I wanted to figure out why the cow turned upside down."

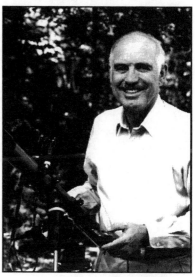

PHOTO BY AUDREY MUNNERLYN

Charles R. Munnerlyn, Ph.D

"Well, Why did it?"
"The lens inverts the image. When you're just looking through glasses, the artificial lens works with your natural lens to project the image upside down on the retina, and then your brain reinverts it. When you look through a terrestrial telescope, like the kind in pirate movies, the inverted image is projected by the front lens and then relayed by another lens which reinverts the image and relays it to the eyepiece lens, which magnifies it. That's why the tube is so long. My first telescope was like most astronomical telescopes—it didn't have the middle lens to reinvert the image, so the cow was upside down.

"But this only happens with lenses for farsightedness. With nearsighted lenses you get a 'virtual' image—it's not inverted. It's a good thing my grandmother hadn't been nearsighted or I would never have become interested in optics!

"But I went to Texas A&M where the physics program only had one course in optics. One day I was looking at a bulletin board and saw a notice for the Institute of Optics at the University of Rochester. I got my Ph.D. there and that got me started."

From those two coincidences: a grandmother's spectacles and a college bulletin, Dr. Munnerlyn went on to invent the first microprocessor-controlled autorefractor which automatically calculates a patient's vision problem, developed a machine to test for glaucoma, and designed a laser that worked like "magic scissors" to break down haze after cataract surgery.

TRY THIS AT HOME!   To see the effect Dr. Munnerlyn saw through his grandma's glasses, simply hold a magnifying glass out at arm's length and look through it out a window to some object in the distance. I won't ruin the experiment by telling you what happens, but here's why: The farther the magnifying lens gets from your natural lens, the less the two lenses can work together to form a single image. As a result, the magnifying lens creates one image, which is inverted in front of your natural lens, and then your lens inverts that image on your retina. The brain does its job by flipping the image one last time. Surprise!

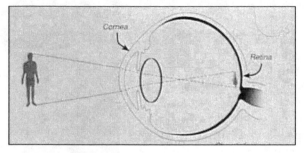

The eye inverts images because light coming from the top of an object is bent to the lower part of the retina and vice versa. The brain reinverts the image so what you see is rightside up.

Hocked Houses

In October of 1983, Dr. Munnerlyn and Terrance Clapham were working for a surgical division of CooperVision. After seeing Dr. Trokel's work with the industrial excimer, they began developing an excimer system that would reshape the eye to correct any degree of nearsightedness.

By 1985 they had developed a prototype: the first PC-controlled ophthalmic excimer laser. "It was a complete delivery system with the computer controls and the safety features to deliver the laser energy to the eye in the exact number of pulses necessary to correct any given amount of myopia," Dr. Munnerlyn said.

"But CooperVision wanted out of the surgical business, so Terry and I hocked our houses and bought the system from Cooper. That's how VISX got started. As exciting as this technology was, can you believe we were unable to raise venture capital in Silicon Valley because nobody believed in it? So to raise money we ended up going public in 1989 with only seven employees."

VISX now has over $100 million in assets, worldwide sales and nearly half a million grateful patients—all thanks to a curious boy with a far-sighted grandmother.

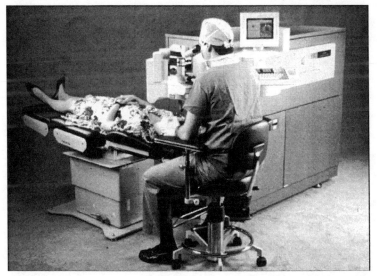

COURTESY OF VISX, INCORPORATED

A patient is receiving PRK with the VISX Star laser, the great-grandchild of Dr. Munnerlyn's first prototype laser for PRK. The Star was approved by the FDA in March of 1996.

◆ **7** ◆

Finding the Right Doctor

*I*n the U.S. there are about 12,000 practicing ophthalmologists—at least 8,000 of whom specialize in refractive surgery of one type or another. Less than 10% of these doctors are trained and highly experienced in PRK. Your mission is to find one of them.

Unless your case is unusual, falls outside the FDA limits, or you have health conditions which could pose problems in healing, you don't need one of the leading experts in PRK. A well qualified eye surgeon who has *enough* experience will serve you just fine, and be much easier to locate. Table 7.1 outlines the minimum qualifications. At the end of this chapter, I provide a list of doctors who meet all these criteria and are part of the elite group of the world's experts in PRK and other vision correction procedures.

PROFILE OF THE RIGHT DOCTOR FOR PRK   Table 7.1

Education
- Medical degree
- Specialty in ophthalmology—an ophthalmologist
- Subspecialty in cornea and/or refractive surgery.

PRK Experience
- At least six months of experience performing and following PRK procedures on at least 100 eyes.* Other types of refractive surgeries don't count here.

Other Experience
- Can perform, or is willing to refer you to other surgeons who can perform, the procedures mentioned in Part Three which are relevant to your vision problem.

*A few cases short of 100 is not likely to make a difference in your outcome, but research indicates that six months of follow-up on a large number of cases is the minimun requirement for a doctor to obtain consistently good results. Be aware that some doctors brand-new to PRK advertise they have performed "thousands of procedures," but they are counting RK and other refractive or corneal surgeries that have no bearing on their experience with PRK.

THE THREE TYPES OF EYE-CARE PROFESSIONALS

Ophthalmologists

Ophthalmologists are medical doctors trained to treat diseases and conditions of the eye. They can perform surgery and prescribe drugs and other treatments. They might also prescribe glasses and contacts. *Minimum* training required for ophthalmologists:

- Four years of college (pre-med)
- Four years of medical school
- One year of internship
- Two years of residency specializing in ophthalmology

Add this up, and your local ophthalmologist has had *at least* 11 years of training. In addition, cornea and refractive specialists usually have at least one or two years of second residency or fellowships in their area of specialty.

Optometrists

Optometrists are not medical doctors. They are trained in the physiology of the eye and the human visual system. Optometrists can examine eyes for refractive errors and screen for diseases, prescribe glasses, contacts, non-medical therapies and limited medications, and refer patients to ophthalmologists.

Many large laser centers are training optometrists to conduct the pre-examinations necessary for PRK and to handle follow-up care in close coordination with the surgeon. In a few states optometrists might be able to perform PRK themselves—but I haven't spoken to anyone—even other optometrists—who recommends that patients receive PRK treatment from an optometrist. *Minimum* training for optometrists:

- Two years of college
- Four years of optometry school

The Role of Optometrists in PRK

Since prescribing glasses and contact lenses are an optometrist's primary business, some might be reluctant to refer patients out for a permanent solution. Many optometrists are getting involved in PRK, however, and are being trained by ophthalmologists to handle pretesting and follow-up care.

As a result, patients can find a PRK surgeon through their optometrist. One advantage of working through your optometrist is that he is familiar with your vision and any vision changes over the past few years. He probably is local and his volume of PRK cases most likely is low, so he can focus a great deal of attention on yours.

If the optometrist has participated in training with the surgeon—observing PRK cases at various stages of recovery, for example—the surgeon can provide detailed instructions for post-op procedures and require regular reporting and immediate consultation on any problems.

If you plan to work through your optometrist, be sure to find out how much training the optometrist has had, how the surgeon and optometrist work together, and what the surgeon's experience level is. Remember, an optometrist is not a medical doctor. If you have complications, your optometrist should refer you to the surgeon who treated you or to another ophthalmologist experienced in following PRK cases. Be sure you know in advance who will provide, and whether you will be charged for, any necessary medical care during the follow-up period.

Opticians

Opticians are technicians trained to fill lens prescriptions for glasses and contacts and to fit glasses on patients. In most cases, they don't actually make the lenses—they are purchased from optical labs.

Opticians are not qualified to perform PRK procedures or handle pretesting and post-op care.

WHERE TO GO FOR PRK?

Dr. Roger Steinert summed it up: "Patients can pick a surgeon or pick a site." He is referring to the fact that you can choose a doctor and let him choose where you have the procedure, or you can go to a medical center or commercial laser center and let it choose the doctor.

I would add two more methods of picking a doctor: Ask your optometrist, as described above, or ask a friend who has had a successful PRK.

The "Pick a Surgeon" Method

With this method, you choose the surgeon and the surgeon determines how, where and by whom your pretesting, PRK procedure, and post-op care will be handled. The surgeon might have a laser in his own office, might use a laser at a local teaching university, might be part of a group of doctors which has jointly purchased a laser, or might have operating privileges at a surgery center or hospital which owns a laser.

The surgeon who does your procedure will have a great deal to do with your final outcome. "We went through a period where the perception was that

PRK is a no-brainer," Dr. Steinert said, "but there's more to PRK than meets the eye, so to speak. Subtle skills that only come through experience can make a huge difference."

Dr. Robert Maloney agrees. "There are a few aspects of PRK that only a surgeon experienced in it can control. One of these is hydration." Dr. Maloney went on to describe a study he was part of[1] which showed that the drier the cornea becomes during surgery, the more likely the patient will end up over-corrected. "But if the eye is too wet, she'll be undercorrected. The key is to know how to perform each step of the procedure at the right pace so that you can consistently control variables like wetness. The only way to learn how to do that is by doing it."

Another ophthalmologist wrote, "It appears that there is a significant difference in the results of doctors new to PRK [compared to] experienced doctors...their first cases will not be as good as their later cases...The same thing appears to be true with the complication rate. The greater the surgeon's experience and commitment to understanding all the effects of the procedure, the lower the incidence of complications. The bottom line is: Laser surgery is just that, surgery."[2]

Mark Logan, CEO of VISX Corporation, one of the two laser makers with FDA approval, said, "The laser is not entirely surgeon-dependent. You input the prescription, step on the pedal and the laser does its job. But the reason the surgeons are there is that if something does go wrong, they're going to catch it. I would always go to the highly experienced surgeons. They can recognize when something is not quite right and that's important."

Personally, I wouldn't trust my eyes to anyone who had performed and followed PRK procedures on less than a hundred eyes for at least six months. A doctor needs time to see the effects of her treatments on a wide range of patients so she can finetune her methods to achieve the best results.

How Do Doctors Gain Experience?

Just like anyone trying to enter a new field, it's more difficult for doctors to get experience when they don't have experience. Doctors wanting to become proficient in new procedures need patients willing to go first.

Luckily for you, a great many doctors became highly experienced in PRK long before the FDA issued their approvals. They gained their experience through their own expense and effort by:

- Buying a laser and participating in the U.S. clinical trials.
- Buying a laser and performing PRKs in Canada or other countries.

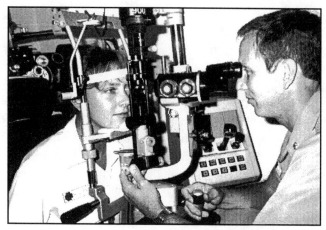

COURTESY OF U.S. NAVAL MEDICAL CENTER, SAN DIEGO

Dr. Steven Schallhorn examines Tiffany Baisden's eye five days after her PRK during FDA trials.

- Being part of the staff of a teaching university or hospital which bought a laser in order to participate in the FDA clinical trials or as part of manufacturer testing programs. Doctors sacrifice income from private practice to be part of teaching programs.

In addition to (not instead of) the above, some ophthalmologists in the U.S. have spent vacation time and weekends traveling to Canada and other countries to work with highly experienced surgeons who were developing state-of-the-art procedures. They have attended medical conferences and compared their results with other researchers.

By contrast, ophthalmologists who became involved in PRK just prior to, or after, FDA approval are still moving up the learning curve. Some have accelerated their own progress by apprenticing themselves to the more experienced doctors. Some are learning on their patients. But none of them will learn by treating *you*, now that you've read this chapter.

For Americans, Equipment Can Make a Difference

If your vision or age falls at the borders of FDA approvals, you might have to look specifically for a doctor who uses either a VISX or Summit laser. These limits don't say anything about the quality or capabilities of the lasers—they simply are what the manufacturers included in their clinical trials.

Age
- VISX equipment is approved for treating patients 18 years and older.
- Summit equipment is approved for treating patients 21 years and up.

Refractive Error
- VISX's initial approval was for treating patients with up to -6.0 diopters of nearsightedness with up to 1 diopter of astigmatism. As this book went to press, VISX's application for approval to treat up to 4.5 diopters of astigmatism with PRK had received expedited consideration and a final approval was expected soon.
- Summit is approved for treating up to -7.0 diopters of nearsightedness with up to 1.5 diopters of astigmatism.

Patients in clinical trials are treated outside these limits and some doctors will perform "off-label" PRKs, as described in Chapter 13. If you know your vision falls within FDA approval boundaries and the doctor you are talking to can't treat it, ask which laser she is using and then try to find a doctor with the other type of laser or go to Canada for treatment.

How Many Alternatives Does the Doctor Offer?

If you choose a doctor who can offer most or all of the procedures that you consider relevant to your vision problem, chances are you'll receive an unbiased discussion of your alternatives. There's no need to look for one doctor who can do it all, however, as long as he can do what you need.

If you choose doctors known for their participation in research and experimental procedures, you have a better chance of being offered new solutions or being referred to other surgeons who can offer them. This could be especially important if your case is unusual in any way.

"I think what the world sorely needs is more *pure* refractive surgeons—not ones who only promote one procedure or another," Dr. Vance Thompson said. "The doctors should review all the alternatives with the patients and not let their personal biases, or limitations, enter into it."

Medical Board Certification for PRK?

At this time there is no specific certification procedure for PRK except that doctors must go through FDA-required training programs. Gary Jonas, CEO of 20/20 Laser Centers says that the FDA requires ophthalmologists to complete two training courses in PRK before performing the surgery on their patients: A six-hour lecture and then a surgical lab where they operate on nonliving animal eyes. finally they must perform one supervised PRK procedure.

Manufacturer-Certified Training

In the U.S. the FDA has required the laser manufacturers to be the primary source of training for doctors who want to learn PRK. Both manufacturers have set up "centers for excellence" at major regional medical centers and hospitals. Doctors attend the lectures, receive laboratory instruction and are supervised during the first few procedures. Importantly, the regional center becomes a resource for doctors who need advice as patients proceed through recovery.

"The VISX training is much more intensive than the FDA minimum requirement," Mr. Logan said. "In addition to the lecture and lab, we train each doctor on his own laser. The surgeon responsible for training will perform a few procedures while the new doctor observes. Then the new doctor's first few PRKs will be supervised by the experienced surgeon. As the new doctor begins to perform PRK on his own, the training surgeon provides consultation."

One of Summit Technology's centers is at the Jules Stein Eye Institute of UCLA and it is supervised by Dr. Maloney. "I can tell you that the centers work. I not only have the chance to teach the doctors, but I spend a great deal of time on the phone every day answering their questions and consulting with them on follow-up issues. Doctors who take the time to go through the program and take advantage of the help available to them can accelerate their progress up the learning curve."

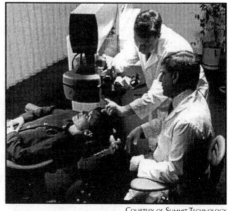

Experienced surgeons train doctors by demonstrating and then supervising several PRK procedures.

COURTESY OF SUMMIT TECHNOLOGY

WHO CAN BE TRAINED?   No matter how good the training program is, ultimately your outcome will depend on the background and experience of the doctor. The only problem is, there is nothing in the FDA regulations to prevent doctors who have no experience in eye surgery, such as dermatologists, dentists, or even, in some states, optometrists, from taking the PRK training and offering the procedure to their patients. Only patients can make sure they get qualified surgeons by refusing treatment from anyone other than a corneal specialist certified by the local medical board.

Mr. Logan added, "You have to remember that these are corneal specialists we are training, not people off the street. We don't have to teach them how to do eye surgery—only how to use the laser. They are familiar with the other components of PRK, such as centration of the eye and medications, because these are part of many other eye surgeries."

TYPES OF PRK TREATMENT CENTERS

There are many different types of centers offering PRK as well as other vision correction procedures, and all are available in both the U.S. and Canada. Each type of center has advantages and potential drawbacks. It might be possible to "pick a surgeon" at any of these centers if you know in advance which surgeon you want (see Table 7.2).

The "Pick a Site" Method

Looking up a laser center in the phone book or responding to a television or direct-mail ad are ways to "pick a site." There's nothing wrong with this approach as long as you are sure that the doctor(s) who will be performing your procedure and follow-up care are fully qualified.

Dr. Steinert, who is an academic ophthalmologist with a private consulting practice and uses a laser at a university center, acknowledged his bias toward the "Pick a Surgeon" method, but continued with his description. "When you pick a site just because it has a laser, you might not get to choose your doctor, you develop no relationship with the doctor, you might not know about the individual doctor's skill or experience, and you don't see the doctor for post-op care. There are quality treatment centers, but my advice is: *buyer beware.*."

What are the advantages of going to a "site" rather than a doctor?

TYPES OF PRK TREATMENT CENTERS		Table 7.2
Type of Site	Possible Advantages	Cautions
University Medical Centers, Teaching Hospitals		
PRK treatments usually are performed in the "Refractive Surgery Unit," "Eye-Care Institute" or "Eye Clinic."	• Highly experienced supervising surgeons • Advanced treatment methods • Access to clinical trials • Possible lower cost if you can be part of a clinical trial.	• Professors supervise interns and residents, so your procedure might be performed by a doctor in training. • A clinic atmosphere can result in long waits, little personal attention. • If the center is far from your home, it might be difficult and expensive to get after-hours care in an emergency, and follow-up appointments could be inconvenient. • Probably won't help you with insurance billing. • Credit terms are unlikely.
Centers that Employ or Retain Surgeons		
a) Centers dedicated to PRK which do the procedure and handle all the pre- and post-op care b) Centers that handle only the PRK procedure and accept referrals from optometrists whom they have trained in pre- and post-op care	• High volume of PRK procedures gives most surgeons in these centers much experience. • Costs might be lower. • More emphasis placed on patient convenience. • Experienced staff can spend time answering questions. • Insurance billing can be handled for you. • Credit terms are likely to be available.	• How experienced is the surgeon who will perform your PRK ? • What is your own optometrist's level of experience in following PRK cases, if he will be involved in your aftercare. • How will medical emergencies be handled; is the cost is part of the package?
Centers Providing Laser Facilities		
a) Laser centers owned and operated by several surgeons in different private practices, for the use of those surgeons and other doctors. b) Private hospitals and outpatient centers provide the laser, facility and training for local surgeons who want to perform PRK but don't own a laser.	• Pre-and post-care will be handled by the doctor who did your procedure. • Local emergency care is more easily arranged and might be part of the fee. • Center probably is local, reducing travel expense. • Can handle insurance billings. • Credit terms are likely.	• Is the laser maintained by a full-time staff technician? • Does your ophthalmologist have adequate PRK experience? • What are the qualifications of the person who will take care of you through the post-op period, if it is not the surgeon?
Lasers Used in Private Practices		
The laser is owned and used exclusively by a doctor or several doctors in a single practice.	• Your doctor probably will handle your PRK and your follow-up care. • You have a local resource for emergency care, probably at no extra charge. • Might handle insurance billings.	• Is there adequate technical staff to maintain the laser? • Credit terms are less likely to be available. • The cost might be higher.

Cost and Financing

Large laser centers are more likely to offer attractive prices and financing arrangements than individual doctors, small practices or medical centers. The average cost today is about $2000 per eye.

In Canada, both individual doctors and laser centers currently offer an automatic discount to U.S. patients because of the favorable exchange rate. A procedure that costs $2000 Canadian dollars today only costs $1600 U.S. dollars, and most Canadian doctors accept payment in U.S. currency. This might be a good bargain for Americans, but travel, lodging and meals usually are not covered by the fee, and your local doctor might charge an additional fee for pretesting, follow-up care and any emergency care. In addition, exchange rates can change rapidly, so check the U.S. -to-Canadian exchange rate at the time you are creating your budget (the easiest way to do this is to call your bank or look up the rates in the business section of the Sunday paper or Wall *Street Journal*).

Access to Other Treatments

As we've already discussed, the FDA limits the degree of myopia which is approved for treatment with PRK and has not yet approved treatments for astigmatism by all laser or hyperopia. Canadian laser centers which have gained experience in these areas can be the solution, as can any doctors or centers in the U.S. which are involved in clinical trials.

The "Ask a Friend" Method

About half of the patients I spoke with learned about PRK and their doctor from a friend who was ecstatic with his or her results. This is a good idea—as long as the doctor meets the qualifications listed in Table 7.1. Your vision problems, your overall health and your own healing patterns might be quite different from those of your friend, so you need a doctor equipped to handle any eventuality.

FIX WRINKLES AND VISION IN ONE TRIP? If you're into super-efficiency, why not get your wrinkles removed at the same time your vision is fixed? Two companies, The Medical Laser Institute of America and Vision Sculpting of Alberta, jointly announced plans to open a chain of clinics that will offer a combination of PRK and "laser skin rejuvenation," giving patients a "one-stop location for most of their cosmetic surgical needs." Tempted? Just remember: the outcome (of your vision or skin) will depend on the skills and experience of the individual surgeon who performs each procedure.

EXPERT RESOURCES

The doctors listed in the Resource Guide on the following pages are all ophthalmologists with specialties in corneal and refractive surgery who have become some of the world's leading experts in laser vision correction. All the U.S. surgeons were investigators in the FDA clinical trials for the two lasers approved for PRK. All the Canadian surgeons have been involved with PRK for at least five years and have tested most of the lasers in use in the world today. Each has agreed to be a potential treatment resource for the readers of *Beyond Glasses!*

In addition to years of experience with PRK and some of the other procedures, these surgeons were considered top-of-their-class *before* they became involved in PRK. That's why the laser manufacturers chose them. If you have millions of dollars riding on the outcome of an FDA trial, you want the very best doctors developing and refining the procedures. The Canadian surgeons were chosen as test sites for the same reason, and because they were less regulated by their government, they have developed and taught their colleagues the U.S. many of the laser vision correction techniques being used today. The doctors are listed alphabetically by state or province.

I have also indicated which of these doctors are currently involved in investigating procedures such as PRK for astigmatism, hyperopia and high myopia, LASIK, the intrastromal ring, the implantable contact lens and the holmium laser treatments for hyperopia/presbyopia. All these procedures are described in Part Three.

Before You Call...

You will need to know your vision prescription (see Chapter 4) and whether you have any of the physical or lifestyle conditions which might be a barrier to laser treatment (see Chapter 3).

When you call, ask for the patient care manager or new patient administrator and tell him that you were referred by *Beyond Glasses!* specifically to the doctor listed.

Because of the high level of expertise of the doctors and facilities on this list, their staffs are overtaxed and their lines often busy. Be patient when you try to get through and, as a courtesy to these doctors who have agreed to be of service, please do *not* call them to request referrals to doctors in other areas.

What if There's No Listing for Your Area?

I am living proof that traveling for PRK is not a problem—although it can be more expensive. If there's no doctor in your area, call the nearest facility that offers the treatment you are interested in, tell them you are interested in being a patient but live out of the area, and ask if they can suggest an optometrist or ophthalmologist nearer to you who could do the pretesting and follow-up care.

Living a long distance from the treatment facility might prohibit you from participating in clinical trials, but it never hurts to ask.

What if a Doctor Isn't on This List?

This list contains only the principal U.S. investigators for the two FDA-approved laser manufacturers plus Canadian doctors who have been involved with PRK for at least five years. There are other ophthalmologists who are skilled and experienced in PRK who would be good sources of treatment. Just be sure the doctor you choose fits the qualification profile at the beginning of this chapter.

PROCEDURE CODES   In June of 1996 all the doctors on the list performed PRK as well as other vision-correction procedures. In addition, each reported which procedures, if any, they were currently investigating. The procedures are described in Part Three. These are the codes used for all the procedures:

Code	Procedure
AK	Astigmatic Keratotomy
APRK	Astigmatic PRK
CLE	Clear Lens Extraction for Hyperopia
HH	Holmium Laser for Hyperopia
HLSK	Hyperopic LASIK
HPRK	Hyperopic PRK
ICL	Implantable Contact Lens
ICRS	Intrastromal Corneal Ring Segments
LSK	LASIK
MZ/PRK	Multizone PRK
RK	Radial Keratotomy

BEYOND GLASSES! RESOURCE GUIDE

ALBERTA
Howard Gimbel, MD
Gimbel Eye Centre
4935 40th Avenue NW, Suite 450
Calgary, AL T3A-2N1
403-286-3022
Current trials: MZ/PRK, HPRK, LSK, HLSK
Other procedures: PRK, APRK, ICL

BRITISH COLUMBIA
Donald G. Johnson, MD
London Place Eye Centre
918 Twelfth Street
New Westminster, BC V3M 6BI
604-526-2020
Currently offers: MZ/PRK, HPRK, PRK, APRK

David T.C. Lin, MD
Pacific Laser Eye Centre
1401 W. Broadway, 5th floor Vancouver, BC
800-818-3937
Currently offers: PRK, LSK

CALIFORNIA
Richard L. Abbott, MD
Beckman Vision Center
University of California, San Francisco
10 Kirkham Street, K301
San Francisco, CA 94143-0730
415-502-6265
Current trials: PRK, ICRS
Other procedures offered: RK, AK, LSK, ALK

Christopher L. Blanton, MD
Inland Eye Institute
1900 East Washington Street
Colton, CA 92324
909-825-3425
FDA trials for: PRK
Current trials: Steroids and analgesics during PRK
Other procedures: RK, AK

Michael Gordon, MD
Vision Surgery and Laser Center
8910 University Center Lane, Suite 800
San Diego, CA 92122
619-455-6800
FDA trials for: PRK, PTK
Current trials: MZ PRK, APRK, HPRK, LSK
Other procedures: RK, AK, ALK

Robert K. Maloney, MD
UCLA Laser Refractive Center
University of California, Los Angeles
100 Stein Plaza
Los Angeles, CA 90095-7003
310-206-7692
FDA trials for: PRK, PTK
Current trials: HPRK, MZ/PRK, LSK
Other procedures: RK, AK, ALK

Peter J. McDonnell, MD
Doheny Eye Institute, University of Southern California School of Medicine
1450 San Pablo Street, Box 5K
Los Angeles, CA 90033
213-342-6377
FDA Trials for: PRK, PTK
Current trials: APRK, HH

James J. Salz, MD
American Eye Institute
Cedars-Sinai Laser Vision Center
8635 W. Third Street
Los Angeles, CA 90048
310-652-1133
FDA trials for: PRK, PTK
Current trials: HPRK
Other procedures offered: RK, AK, CLE, ICL

Steven C. Schallhorn, MD, CDR USN
(U.S. military personnel only)
Naval Medical Center
San Diego, CA 92134-5000
619-532-6700
FDA trials for: PRK
Current trials: PRK, APRK as they apply to functional vision in the military.

ILLINOIS

Randy Epstein, MD
Chicago Cornea Consultants, Ltd.
Illinois Cornea Center
1585 N. Barrington Road, Suite 502
Hoffman Estates, IL 60194
847-882-5900
FDA trials for: PRK, PTK
Current trials: APRK, HPRK
Other procedure offered: ALK

Robert J.S. Mack, MD
Rush Medical College
1725 W. Harrison Street, Suite 928
Chicago, IL 60612
847-882-5900
FDA Trials for: PRK, PTK
Current trials: APRK, HPRK, LSK, MZ/PRK
Other procedure offered: ALK

Manus C. Kraff, MD
Kraff Eye Institute
25 E. Washington Street, #606
Chicago, IL 60602
312-444-1111
FDA trials for: PRK, PTK
Current trials: APRK, HPRK, LSK,
MZ/PRK, HH

LOUISIANA

Marguerite B. McDonald, MD
Refractive Surgery Center of the South
Eye, Ear, Nose & Throat Hospital
2626 Napolean Avenue, 4th Floor
New Orleans, LA 70115
504-896-1250
FDA trials for: PRK
Current trials: HPRK, APRK, LASIK

MASSACHUSETTS

Michael Raizman, MD
New England University Eye Center
Tufts University, 750 Washington Street
Boston, MA 02111
617-636-7625
FDA trials for: PRK, PTK
Current trials: APRK, HPRK, LSK,
MZ/PRK, HH
Other procedure offered: ALK

Roger F. Steinert, MD
Ophthalmic Consultants of Boston
50 Staniford Street
Boston, MA 02114
617-367-4800
FDA investigator for: PRK
Current investigator for: APRK, MZ/PRK,
HPRK, LSK
Other procedures offered: RK, AK

Jonathan H. Talamo, MD
Cornea Consultants
100 Charles River Plaza
Boston, MA 02114
617-523-2010
FDA trials for: PRK, PTK
Current trials: APRK, HPRK, LSK, MZ/
PRK, HH
Other procedures offered: RK, AK

MARYLAND

Walter J. Stark, MD
The Wilmer Institute
The Johns Hopkins Hospital
Maumanee Building, Room 327
600 N. Wolfe Street
Baltimore, MD 21287-9238
410-955-5490
FDA trials for: PRK, PTK
Current trials: APRK, HPRK, LSK, MZ/PRK

MINNESOTA

Richard L. Lindstrom, MD
Lindstrom, Samuelson & Hardten
Associates
710 E. 24th Street
Minneapolis, MN 55404-3810
612-336-5792
FDA trials for: PRK, PTK
Current trials: MZ/PRK, HPRK, LSK,
ICRS, HH, PRK, ICL
Other procedures offered: RK, AK, ALK

MISSOURI

Timothy B. Cavanaugh, MD
Daniel S. Durrie, MD
Hunkeler Eye Centers
4321 Washington
Kansas City, MO 64111
800-753-4580
FDA trials for: PRK, PTK
Current trials: APRK, HPRK, LSK,
MZ/PRK, HH, ICRS, ICL
Other procedures offered: RK, AK, ALK

Charles H. Cozean Jr., MD
56 Doctor's Park Cape
Girardeau, MO 63703
800-456-4401
FDA trials for: PRK, PTK
Current trials: APRK, ICRS

Larry W. Piebenga, MD
University of Missouri—Kansas City
4400 Broadway
Kansas City, MO 64111
816-561-1136
FDA trials for: PRK, PTK

NEW JERSEY

Peter S. Hersh, MD
Cornea & Laser Vision Institute
Hackensack University Medical Center
300 Frank W. Burr Blvd. Glenpointe Ctr
East
Teaneck, NJ 07666
210-883-0505
FDA trials for: PRK, PTK
Current trials: APRK, HPRK, LSK, MZ/PRK,
ICL
Other procedures offered: RK, AK, ALK

NEW YORK

Claus M. Fichte, MD
Eye Care of Niagara, PC
2400 Pine Avenue
Niagara Falls, NY 14301
716-438-2071
FDA trials for: PRK
Current trials: APRK, HPRK, LSK,
MZ/PRK, HH
Other procedures offered: ALK, RK, AK

Lewis R. Grodin, MD
Montefiore Laser & Eye Center
220 Westchester West
White Plains, NY 10604
914-328-5300
FDA trials for: PRK, PTK

Stephen Trokel, MD
Laser Vision Center at Columbia-
Presbyterian Eastside
16 East 60th Street
New York, NY 10022
212-305-5477
FDA trials for: PRK, PTK
Current trials: MZ/PRK, HPRK
Other procedures offered: AK

NORTH CAROLINA

Steven A. Dingledein, MD
1214 Vaughn Road
Burlington, NC 27217
910-228-0254
FDA Trials for: PRK, PTK
Other procedures offered: RK

OHIO

Thomas F. Mauger, MD
Ohio State University
456 West 10th Avenue
Columbus, OH 43210
614-293-5635
FDA trials for: PRK, PTK
Current trials: APRK, MZ/PRK
Other procedure offered: RK

Jeffrey Robin, MD
NuVista Refractive Surgery and Laser Center
3755 Orange Place
Beachwood, Ohio 44122
216-514-3937
FDA trials for: PRK, PTK
Current trials: PRK, LSK

ONTARIO

W. Bruce Jackson, MD
University of Ottawa Eye Institute
Ottawa General Hospital
501 Smyth
Ottawa, K1H 8L6
613-737-7777
Current trials: HPRK, MZ/PRK
Other procedures offered: PRK

Jeffrey Machat, MD
TLC - The Laser Centers Inc.
3200 Desziel Drive, Suite 208
Windsor, ONT N8W 5K8
1-800-463-2020
Procedures offered: PRK, LSK

Raymond M. Stein, MD
Beacon Eye Institute
BLE Place
181 Bay Street, Suite 150
Toronto, Ontario M5J 2T3
800-265-4777
Current trials: HPRK, LSK
Other procedures offered: PRK, MZ/PRK,
APRK

PENNSYLVANIA

Daniel M. Kane, MD
Daniel M. Kane, MD and Associates
30 Hampden Road
Upper Darby, PA 19082
610-352-1166
FDA trials for: PRK, PTK
Current trials: APRK

QUEBEC

Mihai Pop, MD
Michel Pop Clinics
90001 boulevard de l'Acadie Nord
Montréal, Québec H4N 3H5
514-381-2020
Procedures offered: PRK, MZ/PRK,
APRK, HPRK

SOUTH DAKOTA

Vance M. Thompson, MD
Ophthalmology Ltd.
1200 South Euclid Ave., Bldg. 1
Sioux Falls, South Dakota
800-888-1433
FDA trials for: PTK, PRK
Current trials: PRK, MZ/PRK, APRK, LSK,
HPRK, HH
Other procedures: RK, AK, ALK

TEXAS

Daniel H. Gold, MD
The Eye Clinic of Texas
University of Texas Medical Branch
1100 Gulf Freeway, Suite 114
League City, TX 77573
800-423-3937
FDA trials for: PRK, PTK
Current trials: APRK, MZ/PRK

WISCONSIN

Stephen S. Dudley, MD
The Eye Clinic of Fox Valley, S.C.
503 Doctors Court
Oshkosh, WI 54902
800-263-0404
FDA trials for: PRK, PTK
Current trials: APRK, MZ/PRK
Other procedures offered: RK, AK, LSK

8

Getting Ready for PRK

*T*he most important part of getting ready is, of course, finding the right doctor. Assuming you've found a doctor as experienced as the ones listed in Chapter 7, this chapter will help you arrive at PRK day prepared for the best.

If you are over 40 be sure to read Chapter 17 on Monovision *before* your initial office visit. In fact, reading all the chapters in Part Three which apply to you will help you prepare your questions for the initial consultation.

STEP ONE: PICKING YOUR TIME

When you have PRK can have a dramatic effect on your recovery experience:
- Pick a time when you have the time to take care of yourself properly.
- Allow yourself a couple of days of break from routine.
- Expect that you'll be back into your normal activities in a day or two, but leave room for the unexpected.
- Choose a time when your schedule is predictable so you can make all your follow-up appointments.
- Try to pick a week when someone is available to drive you back and forth to your doctor if necessary.

"Better one word before than two words after."

—Welsh Proverb

STEPS TO GETTING READY	
1. Pick your time carefully	6. Set the date
2. Make an appointment	7. Stop wearing contact lenses
3. Stop wearing contact lenses	8. Make arrangements
4. Have the exam	9. Pick up some essentials
5. Review your options	10. Enjoy PRK day
——Decision Point——	

The Best of Times

I didn't have the luxury of choosing any of these times, but they would have been wonderful:

- Between jobs
- During a leave of absence
- The day before a 3-day weekend
- During vacation
- Thursday or Friday if Saturday and Sunday are not work days.

The Worst of Times

My first appointment for PRK was canceled, much to my utter dismay. To make it up to me, the office called with a sudden opening—two days before I was throwing a Christmas party for 78 people. As tempted as I was to have my new vision in time for Christmas vacation, I decided to pass because of the travel time to Canada.

Now I know there was no way I could have held the party right after the procedure, and with red, burning eyes and the inability to wear makeup, I would not have been in a festive mood. Other exceptionally bad times:

- During allergy season if you rely on antihistamines or anti-allergy eyedrops
- When you have an infant to take care of
- The week before you start a new job or go on vacation
- Right before your wedding
- Right before *any* significant event in your life
- Right *after* a particularly stressful event.

What's the hurry? You've been wearing glasses and contacts this long—why not give yourself the gift of at least two weeks between your procedure and anything that could add to the stress of recovery.

STEP TWO: MAKE AN APPOINTMENT

The only thing to say about this step is that the world isn't yet overpopulated with gifted refractive surgeons who are highly experienced in PRK. The ones that exist are booked up well in advance, so be ready with a few alternate dates for the procedure.

The good news is that many doctors, and certainly all of the medical centers, have well-trained support staffs who can handle pre-op exams. Once you've chosen the doctor, call the office and ask:

- How soon can I schedule an initial exam?
- How long will I have to wait between the exam and the procedure?
- If you have a target PRK date in mind, ask if it is likely you will be able to meet it. The office probably will send you some reading material and disclosure statements plus instructions for the first appointment including:
- How to obtain and communicate the results of your last eye exam, so the doctor can tell if your vision is still changing.
- The cost of the initial exam, which usually is credited toward the procedure, if you have it.
- The cost of the procedure and any available credit terms.

STEP THREE: STOP WEARING CONTACT LENSES

If you wear contacts, you have to take time off from wearing them before the initial eye examination, because contacts can alter the physical shape of your cornea. This could produce false symptoms that would prohibit you from having the procedure, and it could change the results of your refractive exam. Your doctor will give you specific instructions, but typically:

- If you wear gas permeable or other **rigid lenses**, you will need to stop wearing them at least three weeks before the initial exam.
- If you wear **soft lenses**, you'll need to stop wearing them two weeks before the initial exam.

Don't cheat during this period: Even a few hours in lenses could alter the results of your tests, and therefore the quality of any decisions that are made.

STEP FOUR: THE INITIAL EYE EXAM

The initial exam has two purposes: to screen out any conditions which would make PRK an inappropriate solution for you, and to determine the nature and extent of your vision problem. Happily, all the tests are completely painless.

In addition to the physical exams, you will be asked to answer a series of questions about your health, past vision problems, history of wearing glasses and contacts and other factors which could influence your candidacy for PRK or other vision-correction surgery.

The last thing you would want is to have a procedure that is not right for you, so answer every question honestly, please! In Part Three I briefly describe some exciting new procedures that are in clinical studies right now and might only be a few years away from FDA approval. If PRK isn't the answer, one of these other options might well be.

Unless you've had eye surgery or eye problems in the past, you probably have never had an eye exam as thorough as the one you'll get before PRK. Allow a couple of hours for this, or even longer if you're going to a medical center or teaching hospital. Your eyes might be dilated when you leave, so bring along some dark UV-protected sunglasses.

The Physical Exams
- A check of the outside of your eyes and eyelids for infections and other abnormalities
- A test and measurement of your pupils
- A glaucoma test to determine the internal pressure of your eye
- A *videokeratography* (also called *corneal topography*) test which visually depicts the surface structure of your cornea.
- An examination of the inside of your eyes for cataracts, retinal and macular problems. This is done after the pupil has been dilated.
- A detailed refractive exam with and without drops that temporarily make it impossible for your focusing muscles to help finetune your vision. This test determines the degree of your refractive error, your current vision prescription and your best-corrected acuity.

HOW HARD SHOULD YOU TRY?   It always worried me that doctors would test my eyes by asking me to read a line I could hardly see. I would squint, struggle and finally guess and they would say "good, now read the next line down." I wondered if they would think I could see better than I really could and give me the wrong prescription. Right before PRK this worry turned into anxiety.

It turns out, I shouldn't have worried because this is method of testing standard practice. "We have to do it that way," Dr. Christopher Blanton said, "to be able to see the absolute limits of your vision. Even if you are guessing, we can assume you are seeing something on which you base your guess."

What is a Corneal Topography?

One of the technologies that microcomputers made cost effective enough for every eye doctor to use is videokeratography—or corneal topography. Like an aerial topographic map, the corneal topography printout shows the peaks and valleys of your cornea in full color (sme examples are shown in Chapter 16).

The test is easy: you simply rest your forehead on a curved support and look into the center of the equipment. The computer quickly maps your cornea and creates a color printout.

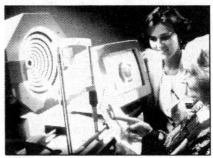

COURTESY OF GIMBEL EYE CENTRE

A corneal topography exam is quick and painless.

The corneal topography lets the doctor see exactly what kind of astigmatism you have, if you have any, and where it is positioned on each eye. It also can show early forms of conditions, such as irregular astigmatism and keratoconus, which deserve special consideration.

Most important, the first topography provides the doctor with a baseline against which to compare the effects of your PRK treatment. After PRK a second topography test will be performed which will show the newly shaped cornea. Then the computer can generate a third map showing the difference between the before and after topographies.

STEP FIVE: CONSULT WITH YOUR DOCTOR
AND REVIEW YOUR OPTIONS

During this consultation your doctor will review all the test results and discuss your options with you. If you are mildly nearsighted, your options might include RK (see chapter 14). If you have high myopia (over -7.0), astigmatism or hyperopia, other options will be discussed (see Part Three).

For each option, the doctor should provide a concise explanation of the risks and benefits along with information about recovery times, outcomes and his or her own experience performing the procedure. If an option described in this book is not presented, be sure to inquire about it if you feel it might be relevant. Take notes.

This is your chance to get everything out on the table: what you hope and expect from a vision-correction procedure; what kinds of vocational or lifestyle factors might be influenced by the results, and any fears or doubts you might have. If there is anything that worries you or you feel needs explanation or further discussion, be sure to bring it up during this consultation.

In addition to determining which procedure, if any, you should have, you should also discuss whether your doctor recommends treating both eyes simultaneously, within a few days of each other, or after a three-month waiting period.

Should You Have Both Eyes Treated at the Same Time?
In the U.S. the FDA has approved PRK for treatment of one eye at a time with a delay of three months between eyes unless there is a "compelling" reason to do it sooner. The three-month delay is only a guideline, not a law, and the doctor and patient can choose to shorten the time between procedures. Compelling reasons might include:
- The difference in vision between the treated and untreated eye makes it difficult for you to function. Most people can get along with glasses that have one lens removed or a plain glass lens in its place if they can't tolerate a contact lens in the untreated eye. If you can't, the date of the second surgery could be moved up.
- You have to travel a long distance for the procedure.

Why Wait?
The FDA's recommendation took into consideration several factors:
1) When the U.S. clinical trials began, simultaneous treatment was not allowed because doctors were still working out the fine details of the procedure and investigating various treatment methods. As a result, the data collected were based on three- or six-month delays between procedures. The FDA cannot issue new guidelines until new data have been presented.
2) Earlier procedures for correcting myopia (such as RK) involved incisions which carried with them long healing periods and the risk of infection.

While we know that after PRK the epithelium heals within the first week and there has never been a serious infection reported, many doctors feel that the conservative approach is to wait between procedures.

3) During the period in which doctors outside the clinical trials buy lasers and learn how to treat and follow PRK cases, there is a greater risk of under- and overcorrection and off-centered treatment. Many of the clinical trial doctors I spoke with felt that these doctors would do their patients a favor by waiting to see how the individual patient's eye responds to the first treatment before doing the second eye.

4) Each person's healing response is unique and there is no way of predicting it. The one person in the Navy study[1] who elected not to have her second eye treated had an unusually aggressive healing response which resulted in significant glare. The second eye could have reacted completely differently to the procedure, but not having both eyes treated together gave her the option of opting out of the second treatment.

5) If you have blurred vision for a week or two, having it in only one eye is less limiting than having it in both.

6) There is less likelihood of short-term presbyopia between the first and second eye because you can use the untreated eye for reading. After the second eye, you might need mild readering glasses for a few weeks.

On the Other Hand...

In Canada and other countries, both eyes are treated routinely in a single visit. This makes sense, too: Once the patient is prepped with eyedrops, and the laser has been tested for alignment, moving from one eye to the other is just a matter of entering a new prescription into the laser computer. Throughout the next year both eyes are checked during each post-op visit, and there is only have one regimen of eyedrops to follow.

Dr. David Lin tells other doctors, "When you've done over 1,000 cases you know how to check your calibration and you can better predict your results, so doing both eyes at the same time makes a lot of sense. But if you're just starting out, and you're not sure of the results you're going to get, you're better off doing one eye at a time." What's the payoff from having both eyes done simultaneously or a day or two apart?

1) Most likely in 2-4 weeks you will have 20/40 vision in both eyes and you can give your glasses and contacts to your local Lion's Club.

2) You don't have to deal with the awkward visual period between treatments if you can't wear contact lenses.

3) There is less downtime because you have only one healing period and then you're back to the races.

4) There is less inconvenience: fewer office visits both pre- and post-op, less time on medication and eyedrops, less travel, if that's necessary, and less time off work.

Balancing the Pros and Cons of Simultaneous Treatment

Deciding whether to have both eyes treated at the same time is a decision you should make with your doctor. For people who don't have a compelling reason for simultaneous surgery, the three dominant factors in the decision are:

1) Your doctor's experience. If she or he has performed PRK on fewer than 200-300 eyes followed for less than six months, I believe you are better off getting one eye done at a time. Your doctor needs time to see the outcomes of her particular procedures.

2) Your personality/lifestyle. If downtime and multiple office visits aren't a major problem for you, go the conservative route.

3) Your risk factors. If your doctor feels you have any risk factors at all that could make your healing response unusual, you should test PRK on one eye first.

"U.S. guidelines tell us to wait," Dr. Robert Maloney said, "and I usually follow them; but having simultaneous PRK is fine in selected cases. It's very safe."

Dr. Salz believes PRK is "incredibly safe and predictable" but still wants patients to wait at least a month between eyes. "There's no way to know if an individual is going to be the one case in 500 who responds with an unusual degree of corneal haze. If this happens in both eyes, the patient can be out of work for awhile until it clears. If the doctor waits a month and there's no significant haze, chances are it won't develop."

Which Eye to Treat First?

If you decide to have your eyes treated separately, which eye should be treated first? Dr. Roger Steinert said that most of the time he treats the nondominant eye first (See Chapter 17 on how to test your own eyes to see which one is dominant). "Patients usually can tolerate a little less than perfect vision in the nondominant eye," he said, "so treating that eye first can help finetune our approach to the dominant eye, where having the best acuity is more important." He described several exceptions to this rule:

- If you are more contact-lens intolerant in your nondominant eye, you will be more comfortable between procedures if you have that eye treated first. Then you can wear a contact in your dominant eye until it is treated.
- If your dominant eye is much more nearsighted than the nondominant eye, you will be more visually comfortable between treatments if the dominant eye goes first, because there will be less difference between your two eyes.
- If your nondominant eye is 20/25 or 20/30, you might consider not treating it at all and having monovision (see Chapter 17). Dr. Steinert would treat your dominant eye first, zand let you live with monovision for a little while. You might like it and save the cost, time and effort of a second procedure.

DECISION POINT

You do *not* have to make a decision during the initial exam and consultation. In fact, unless you have completely made up your mind before the exam and your doctor confirmed that all systems are "go," you will benefit by going home and thinking over everything you have heard.

If your doctor does not offer options you feel would be beneficial to you, you should get a second opinion. If you are a U.S. resident and are wondering about treatments available in Canada you might ask for a referral to a Canadian facility or refer to the list in this book. Most Canadian doctors have patient care managers who can speak with you over the phone. In most cases the results from your initial eye exam can be sent and an evaluation made without your physical presence.

If you trust the first doctor, take the information gained from the second opinion and return for a follow-up consultation.

If you are still uncertain, make the decision to wait.

STEP SIX: SET THE DATE

Between the decision and PRK day, you will need to allow two to three weeks without contacts.

STEP SEVEN: STOP WEARING CONTACT LENSES

Yes, again, and for the same reasons. Rigid lenses have to be off three weeks, at least, before PRK. Soft lenses should be off at least two weeks. Just think of all the money you'll save on cleaning solutions! Of course, if you are only treating one eye, or one eye first, you may continue to wear a contact in the other eye, if this gives you adequate vision.

STEP EIGHT: MAKE ARRANGEMENTS

If you are having the procedure done within driving distance, you will need someone to drive you home after the procedure, back to the doctor the next day, and possibly one more time the first week. If you are flying to the treatment facility, you'll need transportation home from the airport.

If you are traveling any distance, you also will need air and hotel reservations. Unless you plan to make a vacation out of the trip, basic accommodations are all that are necessary. You won't be using pools, weight rooms or discos, so save your cash for some flashy new sunglasses. If you are traveling alone, try to find a hotel within walking distance of the doctor's office. The office staff should be able to help with this and many major hotel chains give discounts to people traveling for surgical reasons.

If you live alone, it would be optimal to have someone on call, or staying with you, the first night.

Tips for Women

Because you should keep anything except the prescription eyedrops away from your eyes right after treatment, you will not be able to wear any makeup except lipstick and a non-powder blusher from the day of the procedure until the epithelium of your cornea is healed (2-5 days, on average).

If the thought of going out in public without mascara makes you want to wear a mask, consider having your eyelashes and/or brows dyed the week before the procedure. I did and it gave me a little extra boost—especially since, for the first time, I could see my eyes from more than a foot away.

Keep your hairdo simple, too, because you might not be able to do much with it the next day. While your cornea is healing, hairspray should be used sparingly, if at all. If you need color or a perm, have it done ahead of PRK or plan on waiting at least a week after.

STEP NINE: PICK UP A FEW ESSENTIALS

These things are only essential if you need them, and you can get them after the procedure. However, having them at hand might make your first two days easier, especially if you live alone.

Medications

Ask your doctor or the nurse whether they will provide prescription pain medication or sleeping pills as a part of the procedure. Many doctors do and most patients don't need them. If your doctor doesn't, ask for a prescription that you can get filled ahead of time so you won't have to worry about it the first day. Two or three pain pills and two sleeping pills should be the most you will need.

While you are at the drug store, get a bottle of extra-strength acetamenophin (Tylenol or similar). During the procedure, and perhaps after it, your doctor will give you non-steroidal anti-inflammatory drops (NSAIDs) so you should not take other anti-inflammatories such as aspirin, ibuprofen (Advil or Motrin) Naprosyn (Aleve), or ketoprofen (Actron).

Sunglasses

Your doctor probably will provide post-surgical wrap-around sunglasses which you will appreciate the first couple of days. These are not fashion-forward, however, so you might want to buy a nifty pair of non-prescription sunglasses ahead of time. Make sure they are dark and UV filtered. Polarization would be an extra help if you can afford it.

Reading Glasses

Even though I recommend you avoid recreational reading the first few days (you'll learn why in Chapter 11), you might need reading glasses for essential activities, such as reading the labels on your prescription drug bottles, especially if you are traveling. Glasses with +3.0 magnification will carry you through. If you find you still need readers after the first week, go back to the drugstore, test various magnifications, and buy the weakest one that allows you to read newsprint type or business cards.

I didn't know that wearing too-strong magnifying glasses can make it even harder to read, so there I was, three weeks after PRK, with my nose in my phone file trying to read the numbers through +3.0 magnifiers. Then one day I found myself standing next to some reading glasses in a department store and I started trying them on. I was amazed at how well I could see with +1.50s. Two weeks later, I cut back to +1.25s. Now, I have +1.00s to wear when I have to read in very dim light. I could actually use weaker ones, but I'm too stubborn to pay money for prescription readers when I only need them 30 minutes a day.

Magnifying Make-up Mirror/Shaving Mirror

If you've been nearsighted all your life, you probably take it for granted that when you look in the mirror you'll see your eyelashes. This is not so for the farsighted, and for the first month or two after PRK you might be slightly farsighted. I had to put mascara on by touch for at least six weeks and I shudder to imagine how I probaly looked, even with the use of a good illuminated magnifying mirror. If you don't have one, you might want to get one. Buy one with 3x magnification—you'll find uses for it for the rest of your life.

A TWELVE-STEP PROGRAM FOR ENJOYING PRK DAY

I got up on the morning of January 9, 1995 and, being someone inclined to drama and cliché, said to myself, "Well, Franette, this is first day of the rest of your *sight!*" If you're like me you'll be feeling anticipation mixed with anxiety: I wasn't worried so much about the procedure itself, I just couldn't *wait* for the results. These twelve steps will help take the stress out of PRK Day:

1. If you regularly take medications, clear them with your doctor *before* the day of the procedure.

2. Wear comfortable clothes. You won't have to change out of them for PRK.

3. Wear a simple hairstyle that can take care of itself if your vision is a little fuzzy for 24 hours.

4. Eat a good breakfast.

5. Take it easy on caffeine so you won't be awake when you want to sleep.

6. Stay conscious: no alcohol, tranquilizers, antihistamines or any other medication that can make you drowsy. If a tranquilizer is necessary, your doctor will give it to you just prior to the procedure.

7. Take someone with you to keep you company in the waiting room. Some doctors have the space to allow a spouse or friend to stay with you throughout the entire procedure. I would have loved this!

8. Stay busy before you go and take something with you to keep your mind occupied in the waiting room.

9. Eat a good lunch if you are still waiting for the big moment.

10. Afterward, have a light dinner. Drink *lots* of water, but little or no alcohol.

11. Go for a short walk if you feel like it and if it's not too dry or windy.

12. Take a sleeping pill, your prescribed eyedrops, some vitamin C, and get a good night's sleep.

9

The PRK Procedure

*I*t has been estimated that well over 600,000 eyes have been treated by PRK worldwide, and in survey after survey nearly 100% of the patients say they would do it again. That's not only because PRK works, but because it is fast, painless and effortless.

"My entire staff works together to keep things moving," Dr. Robert Maloney said, "so patients don't have time to sit around and worry. Everyone who deals with our patients is knowledgeable and I think that's very reassuring. It gives patients confidence."

So, you're finally with the right doctor, at the right time, and you're being moved right along. What will the next hour be like?

THE COUNTDOWN

PRK -60: Check-in and Final Exam

After you check in, your vision will be tested one final time to ensure a consistent result. If the doctor finds too large a difference between the first exam and this one, you might be asked to wait another week or two.

This rarely happens, but if it does, it is in your own best interest to wait: The single most important component of the PRK procedure (aside from a properly working laser, of course) is an accurate refractive exam. This is what determines how much tissue will be removed from your cornea.

Test results can vary from one exam to another for a wide variety of reasons, including pregnancy. Regardless of the reason, though, your vision must be stable before you have PRK.

WHO CAN HAVE PRK?   At this writing two lasers for PRK have been approved by the FDA for treatment of -1.0 to -7.0 myopia with less than one diopter of astigmatism in people over the age of 18. Other procedures described later in this book are still in clinical trials. The Canadian Health Protection Branch still classifies PRK as investigational for nearsightedness over -6.0, but for five years PRK has been widely used in Canada for treatment of all degrees of nearsightedness and astigmatism and, to a lesser extent, farsightedness.

PRK -30: Preparation
This is the part that makes PRK painless. Eyedrops are instilled in your eye at regular intervals:
- Anti-inflammatory drops to reduce swelling after procedure
- Antibiotic drops to reduce risk of infection
- Anesthetic drops to numb the cornea. The first few drops might sting or burn a little until your eye is numb.

If you are nervous, you might be given a mild tranquilizer, but don't take your own ahead of time. You need to be alert enough to focus on a light when the time comes.

PRK -5: Pre-Op
Now it's time to go into the laser room and the pre-op steps begin:
1) You are seated in a reclining chair like a dentist's and a pillow might be placed on either side of your head to keep it stationary.
2) The eye that won't be treated is covered to help you better concentrate during the procedure.
3) Final anesthetic drops are placed in your eye.
4) Your chair is reclined and the light in the room might be dimmed. I found the darkened room to be very helpful emotionally—perhaps because it brought my attention right down to the doctor and what he was saying. There was no temptation to look around at the equipment or make myself nervous in other ways. My doctor had a nice, calm voice, as did his assistant, and that helped, too.
5) A small instrument is used to hold your eyelids apart. You might feel a slight "opening" sensation, but nothing else.

THE PRK PROCEDURE

Step One: Removing the Epithelium

As we learned in Chapter 5, the cornea is covered with an outer "skin" called the epithelium which protects it from injury and the elements. Because the composition of the epithelium is different from the cornea, it vaporizes at a different rate and must be removed separately before the cornea is treated by the laser.

There are two ways to remove it, but with either method the process takes less than a minute and is completely painless.

The Manual Method

The method that was used in the clinical trials, and therefore is part of the FDA approval, was the manual method where the epithelium is gently scraped off the area to be treated.

The Laser Method

An alternative method, which Dr. Donald Johnson terms "the no-touch technique," is popular in Canada and with some doctors in the U.S. With this method, called *transepithelial ablation*, the laser is set up to remove the epithelium in the 6mm PRK zone. It only takes a few pulses. Then the laser is reset to perform the PRK.

"By looking through the microscope while the laser removes the epithelium I can tell exactly when it's all gone. The epithelium has an iridescence to it that is quite distinctive," Dr. Johnson said. "This method leaves the surgical zone completely clear and smooth and a smoother cornea means a smoother ablation, which in turn can shorten recovery time and produce less haze after surgery."

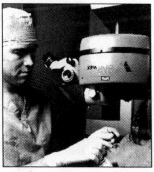

Dr. Robert Maloney places anesthetic drops in a patient's eye just prior to PRK. The drops make the procedure painless.

CHARLIE MARTIN, JULES STEIN EYE INSTITUTE

Some doctors feel that the laser method is superior because it removes only the exact amount of epithelium necessary for the treatment, so less has to grow back during recovery, whereas the manual method is less precise by nature. "Current FDA guidelines state that we should remove it manually," Dr. Lindstrom said, "but we can do what we think is best for our patients. We just can't go out and advertise, 'don't have it that way, my way is better.' He uses both methods, "but I have found that transepithelial ablation is more attractive to patients. You need additional training and have to reprogram the laser in order to do it, though."

Both Dr. Johnson and Dr. Lindstrom said that the laser method is superior for retreatment procedures because it tends to induce less haze, but in a study led by Dr. Howard Gimbel comparing the two methods, there was no statistical difference at six months between eyes treated with the manual and laser removal techniques.

Step Two: Reshaping the Cornea

Once the epithelium is gone, the cornea is ready for PRK. If the epithelium was removed manually, the doctor pivots your chair under the laser—the part that is above your head is about the size of a dental lamp—and asks you to look at a red or green light (Figure 9.1). You probably will have a practice run with no actual treatment to familiarize you with the sound the laser makes.

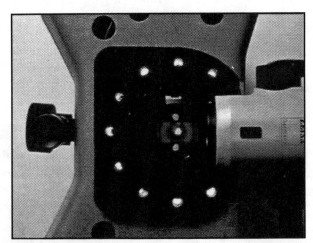

COURTESY OF SUMMIT TECHNOLOGY, INC.

FIGURE 9.1 This is similar to what what you will see when you look up at the PRK laser. The light in the center is the fixation light.

When you are ready, the treatment begins. You'll hear some sounds (see inset) and smell an acrid aroma much like burning hair as tissue from the cornea is vaporized. Don't worry, though: the underlying tissue is not affected.

Total laser time is about 20-40 seconds per eye, but this might be divided into several steps if you are part of a clinical trial or having your treatment in Canada where multizone treatments are common (these are described in Chapter 15). If you are having astigmatism treated at the same time, there might be some delay between portions of the treatment.

Whatever happens, all you'll see is the red light fading in and out of view. Don't be concerned if you lose track of it briefly—that is common during treatment. Just keep your gaze fixed straight up and breathe naturally. You'll be amazed at how fast the procedure goes. Reading this section takes longer than an actual PRK.

Step Three: Finishing Up

Now the doctor simply removes the eyelid support, places a bandage contact lens over the eye, adds a few drops of anti-inflammatory, takes the patch off your untreated eye and moves the chair away from the laser.

If you're having the other eye treated, it will take a few minutes for the doctor to enter that eye's data into the computer, so relax. When the laser is ready, the newly treated eye will be covered and the doctor will begin again at Step One. The doctor won't kick you out of the office if you remind him to double check the programming for the second eye. I've never heard of anyone making a mistake and reversing the corrections, but I suppose it could happen.

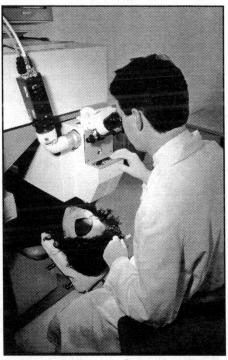

FIGURE 9.2   Dr. Raymond Stein treats a patient with PRK. "Having PRK is *much* easier than getting your teeth cleaned," he said. "All you have to do is relax and look at a red light."

THE SIGHTS AND SOUNDS OF PRK

Because the doctor who performed my initial exams was in California, and a staff member did my pre-op refractive exam in Canada, I didn't meet my doctor until I entered the treatment room. By then, I must confess, my knees were a little wobbly. "Is everyone as nervous as I am?" I asked.

"Yes...and everyone asks me that question!" he replied. For some reason, this answer put me at ease.

I reclined in the chair and room was dimmed. One of my pre-op worries was that it would be like having an MRI—I am claustrophobic—but the part of the laser that came over my face was so small, this was never a problem.

Next I saw a foggy, gauzy, in-and-out image of the light on the laser lamp as my eyelid was propped open and the epithelium was manually removed. There was no feeling at all in my eye or eyelid except a circular rubbing sensation. If my eye were a car fender being polished, it probably would have felt about the same.

When the doctor told me to focus on the red light, I noticed the white lamplight behind it. At first I wondered which I should look at. I also felt like I had to push back my hair and scratch my nose so I bumped the laser not twice, but three times. He said this was common and to relax and keep my arms at my sides. (Later he told me that every now and then a patient bumps the laser so hard that it activates the equipment's shut-off mechanism and a service rep has to be called.)

When the procedure started it sounded like a marble being rattled rapidly in a hollow can, but there was no sensation of seeing a beam of light: All I saw was the red light fading in and out. Since I was having my astigmatism treated at the same time, the doctor would start the laser, do a few pulses, and then reprogram it and do a few more. This went on for several minutes.

When the laser was operating I heard a snapping sound that reminded me of an electrostatic air filter. Other patients have described it as sounding like a wet towel being snapped. I also smelled an odor like burning hair—the scent of collagen molecules exiting my cornea.

During the delays between laser sessions, the experience seemed otherworldly. The dark room, my reclined position, the lights in the lamp above my face and the quiet, calm voice of my doctor and his assistant murmuring phrases to each other: "20 47, OK 375, give me a little more on 238" —all combined to make me feel more like a space capsule being landed than a patient being operated on.

The procedure took about 20 minutes from beginning to end, but I only had to fixate my eyes on the light for a few seconds at a time. I'd hear the rattling can sound, smell a burning odor and then get to relax. In the U.S., unless you're part of clinical trial, your treatment will take under a minute and there will be no stopping once the laser is started unless the doctor detects an eye movement.

When I sat up and the lights came back on, I felt a little dazed. Again, I slipped right into B-movie dialogue. "Is that all there is to it?" I asked. Then I noticed that I could see an exit sign way down at the end of the hall...and the ducks on the doctor's tie...and the numbers on an instrument dial several feet away. It was the kind of sudden relief you feel when you come around the last fast bend on a roller coaster and it abruptly stops: You survived and it was worth it.

The thrill of a lifetime doesn't *begin* to describe it.

Step Four: Sitting Up

I know this doesn't sound like much of a step, but that's all that's left to the procedure. Most likely, you'll be able to see somewhat foggily out of the treated eye. The amount of vision you have immediately after PRK depends on how much and how fast your cornea responds to the stress of the treatment. Some lucky patients, like me, see very clearly for the first few minutes after PRK and are utterly amazed by their sudden vision. Dr. Maloney said that he never tires of hearing the patient's exclamations when this happens, but most people find their vision foggy or cloudy for the first day or two.

Step Five: Getting Ready to Go

Your doctor most likely will give you a care kit which will include supplies such as eyedrops, and an instruction sheet for using them, pain medications, artificial tears, sunglasses and a phone number you can call if you experience problems.

If you wore glasses into the office and only had one eye treated, you might ask to have one lens removed from the glasses frames. I tried this, but found it very disorienting. By the next day, I was able to get around fine using only my newly treated eye. I wasn't driving, however. If you intend to drive with only one treated eye and no lens on the other, be sure to check your depth perception before heading out on the road—and don't plan on driving at all until your vision clears.

Step Six: A Final Lens Check

As Dr. Maloney describes in the next chapter, fitting a patient with a bandage lens involves some trial and waiting. It is worth your time to sit with the lens for at least 20 minutes and then ask the doctor or his assistant to check the fit one last time before you leave. According to Dr. Maloney, about 15% of his patients need a larger lens because the eye continues to swell a little after the first lens is applied. A too-small lens can lead to Tight Lens Syndrome, which is to be avoided if at all possible. The next Chapter has more information about dealing with tight lenses.

Step Seven: Enjoying the Next Hour

Whether you are going back to a hotel or your own home, you have about an hour before the anesthesia wears off and you begin experiencing any discomfort. This is a good time to eat a light meal, drink plenty of water, take some vitamin C, and get settled. Recovery is the subject of the next chapter.

WHY IS VISION CLOUDY AFTER PRK?

Most people experience foggy or cloudy vision for the first few days after PRK. The cloudiness can occur immediately, or gradually over the first few hours. This is not something to worry about, and certainly not an indication that your PRK "didn't take."

Physiologically, here's what's happening: The epithelium, which protects your cornea, has been removed over the treatment zone and a hairbreadth of tissue has been vaporized off the cornea surface. This exposes part of the cornea that usually doesn't come in contact with the tear film. The tissue of the cornea absorbs the tear film and puffs up a little from the extra fluid. This swelling lifts the tear film—and remember, it's the tear film that refracts light through the cornea to the retina— and so that light rays aren't bent properly and therefore the image isn't focused on the retina.

After the epithelium grows back, the swelling of the cornea subsides, so the tear film returns to its normal thickness and to its new, flatter position on the cornea. When this happens your vision will begin to be as you imagined it would be—usually on the third or fourth day after PRK.

FDA TRIAL DOCS TREAT THEMSELVES TO PRK

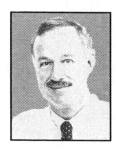

Name
Roger Steinert, MD, 45

Occupation
Corneal Surgeon, Mass.

Pre-Op Vision
-4.0

Procedure
PRK

Post-Op Vision
20/15 (at 13 days)

For Dr. Steinert, excimer lasers were no mystery: He had been experimenting with them since 1983. He was involved in testing some of the very first ophthalmic lasers and he was a principal investigator for Summit Technology's FDA trials. Dr. Gordon wasn't a stranger to lasers, either. As the first doctor to use a Summit laser for PRK, in 1989 he treated the first human blind and sighted eyes, and he was the principal surgeon for the Navy's FDA trials.

During all these years of developing PRK procedures and treating patients with them, neither doctor could have the procedure himself. "It just wouldn't have been right for an investigator to bias himself by becoming part of the trials," Dr. Steinert said, "and when FDA approval finally came, we were both too busy treating patients to do anything about our own eyes."

Finally, in May of 1996, Dr. Gordon flew to Boston to have one eye treated by Dr. Steinert. Three days later, Dr. Gordon returned the favor and treated Dr. Steinert in San Diego. I spoke with them both about two weeks later.

From the Atlantic....

Three years ago Dr. Gordon considered having PRK in Germany but couldn't work it into his schedule. When he went to Dr. Steinert he said, "Now, I want you to treat me exactly the way you do your patients. Don't do anything special."

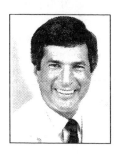

Name
Michael Gordon, MD, 47

Occupation
Corneal Surgeon, California

Pre-Op Vision
-3.5, -4.0

Procedure
PRK

Post-Op Vision
20/25 (at 16 days),
20/30 (intentionally
undercorrected)

"It was very strange for me to go through it. If felt kind of like an out-of-body experience. I was lying there watching everything as if it were happening out in the room, but it was happening right there on my cornea and I really couldn't feel a thing."

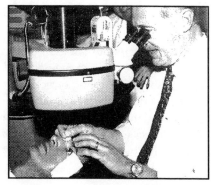

In his Boston office, Dr. Steinert treats Dr. Gordon to PRK

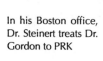
COURTESY OF SUMMIT LASER VISION CENTERS

"I never lost a single day from work. I had my eye done on Tuesday, flew home that night, and performed an RK on Wednesday. So far, I haven't even had any side effects and I keep checking, of course. In fact, I have more night glare with the eye that's still wearing a contact than with the PRK-treated eye."

...to the Pacific

"I thought I pretty much knew what to expect," Dr. Steinert said, "but I learned a great deal from going through the experience myself.

"I had a much stronger foreign-body sensation than I expected, for one thing. About 20% of my patients would tell me they felt the bandage lens—even after I had removed it. I couldn't understand it. Now I've had the same feeling in my own eye. I changed lenses about

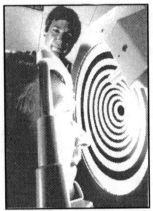

COURTESY OF SUMMIT LASER VISION CENTERS

Dr. Gordon tests Dr. Steinert after his PRK.

four times and even—very briefly—tried it without the lens. I think I've proven to myself that it's the edge of the treatment zone that we are feeling, not the lens."

That sensation lasted for about two days, then disappeared. "There was much less disruption to my life than I expected," he said. "I thought I might be off work for a couple of weeks, but I had PRK on Friday and was back to work on Monday. I performed several PRKs on Tuesday and did 6 microsurgeries on Thursday—less than a week after my treatment!"

Patients should note that doctors can fine-tune their microscopes before surgery to compensate for a difference in vision between two eyes or for a slight lack of acuity. Those who need fine acuity at work and can't use a microscope might experience more downtime.

UPDATE   A month later Dr. Gordon again flew to Boston to have his second eye treated by Dr. Steinert and returned home the same day. That eye was deliberately undercorrected for reading (see Chapter 17). Five months later his "distance" eye was 20/15, his "reading" eye was 20/30, and he could read the smallest type on the reading test card. At six months post-op Dr. Steinert's treated eye was still 20/15 and he was waiting for a break so he could have his second eye treated.

A DRIVING NEED FOR PRK

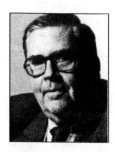

Name
Henry Walker, 74
before his PRK

Occupation
Retired business executive,
Hawaii

Pre-Op Vision
20/60; 20/80

Pre-Op Vision
20/15; 20/20

Surgeon
David Lin, MD

Henry Walker recently bought a Ferrari—his sixth. He's had all colors, but this time he got blue. "It attracts less attention," he said, meaning attention of the red light/ screaming siren type.

"At my age, driving a red car fast just isn't the thing to do. So I have a nice blue one now and I drive it as fast as I can.

"I heard a man making a presentation on financial management and he mentioned that he was seeing without glasses for the first time in his life. He was so excited about it that he treated both of his sons to PRK as a Christmas gift. This really interested me. I've had glasses on and off for most of my life and I hate them. My nose is poorly shaped for glasses, so they slide down, and my peripheral vision with glasses is terrible. I have always been looking for a way around them.

"I tried contacts once, but I felt it was just too much boiling of stuff and my fingers weren't that clever in dealing with them. I love to drive fast, but going around curves always made me a little nervous because of my bad peripheral vision. That really was the motivator.

"I nearly went to have RK, but my ophthalmologist urged me to have PRK instead. She made all the arrangements for me with Dr. Lin and did all my pretests and follow-up. All I had to do was set forth with my wife for Vancouver.

"After the first eye was done Dr. Lin checked his work to make sure it was right before going on to the other. Then he asked me if I was ready for the second eye. I said, 'Sure, that was nothing.' After he was done he said, 'Now stand up and look out the window.'

"Everything was as clear as could be: the mountains, the trees. He put in the protective contacts and about 12 hours later I started getting a feeling in my right eye like an eyelash was in it, but Tylenol took care of that. He took the contacts out after two days. I went to the movies that night without glasses for the first time in years. It was great fun.

"Now it's been a month and I see very clearly. I drive without prescription glasses. There's no question I see better without glasses now than I ever did before with them. I'm more alert to what's going on around me because I can see out of the sides of my eyes. The colors even seem brighter.

"My ophthalmologist was amazed when she saw my results and now she is getting trained to do PRK. I'm delighted I took advantage of it."

Planning for a Perfect Recovery

*L*et's call this the "empowerment" chapter, because with a little knowledge you can take charge of your recovery. The information falls into three categories:

1) What you *must do* to ensure the best possible outcome for yourself
2) What you *should do* to accelerate your recovery
3) What you *can* do to make yourself as comfortable as possible the first few days after treatment

And while you're recovering remember: Knowing what *can* go wrong does not increase the chances that something *will* go wrong! According to surveys conducted by Dr. Raymond Stein, PRK has the highest patient-satisfaction rating of any refractive surgical procedure. Being prepared and taking care of yourself will make your chances way better than good that you'll find yourself in the "totally satisfied" category.

THE FIRST FEW DAYS

Right after your procedure you might sit up and be able to see the EXIT sign down the hall, as I did. Or, your vision might be cloudy. The cloudiness is caused by a slight swelling of the cornea, which affects vision, but this takes longer to happen for some people than others. Right after surgery and for the first few days, your treated eye might look red and watery.

In about 1 1/2 hours my anesthetic wore off completely and my vision had become cloudy. At this point I felt like there was something under the bandage contact lens. This is normal and usually lasts 12-24 hours. During this time you might also have tearing or your eye might feel a little hot.

The next morning (about 14 hours post-op) my treated eye had very good vision for distance and I was able to function without wearing any glasses at all—even though my other eye was still 20/550. The doctor said my cornea was clear, but slight hazing is more usual at this point. He tested my vision at about 20/40 and said that it would continue to improve. In this measure I was, again, ahead of schedule. Many patients get to 20/40 or better more gradually—especially if they start out very nearsighted. In general, the less myopia you have going in, the faster your vision will stabilize after PRK.

As I mentioned earlier, I spent hours walking outdoors while I waited to have my second eye done. Even though it was a gray day, I noticed that I was much more comfortable wearing the sunglasses the doctor gave me because any strong light made me squint.

Some of the patients I talked to felt nothing after they woke up the next morning. Others continued to feel irritation throughout the second day. All of them had complete relief by the third day, except for me and a patient with extreme light sensitivity. I describe our experiences in more detail in the next chapter.

The bandage lens on my second eye was removed on the third day post-op, but the first eye took a week. With each eye, once the lens was removed there was no sensation of having had the procedure.

Anticipating Downtime
Most patients can return to work and are able to drive in two or three days or sooner. Others might feel they need another few days. If your work involves reading or use of a computer, you might find you need reading glasses for awhile.

Dr. Raymond Stein said that he treated both eyes of a fellow surgeon in the same visit. The PRK was done on Friday afternoon and the patient was performing microsurgery the following Tuesday. "I have treated over 100 optometrists with PRK and almost all were able to do eye exams within a few days," he said.

If your experience is like this, great. My advice is to plan to take a few days off for the procedure and to take it easy in general the first week. You can always do more if you feel like it.

In the Navy study, 29 of the 30 first participants had 20/20 vision within three months of their PRK procedures.

ACHIEVING THE BEST POSSIBLE OUTCOME

The items in this section are *must do's*. Don't even *think* about having *any* type of eye surgery unless you are willing to make these commitments. The quality of your eyesight might depend on it.

Use Your Eyedrops Exactly as Prescribed

As described in Chapter 9, you'll be using eyedrops or ointments for the first 1-7 days to prevent infection and reduce inflammation. "I give patients anti-inflammatory drops (Voltaren or Accular) to take home with them," Dr. David Lin said, "but I tell them to use the drops only if the eye hurts. Overusing anti-inflammatories can delay healing." Dr. Salz suggests that patients pay attention to whether the anti-inflammatory makes the eye feel better. "At the point you notice no difference within five minutes after using them, stop."

After the first week your doctor might put you on a regimen of steroid drops. Other doctors wait a few weeks to see how the eye responds. Steroid eyedrops control the rate your cornea heals to prevent overhealing, which could cause scarring or overcorrection. If you are given the drops, your doctor will develop a gradually decreasing schedule for you which you should follow exactly. The number of drops per day and their frequency will be determined by factors such as your age, the amount of your correction, and your overall health. "The goal," said Dr. Lin, "is to use as little as possible for as short a time as possible, but the doctor has to be the one controlling the dosage."

Notify your doctor if you experience burning when you use the drops, and if you lose a bottle, replace it immediately, without skipping doses, if possible.

Show Up for Your Follow-Ups

Visit your doctor for your follow-up exams without missing appointments. Your doctor knows what kinds of results are normal at certain intervals and what changes are expected from one visit to the next. If you skip a visit or

---

MUST DO's

1. Use your eyedrops as prescribed.
2. Visit your doctor on schedule.
3. Report any significant change in vision.

---

lengthen the time between one visit and the next, the doctor's ability to gauge or alter your progress might be compromised.

In addition, it is extremely important for your eyes to be checked at regular intervals so the doctor can finetune your eyedrop regime according to your individual healing response. Some complications, such as increased eye pressure, have no symptoms at all but can be quickly spotted and treated by your doctor. If not treated, they can lead to serious trouble.

Part of the PRK procedure is making 5-7 office visits over the first year. Don't cheat yourself out of a single one just because you think you're doing fine! You probably are, but wouldn't you like to know for sure?

Report Any Significant Change in Vision

It is normal for your vision to "come in and out" the first few months and fluctuate from one day to another. Try to ignore these normal changes, because your eyes gradually will stabilize.

Other symptoms could indicate the need to change your eyedrops or add medication such as antibiotics or beta blockers. Notify your doctor immediately if you have any of the following:

- *Sudden change* in vision such as cloudiness
- *Progressive blurriness* over a period of a day or two
- *Pain, redness or burning* at any time after the bandage lens has been removed.
- *Extreme discomfort* at any time.

FAST-TRACKING YOUR RECOVERY

The part of the healing process that gets most people's attention is the time it takes for the epithelium to heal. Remember, this is the "skin" that protects your cornea's innumerable and very sensitive nerves from being jangled every time you bat an eye. During the 1-5 days it takes for the epithelium to rebuild its 40-micron layer of cells, you'll feel discomfort ranging from "there's something irritating my eye" to a burning sensation. Most people do not experience actual pain—it's more of a "soap-in-the-eye" feeling of discomfort.

For the vast majority of PRK patients the worst of the irritation is over after 24 hours and disappears completely the second day. The bandage contact lens is removed any time after that, but usually by the fifth day.

SHOULD DO's

- Keep your bandage lens in place.
- Keep your eye clean and protected.
- Avoid touching your eye.
- Use artificial tears.
- Be cautious with anesthetic drops.
- Wear dark UV sunglasses.
- Refuse other people's eyedrops.
- Be careful with alcohol and caffeine.
- Use common sense about driving.

Don't Remove Your Own Bandage Contact!

Reread my case in Chapter 11 or Byron Tucker's in Chapter 16 if you are tempted to take out your bandage contact for any reason at all. Call your doctor first. *Trust me* on this one!

It is remotely possible for the lens to fall out, blink out, or blow off. One patient who traveled to Canada for PRK as part of a group from the U.S. went for a walk right after his procedure while he was waiting for the other patients to be finished. Because his eye was still numb, he didn't realize that the dry wind had blown his contact right off the cornea. When he returned to the doctor's office, the nurse noticed the contact was perched on his lapel. Luckily, she replaced it with a new one before he ever felt a twinge of pain.

To avoid losing the lens or drying it out, protect your eyes from wind and rain while the bandage lens is in place. Wearing wraparound sunglasses helps.

What to Do If You Lose a Bandage Lens

If a lens does fall out, here's what to do:

1) If your doctor is local call the office or the after-hours emergency number and explain that the lens has fallen out. Most likely you will be advised to return to the office as soon as possible.
2) To protect the eye while you're traveling to your doctor, fold sterile gauze into a 1" thick pad and place it over the closed eye. Tape another patch of gauze over it to hold the pad in place with pressure on the eye.
3) Press a towel-covered icepack over the patch for 20 minutes on/20 minutes off to relieve the inflammation which causes the pain.

4) If your doctor's office isn't nearby, try to see another eye doctor who specializes in PRK or corneal surgery.

3) If that's not an option, call an optometrist and tell her you need a disposable contact lens (even if it has a small prescription in it, you can manage with that until you get to your doctor). Then go to your own doctor as soon as possible for the proper bandage lens, because a too-thick lens can delay healing by restricting oxygen flow to the cornea.

6) If it's night or Sunday and you can't reach your doctor, go to your local emergency room and explain that you need the thinnest possible bandage contact lens. The next day go to your own doctor for a checkup.

Keep Your Eye Clean and Protected

Until the bandage lens is removed, your epithelium isn't able to do its assigned task of protecting the cornea from infection. Therefore, you have to step up to the plate and be unusually careful about keeping possible contaminants away from your eyes.

- Keep your hands and the nozzle of eyedrop bottles away from your eyes. If you do have to touch your eyes, wash your hands carefully between touching the eyes to avoid transmitting bacteria.
- Don't wear eye makeup, ladies. See Chapter 8 for alternatives.
- Cover your face before spraying your hair.
- Be careful when you shower or wash your face and hair because soaps and shampoos can be extremely irritating and tap water can contain bacteria.
- Don't use a steam room, spa or a swimming pool until your lenses have been removed. Chlorine and mentholyptus are eye irritants and the steam, spray or humidity can contain bacteria which could cause infection.
- Be careful cooking so that steam or oil spatters don't get in your eyes.
- Avoid smoky, dusty or fumey environments such as bars, construction sites or chemical labs. If you smoke, try to do it outdoors where wind can take the smoke away from your eyes.
- This is not the time to take on a project that requires spray painting, gardening or crawling around under pipes or engines that can drip on your face.
- Delay having your hair cut, colored or permanent waved until the bandage lens is removed. If you go to a dentist, dermatologist, etc., caution them to keep your eyes out of harm's way.

Use Artificial Tears

While your epithelium and cornea are healing, proteins and other chemicals are generated which are sloughed off into the tear film. According to Dr. Louis Catania, these can accumulate and be a source of low-grade chronic irritation.

He recommends using unpreserved, sterile artificial tears as often as you want to flush your eyes and keep the bandage lens moist. These can be continued whenever you need them for the first few months. *Don't* use "redness reducing" eyedrops, allergy drops, saline solutions, boric acid or any homebrewed remedy until your eye is fully healed.

Use Anesthetic Eye Drops Sparingly

At this writing most anesthetic eye drops delay healing, so if you have drops left over from some other procedure, or if your doctor has given you some to take home, be sure to question whether these can or should be used freely and for how long.

For the fastest healing, it would be better to rely on pain medications (see below) than anesthetic eye drops. Most of the doctors I spoke with don't prescribe them.

Wear Dark UV-Filtered Sunglasses Outdoors

After PRK you should protect your eyes from sunlight because they can't protect themselves until the cornea heals.

During the first week, sunglasses have the added benefit of helping to keep out dust and wind, which can dry out the bandage lens—even blow it off your eye—or cause irritation while the epithelium is healing.

Just Say "No" to Other People's Eyedrops

If other people offer you their left-over eyedrops, kindly decline them. You should never use another person's eyedrops, or eye makeup, under any circumstance because it is so easy to transfer bacteria that way.

After you have PRK, your doctor will give you the *only* drops appropriate for your recovery. Others could cause problems.

Be Careful with Alcohol and Caffeine

I haven't seen any PRK patient booklets warning against drinking, but common sense indicates you would be better off drinking water than something alcoholic the first few days. There are several reasons:

- Alcohol is dehydrating and this could exacerbate any dry-eye or tight-lens problems you might have.
- Alcohol should not be combined with *any* pain medication, and can cause liver damage when used with acetamenophin (Tylenol), so if you're taking anything for pain, avoid alcohol for sure.
- A fuzzy head is the last thing you need if your bandage lens falls out or you start to experience a problem.
- Alcohol won't do anything to *help* you recover and it might get in the way.

Coffee, colas and other sources of caffeine can dry your eyes and react with pain medication to make you sleepless—neither of which will help your recovery. Stick to a cup of java in the morning until your bandage lens is out, or switch to decaf.

Use Common Sense About Driving

If you can't see well, don't drive until you can. Test your night vision before getting into the car and taking off. You should be able to drive with no problem by the time the bandage lens is removed, if not sooner.

ENJOYING THE MAXIMUM COMFORT

If you're typical, you'll feel a little irritation the first 24 hours after PRK and then you'll be back to normal. Below are some tips to up the odds that your case will be "typical."

CAN DO's

- Plan to use the first hour well.
- Try an icepack.
- Use pain medication if you need it.
- Protect your eyes from light.
- Rest your eyes as much as possible.
- Watch out for Tight Lens Syndrome
- Help your body heal your eyes.
- Take care of your emotions.
- Take some vitamin C
- Expect your vision to change.

Get Maximum Mileage Out of the Anesthetic

One of the best pieces of advice my doctor gave me was to take advantage of the hour or so before the anesthetic drops wore off to get something to eat and settle into my hotel room. Since my cornea hadn't yet started to swell, I could see very well through my "new" left eye and the doctor simply popped the left lens out of my glasses.

I walked down the street to a restaurant where, it was obvious, they were used to serving people with pink eyes and one lens out of their glasses, and enjoyed a quick dinner. Then I walked to a drug store for reading glasses. By the time I was starting to feel a little scratchiness, I was comfortably ensconced in my room reporting on my miracle by telephone.

Even if your procedure is done in mid-morning, plan ahead about how you will take advantage of that first hour post-op.

Try Chilling Out

Much of the discomfort in the first 1-2 days comes from the swelling of the cornea, which is the reason anti-inflammatory drops such as Voltaren are used. However, these can delay epithelial healing, so the less used the better. Your doctor most likely will place a few antinflammatory drops in your treated eye right after your procedure and might give you some to take with you.

One way to reduce the amount of drops needed is to use ice to limit inflammation. Just place an icepack over the treated eye with a clean, dry washcloth between it and your closed eye. Sports medicine docs say ice is most effective when it is alternated 20 minutes on/20 minutes off. This and some sleep might be all you need.

Caution: Keep both eyes closed when the icepack is on to avoid tracking your treated eye back and forth against its lid by using the other eye.

Use Pain Medication If You Need It

We're not giving out medals for PRK heroism anymore (those went to all the patients who were part of the FDA trials). So take acetamenophin (such as Tylenol) if you feel minor discomfort or take the stronger pain medication your doctor provided if you're very uncomfortable. Avoid NSAIDs such as aspirin, Motrin, Aleve and Actron.

Most patients say the best medicine is going to sleep for the first 6-8 hours (and I will second that), so take a sleeping pill instead of a pain pill if it's night and you can check out for awhile.

One caution: pain medications do different things to different people (Vicodin, for example, makes it impossible for me to sleep, but I can't do anything else while I'm on it, either). If you're feeling jittery, nauseated, dizzy, emotionally sensitive or shaky, the first place you should look for a cause is any medication you're taking, because PRK doesn't have those side effects.

You'll feel better, faster if you take the minimum pain medication that makes you comfortable. Don't redose automatically: wait to see if you really need it (see Joyce Puckett's story in Chapter 16).

Protect Your Eyes from Too Much Light
If you find yourself to be extremely light sensitive, lower the blinds, dim the lamps and wear sunglasses—even inside—and two pairs if you go out. If your doctor gives you wraparound sunglasses, use them. This side effect gradually disappears—usually by the end of the second week.

Give Your Eyes A Break
The layers of the epithelium grow back a few cells at a time. If you scrape off newly generated cells by reading all night, cells aren't going to build up very fast. Dr. Catania has these tips for helping the healing process along.

1) While normal sleeping is good, don't sleep more than 8-10 hours at a time. Too much sleeping can increase swelling of the cornea, which can result in Tight Lens syndrome (see below) and delay healing.

2) If you are having discomfort, try keeping your chin up and looking out from under your lids rather than closing your treated eye. This reduces the pressure of the eyelid on the cornea. Resting your head on several pillows while you watch TV across the room is one way to do this.

3) Read as little as possible and avoid other activities that cause your eyes to track back and forth (such as watching a tennis match or playing video games).

Get a Grip on Tight Lens Syndrome
Tight Lens syndrome is the classic vicious cycle. It begins when your cornea swells a little in response to dryness, irritation or, after PRK, the removal of cells. As it swells, the lens fits more tightly. The tighter lens then causes the cornea to swell even more, and so it goes.

Bandage lenses are extremely thin (they reminded me of Saran Wrap) because they're not designed to correct vision, and so they are much easier to tolerate than average soft lenses. On the other hand, if your eyes are dry or if your cornea swells a little more than average, Tight Lens syndrome could begin. If the lens becomes tight, it can stick to the cornea and every time you blink there can be a slight disruption in the healing of the epithelium.

For this reason, it's important to take care of the problem as soon as you begin to notice it. The symptoms of Tight Lens syndrome are:

- The lens doesn't move freely on your eye when you blink (have a friend check this out for you if you can't see your eye in the mirror.
- Your eye feels hot and burning.
- Your vision is cloudy, like you're looking through Vaseline.

If you have these symptoms, first try some artificial tears and an icepack over your closed eyes. If that brings relief, relax.

If the symptoms persist over the next half hour, call your doctor. She or he might prescribe more anti-inflammatory drops (such as Voltaren or Acular) or might ask you to come to the office. The lens can be removed and replaced with a larger lens which usually quiets everything down and the epithelium heals in a day or two.

Remember, Your Eyes are Part of You

All the things that keep your body strong and resilient also help your eyes: a good diet, regular exercise, ample sleep, and relief from stress. The month before PRK would be an excellent time to start a Yoga class!

Vincent Yeung is a pharmacist who believes vitamin C improves healing; he took 1500 mgs of vitamin C each day throughout the period he was recovering from PRK for high myopia (his case is in Chapter 15). Unless you are allergic to vitamin C, you might consider following suit.

Timed-release tablets allow the C to be absorbed gradually and so more can be used by your body. Most people do better if they take vitamin C after eating. Those of us who take calcium should take it at least 4 hours before or after vitamin C, according to some nutritionists, to maximize absorption of both.

Give Yourself Some TLC

I can tell you from my own experience that having your vision fixed is stressful: if the FUD (Fear, Uncertainty and Doubt) doesn't get you, the excitement will. Add to that any extra traveling, post-procedure discomfort and pain medication, and you could find yourself feeling a little ragged along the edges.

The best remedies for post-op stress combine pleasure with distraction. Here are a few possibilities:

- Unless it's extremely dry or windy outside, grab your dog, your artificial tears and your sunglasses, and get out of the house for a walk.
- Go see a movie (but sit in the back!)
- Snuggle up with someone warm—a dog or cat will do.

- Listen to your favorite CD (on headphones while walking!).
- Go for an easy bike ride (leave the dirt trails to someone else for a week).
- Play a musical instrument.
- Reconnect with a friend on the phone.
- Watch your favorite movies on the VCR.

Don't Try to Out-Snellen Snellen

For the first few months after my PRK, fearing that my new vision was going to disappear at any moment, I gave myself eye tests about six times a day.

Even though I had great acuity almost from day one, I also had a little distortion or blurriness. My personal vision test was to look at the clock on my microwave from across the kitchen (about 20 feet), covering one eye at a time. It took about three months before I could see it without fuzzy numbers.

Many of the patients I talked to had to wait several weeks for good acuity and even longer to arrive at their final vision. Take our advice: Using the McDonald's menu board as a Snellen Chart just causes unnecessary worry. As Dr. Catania says, "relax and get a life," so you can focus on other things besides your vision.

Expect that your vision will take a few weeks to "come in," and that it might change from day to day and during each day for the first few months as it stabilizes. You might have a little glare or halos at night, but these effects should disappear gradually over the first two-to-six months. Even after you reach your final refraction, the quality of your vision—depth perception, contrast sensitivity, night vision—will continue improving for at least two years. PRK is permanent.

Let Good Vision Be the Beginning

Right after surgery my vision was like a hawk's. I could see into the distance better than I ever could with my glasses; birds in the trees suddenly were bigger and in 3-D, colors were much more vivid. I hope this is your experience, too, but don't forget: You might be able to see like Superman but you still have human eyes. The best way to preserve your hard-won eyesight is to begin a lifetime habit of preventing problems from occurring and catching potential problems while they are treatable:

- Don't stop wearing sunglasses just because you can see without them. You still need the UV protection.
- Just because you don't need glasses or lenses, doesn't mean your eye doctor should never see you again. Especially after 40, you should have a complete eye-health check every year to catch glaucoma, macular degeneration and other problems while they can be solved. Glaucoma has

been called "the thief in the night" because it can worsen to the point of being vision-threatening without any symptoms at all, and macular degeneration is the leading cause of blindness in people over 60. Both can be treated if caught early.

- Go to your eye doctor *whenever* you notice a significant change in your vision or if you are diagnosed with a disease, such as diabetes, that can affect your eyes.

11

The Risks and Rewards of PRK

All the U.S. and international studies indicate that the results achieved with PRK are consistently predictable, safe, and permanent. Analysts who claim to know the market for vision-correction surgery expect that over the next five years as many as eight million eyes will be treated with PRK in the U.S. alone. At this writing it is estimated that over 600,000 people worldwide have had PRK and there has never been a report of a single vision-threatening problem.

As Dr. Vance Thompson says, "PRK is King for patients under -7.0 myopia. It's not perfect, but for the right cases, it's close. Personally, I would have it done if I needed it."

So with all that enthusiastic support, is there anything to worry about? And if so, how much should you worry? The short answers are: "yes" and "not much." There are three categories of potential problems:

- Temporary side effects, which are nuisances, not dangers,
- Long-term complications which, if they persist after the cornea has healed, might require retreatment or the continued use of a weaker prescription of glasses or contacts lens, and
- Risks so remote you shouldn't even worry about them as long as you choose a doctor experienced in PRK.

"Deep doubts, deep wisdom; small doubts, little wisdom."

—Chinese proverb

More information on potential side effects and complications is presented here than their frequency justifies because I believe that being forewarned can help all patients become better advocates for their own care. In addition, knowing the relative infrequency of various risks can help relieve the pre-op jitters. First, let's look at some of the FDA trial results.

How Well Does PRK Work?

There have been many different studies of PRK for various levels of nearsightedness, using several types of treatment methods. The FDA's first approval of PRK was based, in part, on Summit Technology's six-month results on 341 eyes:

- 95% were corrected to 20/40 or better. With 20/40 vision most people can drive without lenses.
- 66% were corrected to 20/20 or better.[1]

In the VISX trials, about 90% of the patients had 20/40 vision by the end of the first month after PRK.[2]

A study of 587 patients with mild-to-moderate myopia reported that at the end of six months, 87% had 20/20 or better vision and 94% had 20/40 or better. There were no "severe" complications in any of the 750 cases studied.[3]

Other studies have reported even better results, with up to 98% obtaining at least 20/40,[4] and several have demonstrated that vision continues to improve throughout the first year and beyond.

It's not unusual for people to obtain very high acuity in one eye (20/20 or better) and less in the other. Quite often this is because one eye has more astigmatism to start with. A mild undercorrection can be a benefit to people over 40 (see Chapter 17), but if an eye doesn't reach 20/40 after the first procedure, usually it can be retreated after 4-6 months to take it the rest of the way.

GOOD ENOUGH FOR GOVERNMENT APPROVAL   In the clinical trials of 1600 eyes for the Summit Technology Apex laser, after one year uncorrected acuity was:
- 20/40 or better for 98.8%
- 20/25 or better for 89%
- 20/20 or better for 80.5%[5]

In the Navy portion of the FDA trials, all 30 of the patients treated had 20/20 vision or better at the end of the first year.

Who Gets Better Results?

A very early study indicated that older people had better results than younger people and that higher corrections caused more side effects than lower corrections.[6] More recent studies using newer techniques have demonstrated excellent results in both groups.

Within the mild-to-moderate range of nearsightedness that is approved for PRK in the U.S., there appears to be no indication that any single group is more or less likely to have a better outcome. In fact, results can differ from one eye to the other in the same person, as illustrated by my own story at the end of this chapter.

"Problems are the price you pay for progress."

—Branch Rickey

TEMPORARY SIDE EFFECTS

Most of PRK's side effects are temporary and irritating, not long term or disabling. Some can affect your physical comfort and others can affect the quality of your vision.

Even if you have both eyes treated in the same office visit, each eye can react differently to the procedure. Many patients told me that they had a given side effect with one eye and didn't have it with the other. One patient said that her first eye was absolutely free of discomfort from the start but her second eye, treated just a few weeks later, made her want to take a sleeping pill. There's no way to predict how each eye will react, but you can increase your odds of a smooth recovery by taking care of yourself before, during and after the first week as described in the previous chapter.

Table 11.1 summarizes the possible side effects and the more common ones are described below. I am indebted to Dr. Raymond Stein for providing me with much of the information for the tables in this Chapter.

Pain after PRK? Not today, thanks.

Every seminar I attended by doctors promoting vision-correction procedures described PRK as being more painful than the alternatives such as RK. They are referring to the post-op period, not the actual PRK procedure, which is absolutely painless because the eye is numb.

THESE SIDE EFFECTS USUALLY ARE TEMPORARY
- Discomfort
- Dry eyes and Tight Lens syndrome
- Short-term light sensitivity
- Glare and flare
- Haze and halos
- Side effects from medication

But does this mean that recovering from PRK is painful? In almost all cases, no. The vast majority of patients experience exactly what the patients in Chapter 9 describe: only an irritating sensation of something in the eye. The feeling is like having a speck of dirt under a contact lens or an eyelash in the eye.

Dr. Raymond Stein said that about 80% of his patients rated themselves as "comfortable" after the procedure while the rest said they had "mild" discomfort. Dr. Bruce Jackson said that 90% of his patients were out of their bandage lenses, and therefore any discomfort, by the second day.

Sometimes there's a mild burning or soap-in-the-eye sensation and tearing. Most people take some Tylenol, go to sleep and wake up with little or no discomfort. All discomfort usually disappears during the second day. In rare cases, such as my own (see "Dry Eyes and Ignorance" at the end of this chapter) discomfort can persist until the epithelium heals. Chapter 10 offers suggestions on how to minimize discomfort after PRK.

Dry Eyes and Tight Lens Syndrome

One of the main reasons people are contact-lens intolerant is dry eyes. If the tear film isn't able to regenerate continually, contacts can ride roughly on the surface of the epithelium, leading to irritation, swelling and Tight Lens syndrome.

Even people who have this problem with ordinary soft lenses find the bandage lenses much more comfortable because they are so thin. If the bandage lens dries out, however, it can irritate the exposed cornea. Artificial tears usually solve the problem. If the problem persists, anti-inflammatory drops can be added or increased and the patient can take pain or sleeping medication to get through the first day or two.

"A frequent cause of discomfort after PRK is a poorly fitting bandage lens," Dr. Maloney said. "They're like shoes: You don't want them too big or too small. I generally end up trying several sizes and then letting the patient sit with the lens for 20 minutes or so, just to give the tears a chance to lubricate the lens.

NO MORE PURPLE HEARTS

Part of the PRK procedure is removing the epithelium. After the anesthetic eye drops wear off, the cornea's zillion little nerve endings suddenly are exposed to the outside world, including the eyelid. This can cause extreme pain, but for years cornea surgeons have known that using a very thin, high-water-content contact lens (called a "bandage" lens) and nonsteroidal anti-inflammatory drops after surgeries reduces post-op corneal pain almost to nothing.

Despite this knowledge, in the FDA trials doctors were prohibited from using either the lenses or the drops because the FDA wanted "clean" data. In other words, they wanted to know what effects the PRK procedure had on participants' eyes, without adding other variables which would confuse the analysis. As a result, until October of 1995, trial participants had only a pressure eye patch and pain medication to help them through what, in 7% of the cases, ended up being a pretty rough 48 hours.[7] The FDA is making revisions in its study guidelines to avoid putting patients through unnecessary pain in future trials (see Chapter 13).

"The people who went through the FDA trials deserve a Purple Heart," says Dr. Thompson, one of the clinical trial surgeons. "We all knew early on that using the bandage lens and anti-inflammatory would help with post-op pain but we couldn't do it. Thanks to the patients who went through this, PRK is approved today."

Roger Steinert, also one of the FDA trial surgeons, said he conducted his own search for the ideal bandage lens to use with PRK. "We ended up with the thinnest lens, so it allows more oxygen to the cornea, and it contains about 55% water. Most patients can tolerate it with no problem.

"We knew that using too much anti-inflammatory can delay epithelial healing," Dr. Steinert continued, "but how much was too much? There wasn't a consensus in Canada so these things had to be worked out the first few months after FDA approval, instead of during the studies themselves. Now we use only a few drops of anti-inflammatory right after the procedure, and most patients heal in two or three days without any pain.

"Since we've been able to use the bandage lens and anti-inflammatories, pain is a non-issue," he concluded. "Most people feel nothing more than a mild foreign-body sensation for a day or two."

So, if a Purple Heart is what you want, you're going to have to find another way to get one.

About 15% of the time the eye swells a little more and we have to move up to a larger size."

If the lens fits, wear it, advises Dr. Steinert. "If you just get through the first 24 hours with the lens, you'll feel so much better."

A recent study proved that people with dry eyes have nearly the same tear volume and tear flow as people with "normal" eyes; the difference was rate of evaporation. If you can keep the tears you have where they'll do some good, dry eyes disappear.[8] Dr. Steinert says that before PRK on patients with a history of very dry eyes, he often will place temporary silicone "plugs" in the eye's drainage channels to keep both natural and artificial tears in the eye. This treatment has been so successful in a few cases that the patients discover they can live with contacts and forego PRK altogether.

Short-Term Light Sensitivity

Mild-to-moderate sensitivity to sunlight is possible right after PRK, because the cornea isn't smooth: It scatters light waves until the epithelium heals back over it. For this reason, and because the retina needs to be protected from UV light during the healing period, many doctors give their patients wrap-around sunglasses designed for use after eye surgery. These, or any very dark, UV-filtered glasses, usually provide ample relief.

In far fewer cases light sensitivity extends even to interior light and continues past the first week (see Dr. Hirsch's case in this Chapter). In the VISX trials, only 3% of the patients reported any additional sensitivity to light. Sensitivity gradually disappears without treatment in a week or two, in most cases.

IF THE SHOE FITS...   Dr. Maloney uses a slit-lamp microscope to see how well a bandage lens is fitting right after PRK. "It takes a little extra time to find the right size lens," he said, "but it can make a huge difference in how comfortable patients are that first day." Patients are advised to sit with a lens for about 20 minutes and then are examined to see if the lens still fits.

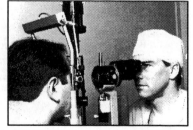

BY CHARLIE MARTIN, COURTESY OF JULES STEIN EYE INSTITUTE

ADVOCATE FOR THE LENS

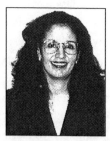

Lisa McKinney before...

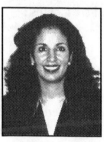

Lisa McKinney after PRK

Name
Lisa McKinney, 36

Occupation
Criminal trial attorney,
Massachusetts

Pre-Op Vision
-3.50; -3.25

Procedure
PRK

Post-Op Vision
20/25 (one month after
second eye was treated)

Surgeon
Roger Steinert, MD

Ms. McKinney's first eye was treated right after FDA approval, while doctors in the U.S. were still experimenting with which brand of bandage lens to use.

"My eyes were so dry I just couldn't wear contacts at all, When my sister was having her second eye done, I decided to try it myself; we went in together. I had an 11-month old baby and the flu right before I had my first eye done, so I was a little run down.

"The procedure was painless. Afterward, Dr. Steinert put a pressure patch on—just a stack of gauze taped on my eye. Of course my baby wanted to play with my eye patch, and I had to keep him away from it. I had a little discomfort and I didn't want to be too knocked out, so I just took Tylenol.

"Three days later, my sister's eye had completely healed, but mine hadn't, so Dr. Steinert put in a bandage contact lens which I wore all day and that evening. But my eye was dry and the lens really bothered me so at midnight I took it out and put the pressure patch back on. The next morning they put another lens in and I made so much better progress after that: I was much more comfortable, it wasn't an attractive nuisance for my son, I got to have vision, and within a day I had healed and I was on my way.

"My second eye was just done a month ago and they used a bandage lens from the start. Everything about this eye went better: I could have driven home after the procedure and I didn't have any discomfort at all.

"The next day I went to court and had no problems, but as soon as I went outside into the sunlight, I started blinking and my eye dried out. So I took myself right into Dr. Steinert's and he said I had Tight Lens syndrome, which I suspected. He numbed my eye, took the lens out and said I was 85% healed. He taped my eyelid shut with no patch and I went home and slept about three hours. When I got up I was fine. I took off the tape and that was it.

"My theory is that my first eye was affected by the flu I had right before the procedure and the pressure patch after it. I was in much better shape with the second eye and the bandage lens just made it that much easier."

Optical Illusions: Glare, Flare, Haze and Halos

These effects usually are temporary and occur at night or in dark environments. Dr. Richard Lindstrom says, "Studies show that all measures of vision improve during the first two years, including contrast sensitivity, glare, ghosting, haloing, and general night vision. People need to know that there is a long-term remodeling of the cornea after PRK which allows the quality of vision to keep on getting better with time, even though the patient's acuity might not change much after the first few months."

Because each of these effects has a different cause, it is unlikely you will have all of them, if you have any. In the Summit Technology clinical trials, all optical illusions disappeared in most patients by the end of six months.[9]

Optical Effects Before *PRK*

One of the factors that many studies, including the FDA trials, do not take into account is whether the patient had any of these optical illusions *before* having PRK. I always noticed a great deal of flare and glare whenever I tried to drive with my contacts in at night, and when I wore glasses light behind me would reflect from the back of my glasses into my eyes. I considered all this "normal," though, and didn't think anything of it until I had PRK, when I was primed to notice every detail about my vision.

Having vision-correction surgery makes most of us much more attentive to the quality of our vision, and much more likely to report optical side effects.

Temporary Glare and Loss of Contrast Sensitivity

It is normal for the cornea to be slightly hazy while it is healing—but the haze is microscopic. You might be seeing 20/20 and still have a little residual haze. The time you will notice haze, if at all, is at night. Like high beams hitting a dirty windshield, when light enters a hazy cornea, it scatters, causing glare.

Dr. Lindstrom says that this isn't a concern except when you're driving because it can diminish your contrast sensitivity—the ability of your eyes to notice, for example, a black cat suddenly crossing the road, or a light-colored car in a snowstorm. "Glare problems are worse in low-contrast environments. Even without glare, contrast sensitivity diminishes naturally as we get older, so this is one of the concerns for senior citizens who drive."

About 10% of the people who have PRK experience glare, but it's usually temporary. Dr. Stein said current thinking is that haze is caused when new collagen fibers are created during the healing process. "At first, the collagen

POSSIBLE SIDE EFFECTS OF PRK   Table 11.1

Side Effect	Description	Treatment(s)
Discomfort	For 1-5 days tearing, burning or an irritating feeling that something is in the eye.	Use Tylenol, antiinflammatory drops or a sleeping aid.
Pain	1-2 days. Usually caused by loss of bandage lens or inflammation.	Replace lens; use anti-inflammatory drops, use stronger pain medication.
Light sensitivity	2-3 days to 2 weeks. Mild to severe discomfort in sunlight or artificial light.	Gradually disappears. Wear very dark, or two pairs of, sunglasses, even indoors.
Tight Lens syndrome	Burning or irritation caused by bandage lens.	Have doctor replace lens; use artificial tears;
Foggy/cloudy vision	Several hours to several weeks. Caused by healing process; usually affects near vision most.	Improves dramatically when epithelium heals, then gradually over 4-6 weeks.
Delayed healing	First 7-10 days. Discomfort might continue for duration.	Doctor might discontinue use of anti-inflammatory drops. Medications are being tested that will accelerate healing.
Blurred vision	2-4 weeks. Images not crisp; usually caused by uneven healing of epithelium.	Doctor can increase steroid drops or, if persistent, can retreat with PRK.
Central haze	2-4 months. Cornea is cloudy under microscope, but except at night, vision usually is not affected.	Doctor can increase steroid drops for a brief period and retreat with PRK if haze persists.
Peripheral haze	2-4 months. A circular haziness around clear images. Can cause overcorrection.	Usually disappears gradually, but doctor might increase steroid drops.
Halos	4-6 weeks. At night, lights appear to have a bright circle around them.	Disappears gradually in most cases. If it persists, retreatment might help
Central "Island"	A tiny bump rises in the center of the cornea during healing. Might cause blurring.	Usually disappears as healing progresses. Can be "polished off" by PRK if necessary.
Temporary presbyopia (difficulty focusing close in for reading or other tasks; especi-ally in dim light)	1-3 months normal, but might be permanent if you are over age 40.	Use the weakest reading glasses that allow you to read newsprint.
Infection	In about 0.4% of cases, occurs in first week. Definite pain, iredness and burning/tearing are symptoms.	Antibiotic eyedrops and (in some cases) systemic medications. Don't take chances if you suspect an infection!

fibers are irregularly arranged, which scatters light. With time, they become aligned with the fibers in the untreated portion of the cornea, and haze clears up."

In a little over 2% of PRK cases, haze persists after the cornea is healed. If it interferes with vision, usually PRK can be used to "polish off" the haze. The good news is, significant haze is rare and getting even more rare with new PRK techniques. In a study of over 2,900 eyes, only 11 (0.38%) had significant enough haze to interfere with vision. Four of the eyes were retreated and all had maintained good results through the two-year follow-up period.[13]

In the VISX clinical trials only 1% of patients experienced mild haze at 3-6 months.[14]

Of the first 30 patients in the Navy's study on PRK, all had 20/20 vision in the treated eye with no retreatment needed. However, one of the patients had significant enough glare in the treated eye to refuse treatment in her second eye.[15] "Even though she had 20/20 acuity after PRK, said Dr. Steven Schallhorn, "she feared that if she had the same degree of glare in her second eye, she would have trouble driving at night."

The good news is that the laser software and PRK techniques are continually being improved and that haze is less of a worry now than it was even during the FDA trials.

If glare is a problem in the daytime during the healing period—when the sun shines on water or snow, for example—polarized sunglasses can help.

Flaring or Ghosting

Flared or ghosted images are slightly different. They are caused by irregular astigmatism which either existed before PRK, or was created as a side effect of PRK. The flaring occurs when light is reflected off an aspherical surface.

SIDE EFFECTS AT SIX MONTHS   In Summit Technology's clinical trials the following side effects were reported at six months post-op. Keep in mind that in all studies, uncorrected acuity and vision quality continued to improve during the first 24 months (percentages rounded to nearest whole number):
- Minor glare: 10%
- Minor halo: 10%
- Undercorrection: 6%
- Overcorrection: 5%
- Haze: 2%
- Increased eye pressure: 2%
- Night vision problems: 1%
- Loss of two or more lines of best-corrected vision: 1% [10,11,12]

JOIN THE NAVY AND *SEE* THE WORLD!

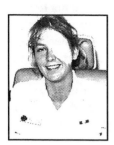

Name
Tiffany Baisden, 29
This photo was taken
right after her PRK.
The eye patch was
used only during the
FDA trials. Today, a
"bandage lens" is
used instead.

Occupation
Patient Administrator,
Naval Air Sation

Pre-Op Vision
-2.75, -2.0

Procedure
PRK

Post-Op Vision
20/15 both eyes

Surgeons
Michael Gordon, MD
Steven Schallhorn, MD
Christopher Blanton, MD

"Am I excited? Are all the other volunteers excited? I doubt any of the alternates will get the chance to fill in for us!"*

This was Tiffany Baisden's reaction in September, 1993 when she learned she had been selected to be the first Navy volunteer to have PRK. She had applied to take part in the Navy study right after she read Dr. Schallhorn's notice in the daily bulletin asking for "a few good people with bad eyesight."

"We got over 15,000 calls from Navy personnel after I ran that notice," Dr. Schallhorn said. "It brought our front desk to a standstill for months. I also received more than 500 letters from active-duty people explaining why vision correction was so important to the Navy. There's no doubt there's a perceived need."

What was Ms. Baisden's need? "I wanted to be able to wake up in the morning and see without having to find my glasses, but also I thought: 'If people don't volunteer, maybe this procedure will never be approved.'"

"I was a little apprehensive beforehand, but not scared. PRK was in the final stage of FDA testing and the success rate had been very good on thousands of eyes. My only disappointment was they couldn't do both of my eyes at once." Volunteers had to wait at least six months between eyes.

"The surgery lasted only about 20 seconds, and was completely painless. My vision was blurry while it was hap-

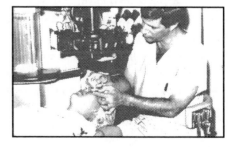

Dr. Gordon places
drops in Ms. Bais-
den's eye moments
before her PRK
treatment.

*From "Experimental Laser Surgery Worked, say Navy Corpsman and Her Doctor," by Pat Kelly, Drydock, September 3, 1993. Photos by Ronald E. Wright, Courtesy of Naval Medical Center, San Diego.

pening, so I couldn't see what they were doing." Because she was part of the FDA trials, she did not receive a bandage contact lens or anti-inflammatory drops—just a pressure patch on the treated eye. "There was a lot of pain the first few days, but it was worth it!" Less than a week after surgery her vision was 20/20 in the treated eye. "On the third day after my first eye was done, I looked out the window and said, 'Wow!' There was a whole world out there. I saw details I had never seen before."

Ms. Baisden had her second eye treated in March of 1994 with the same good results and has participated in an ongoing study since then.

I had both glare and flare the first few months, but neither to a degree that disturbed me. I noticed flare most when I saw white titles against a dark background at the movies: the letters seem to spread out from the centers. The flare, in my case, was caused by residual astigmatism.

If you have astigmatism and wear glasses or contacts, you probably don't notice this illusion because your lenses correct the astigmatism. If the astigmatism isn't treated during PRK, you might experience flare. If flaring doesn't disappear by the time your vision has stabilized, as mine did, you might ask your doctor about astigmatic PRK or AK to correct the problem (see Chapter 16).

Halos

This is a phenomenon unique to PRK because there is a transition zone between the "polished" area of the cornea and the untreated area. Let's say it's night and you're driving behind a car with red tail lights. If your pupil dilates wider than the treated area, it exposes a small ring of the transition zone. The central cornea sees the red light sharply, because it is now flatter and light is focused exactly at the back of the retina. The area in the transition zone is a little steeper—or more nearsighted—so it projects the light in front of the retina in the form of a fuzzy halo. Your brain puts the two images together and you see a clear red light with a fuzzy halo around it.

I had halos in spades the first month—car tail lights looked huge. This didn't disturb my ability to drive (in fact, I felt it was almost a safety feature because other cars were much more noticeable) and the halos were the first optical illusion to disappear.

Whether you see halos and how wide they are depends on the size of your pupils and the treatment zone. Most doctors will refuse to treat you with PRK if your pupils normally dilate substantially wider than the zone their lasers are programmed to treat. As the cornea heals, halos gradually disappear. If they persist after six months or so, the eye might be retreated to enlarge the treatment zone. In a study of 84 patients at the end of the first year, only four still reported "significant" halo effects at night.[16]

Delayed Epithelial Healing

The outer "skin" of the cornea, the epithelium, heals in two or three days for most patients. In rare cases, the healing can take up to a week. From the very earliest studies, though, it has been shown that the rate of healing has no effect on the patient's visual outcome—neither on the amount or types of side effects nor on their final uncorrected acuity.[17]

Reading Glasses for 20/20 Eyes?

As explained in Chapter 5, PRK and other vision-correction surgeries for nearsightedness do not directly affect when or if you need reading glasses—that is a function of the focusing powers of your eye. Getting your nearsightedness corrected without taking reading vision into account can accelerate the need for reading glasses, however, because having good distance vision is just like wearing permanent distance glasses: The natural focal point of the eye moves farther out, so more focusing ability is required to see near images.

Right after PRK you might need reading glasses because doctors aim for a temporary overcorrection in order to allow for regression during healing. In the Navy study, six participants needed reading glasses the first few months after PRK, but five of them were over the age of 35.

If a monovision correction or a multi-focal cornea is achieved with PRK, it can help eliminate or delay the need for reading glasses, as might some of the other treatments that are on the horizon. (Chapters 17 and 18 tell you more about these possibilities).

Side Effects from Medication

The medicated eyedrops you will use before and after PRK have side effects, too, but most are extremely rare under normal use of the drops and even more unusual with PRK because all except the steroids are discontinued during the first day or week. In nearly every case any side effects that do occur are temporary and disappear when you stop the drops. Table 11.2 summarizes these effects.

WHY SEEING AT NIGHT IS A CHALLENGE...FOR EVERYONE

"Darkness is a 20/200 environment in the best of cases," Dr. Lindstrom explains. "Physiologically everyone is more myopic at night because the available light is in the blue spectrum—which means the light waves are shorter than in daylight and therefore come to focus short of the retina in the eye."

"There's also a phenomenon called 'empty-field myopia.' which causes the eye's focusing muscles to work when it's almost totally dark," Dr. Schallhorn added. "The eye moves the focal point in, so even if you can see faintly, images are blurred."

In the daytime both the cones and rods of the retina are activated by light, letting you see color as well as black and white. At night, when light is below the level needed to activate the cones, rod-related vision takes over. Since rods can't perceive color, in dim light you can only see shades of gray, which have less contrast.

To make matters worse, at night the eyes must adjust to periods of high contrast between dark and light such as a neon sign against the night sky, or headlights on a dark road.

When you're in the brightly lit lobby of a movie theater, the rods are washed out by the light and the cones take over. When you go into the dark theater, it takes a while for the rods to regenerate, leaving you temporarily "blind." High beams on a dark highway also can wash out the rods, and it can take a few seconds for your cone vision to kick in. By that time, the car might be past and it's time for the rods to regenerate. This adjustment period between light and dark can take longer as we get older, making night driving more hazardous.

"People with large eyes who are very nearsighted tend to have the poorest dark adaptation because their eye pigment is stretched over a greater area," Dr. Lindstrom said.

PRK can increase myopia slightly at night when the pupil widens to take in more light, because the light that comes through the periphery of the pupil is refracted by a steeper, or more nearsighted, part of the cornea. "This doesn't have much of an effect, though," said Dr. Schallhorn, "because the cones and rods are most sensitive to light that enters through the center of the cornea, not the sides."

"All nearsighted people have a harder time at night, even after surgery," Dr. Lindstrom said, "but this usually isn't a problem. I have a lot of happy patients who keep a pair of glasses in their glove compartment just for night driving."

TWO PROBLEMS, 20/20

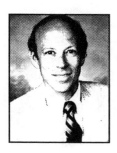

Name
Carl Hirsch, OD, 45

Occupation
Optometrist, California

Pre-Op Vision
-6.50 with 0.75 astigmatism

Procedure
PRK and Astigmatic PRK with bandage lens

Post-Op Vision
20/20

Surgeon
David T.C. Lin, MD

Dr. Hirsch is a good example of someone who knew about all the alternatives for correcting vision and waited for PRK.

"I did my homework by talking to eight or ten other doctors who had been sending patients to Dr. Lin in Vancouver for several years," Dr. Hirsch said, "and they all were happy with the results. I also spent a day with Dr. Lin in his office, watching PRKs and examining patients as they came in for checkups. So after all this, I was pretty relaxed about the whole thing. I went in, got the drops put in and then Dr. Lin did both of my eyes in less than ten minutes. I immediately tested myself on the eye chart at 20/40 and 20/25 but my vision was kind of foggy and I couldn't read anything up close. My eyes looked a little glassy.

"A couple of hours later I felt some irritation and tearing. I noticed that the light from the TV hurt my eyes and I had to close the hotel room curtains—it was pretty severe. But I just took a sleeping pill and went to bed.

"The next day I had trouble going outside, even with two pairs of very dark sunglasses. If my wife hadn't been there, I might not have made it to Dr. Lin's office. He checked me and said that everything was fine. He put in some more anesthetic drops which gave me about 30 minutes of bliss.

"We traveled on to Boston later that day and then to New York. Over the next three days I couldn't drive—especially at night because the headlights killed my eyes. But by Sunday I was home and the light sensitivity was almost gone. On Monday my reading vision was still blurry but I could read the computer screen and my cornea was crystal clear. I got a new lens for my left eye and my local doctor took the right one out.

"On Tuesday I could read the newspaper and the numbers on the telephone, and I could watch TV—that was five days after the procedure. My left eye still felt scratchy, though. On Wednesday I could read the stock quotes and I drove at night for the first time, but my vision was hazy and there were halos around lights. I went to the movies and there was a little flare on some of the images. By Thursday both eyes were fine and my vision was great.

"At the fourth month I went in for a scheduled visit and the doctor discovered that my eye pressure was a little too high. He prescribed a beta blocker eyedrop for a week and the pressure went down. I stopped the drops and two weeks later, the pressure went back up. So I went on the beta blocker for a month. I've been off it for a month now, and everything's still fine.

"I can't say I was ever really worried about any of these problems. I knew there were small possibilities of temporary light sensitivity and increased eye pressure, but I was surprised I got both.

"My vision's 20/20 in both eyes now even though we tried for monovision. I spent the first half of my life needing glasses for distance. Now I guess I'll spend the second half needing them for reading. That's a tradeoff I'm willing to live with!"

POSSIBLE SIDE EFFECTS OF MEDICATIONS FOR PRK	Table 11.3

Medication	Use and Possible Side Effects
Anti-inflammatory eyedrops (ex: Voltaren/Acular)	Used immediately after PRK to reduce swelling. Might cause a stinging sensation when placed in the eye. Continued use can delay epithelial healing. Allergies are rare but reactions include burning, itching, redness and/or swelling.
Antibiotics (ex: Ciloxan, Ocuflex)	Used before PRK and until bandage lens is removed to prevent infection. Side effects can include burning, light sensitivity, tearing, swollen eyelid, itching, redness and bad taste in the mouth right after using. Rarely can cause nausea, skin rash.
TobraDex	Combination anti-inflammatory/antibiotic. Might be used instead of the above. Similar possible side effects.
Corticosteroids (ex: FML, Flarex)	Might be used in a gradually decreasing regimen for a few weeks to several months after bandage lens is removed. Side effects can include temporary blurring right after drops are used and increased eye pressure. Less common reactions are cataract formation, drooping eye lid, and recurrence of any viral infection. All side effects are easily diagnosed during regular office visits and can be quickly treated before problems arise.

COMPLICATIONS

Unlike the side effects described above, the following problems are a little more serious in that retreatment might be necessary to solve them or corrective lenses might still be needed after the surgery. The vast majority (about 95-98%) of the eyes treated with PRK end up within the range of +/-1 diopter of the planned correction after a single treatment: they have 20/40 or better vision, which is good enough to drive without lenses.[18] Another 2-5% might require a fine-tuning procedure. In the Navy study, the only complication found was temporary regression and overcorrection (five eyes) but at the end of a year the vision of all the patients was 20/20 or better.[19] In the VISX trials, about 4% of the patients were retreated, usually because of undercorrection or regression.

As for the worst possible complication—loss of sight—Dr. Lin said the only possibility of blindness "is an undiagnosed infection early on, or prior to the surgery, but this is why we use antibiotics." There has never been a reported case of lost sight from PRK. Out of 909 eyes in the VISX trials, only 3 patients had any form of infection, all occurred during the first week after PRK, and the infections did not affect their vision.[20]

Undercorrection

To avoid overcorrecting vision (so that the patient doesn't become farsighted) in doctors might intentionally undercorrect the eye a little and rely on the patient's healing capacities to further flatten the cornea after surgery. This is one of the reasons vision is often less than 20/20 right after PRK and why it continues to improve over a period of months.

A study of 645 eyes treated with PRK using an older model laser than that approved by the FDA, found that the higher the levels of myopia or astigmatism going into PRK, the more likely the patient would end up needing further treatment to be able to see without lenses. Only 5% of the patients with less than -5.0 diopters of nearsightedness needed retreatment, 13% with pre-op vision between -5.0 and -10.0, and 19% of those between -10.0 and -15.0. The researchers found that the risk of haze was no greater after retreatment than after the initial PRK. In this study retreatment was elected for 39 eyes. At the end of twelve months, most of the patients were within one diopter of perfect vision, but 14 still needed lenses for good distance vision.[21]

POSSIBLE COMPLICATIONS
- Undercorrection
- Regression
- Overcorrection
- Loss of best-corrected acuity

Treatments for Undercorrection

When vision remains worse than 20/30 or 20/40 after three months or so, the doctor might be able to stimulate additional flattening by tapering off the use of steroids. If this doesn't work, after vision stabilizes the eye might be re-treated with PRK. Since less correction is being made in a "finetuning" PRK, the entire experience usually is even easier and the healing much faster than the first time around.

The risk of retreatment is *over*treatment, however, and each patient's case must be evaluated individually before a good decision can be made. Even if the final result is glasses or contacts, patients can be relatively happy because after PRK they are much less visually handicapped without lenses. They can see the soap on the shower floor, and in an emergency they probably could find the exit door.

Regression

Regression is loss of correction after it has been achieved and it is more likely in patients who, before PRK, had a moderate- to high-degree of astigmatism or were very nearsighted. A patient who regresses might have a refraction of -0.50 the first month after surgery and then begin to drop back to -1.0 or less the next month.

In the Navy study, one patient regressed to 20/50 by six months, but at nine months the regression reversed itself with no intervention by the doctors, and the patient had 20/20 vision at the end of the first year.[22]

UV Light and Regression

There is some evidence that exposure to intense UV light during the first six months—such as skiing at high altitudes—can cause regression. To decrease your chances of regression, stay out of those tanning booths and wear dark UV-protected sunglasses whenever you are outdoors—at least until your vision is completely stable.

Treatments for Regression

If caught early, the doctor might be able to reverse the regression process by increasing the steroid dosage. If that doesn't produce good enough results, the eye can be retreated either with PRK or, as some researchers suggest, simply by removing the epithelial layer again to reactivate the healing response.[23]

One study indicated that retreating the eye with PRK provided ample improvement for most patients and that the patients did not regress after the second treatment. At the end of a year 77% had 20/40 vision or better. At the end of 18 months, more than half had 20/20 or better.[24]

In a large follow-up study of 950 PRK treatments, five eyes regressed after a period of good visual acuity. These five eyes experienced "late onset scarring" within five to thirty three months after PRK. The researchers studied the various methods of correcting the problem and determined that scraping the epithelium combined with a course of steroids was the most effective treatment for this form of regression.[25]

In a study of 289 eyes treated with PRK, 8% experienced some regression. These were treated with steroid drops and 12 eyes were then followed for 18 months. At the last exam, 8 eyes (66%) had achieved 20/40 vision or better and about half of the 12 came very close to reaching their vision goals.[26]

Keep in mind though, that all these studies used equipment and treatment techniques which have since been refined, so the results today would be even better.

Overcorrection

In many cases doctors deliberately overcorrect vision (making the eye slightly farsighted) to allow for anticipated regression in the first month or two after surgery. This is another reason why both distance and near vision might be a little blurry for the first couple of weeks after PRK.

If the planned regression doesn't take place, or if the cornea continues to flatten and overshoots the 20/20 target, farsightedness might result. Other causes can include dry eye during treatment, an inaccurate refractive exam prior to treatment, or a calibration problem with the laser.

"In my practice only 0.5% of the patients end up overcorrected and it's usually because the eye doesn't heal the planned amount," said Dr. David Lin. "Wound healing history in other parts of the body doesn't seem to be an indicator of how quickly or slowly the cornea will heal. There's variability in people's healing responses. Some don't heal and end up overcorrected. Others heal too fast and get haze. There's no test at this time to predict who might have these complications, and there are so few cases of overcorrection, we don't have enough data to develop the tests."

At six months four patients in the Navy study were overcorrected by 1.25 to 1.63 diopters, but their uncorrected acuity was 20/20 or better. Because the patients were young, they were able to use their natural focusing abilities to compensate for the farsightedness. As they age, if the overcorrection doesn't regress, they might find themselves needing glasses or contacts.[27]

Overcorrection at six months occurred in less than .2% of the FDA trial cases. As we saw in Chapter 5, mild farsightedness usually isn't a problem in people under age 30 or 35, but it can create the need for reading glasses in those whose focusing abilities are starting to weaken.

Treatments for Overcorrection

If the eye begins to become too farsighted, Dr. Steinert said that doctors can disturb the epithelium a little by lightly scraping it to restimulate a healing response and help the patient regress towards 0.0. Another approach, according to Dr. Lindstrom, is to fit the eye with a soft contact and use an eyedrop to stimulate healing.

PRK for farsightedness, called Hyperopic PRK, can also be used to treat overcorrection. This procedure, in clinical trials in the U.S. and considered investigational in Canada, is described in Chapter 18.

Loss of Best-Corrected Acuity

One of the ways researchers decided that PRK was safe and effective was by comparing the patients' outcomes to their best-corrected acuity before PRK. In the Summit FDA trials, 93% of the patients at six months after PRK, had best-corrected acuity as good or better as it had been before the treatment, and vision continued to improve through the first year or two.[30]

Let's say, for example, that a patient had 20/400 vision before PRK and her glasses corrected her vision to 20/20. Then she had PRK. If, six months or so after the procedure she could read the 20/20 line without glasses or contacts, she would have had no loss in best-corrected acuity and 100% improvement in uncorrected acuity.

QUICK REVIEW   Best-corrected acuity is the line you can see on the Snellen Chart with your glasses or contacts *on*. Uncorrected acuity is what you can see with them off. The goal of all vision-correction procedures is to improve your uncorrected acuity so that you don't need glasses or contacts to function in daily life.

CAN I WEAR CONTACTS AFTER PRK?   Unlike other vision-correction procedures, PRK doesn't involve incisions. Therefore, you most likely could still
wear contact lenses if your vision did not turn out exactly as you hoped. A
study of 13 eyes in Switzerland that had residual astigmatism, regression or
overcorrection after PRK found that all patients could be corrected with rigid
gas-permeable contacts to the same best-corrected acuity they had before PRK.[30]

On the other hand, if she could read only the 20/25 line, even *with the
addition of lenses*, researchers would say that she had a *loss* of best-corrected
acuity. This might sound scary, but it wouldn't mean much to her as long as
she could function without glasses or contacts.

If PRK only took her to 20/60, though, that would be a bigger problem
because she would need to wear glasses or contacts after the procedure. In
that case, she probably would opt for a minor "touch-up" PRK to take her
vision closer to 20/20.

It's important to note that patients whose best-corrected acuity before PRK
was better than 20/20 (such as a few patients in the Navy portion of the trials)
would have been reported as losing acuity if they "only" were correctable to
20/20 after PRK.

As Dr. Christopher Blanton points out, "There are plenty of people running
around without their best possible vision who've never even *thought* of wearing glasses or contacts—they might be 20/30 correctable to 20/20. Almost
everyone could put on a pair of glasses and improve their vision by a line or
two.

"The question patients have to ask themselves is: 'What did the world look
like *without* my glasses *before* surgery compared to after it?' Many studies
demonstrate that PRK improves uncorrected vision 100% of the time. In our
Navy study *none* of the patients had a loss of best-corrected acuity at the end
of the first year."

In Summit's 1600 cases, only 1% of the patients had less than 20/25 best-
corrected acuity and less than 0.2% had vision worse than 20/40.[31]

Patients, Be Patient!

According to Dr. Schallhorn, "Most people experience a rapid gain of vision to
about 20/40 or better with a slower increase in vision over the next 3-4 months
and more gradual improvements throughout the first year. In the Navy's study,

29 out of 30 patients had 20/20 vision by the end of the third month. The other patient reached 20/20 by six months but still had a loss in best-corrected acuity because before PRK her corrected acuity was better than 20/20.[32]

In a three-year study of 161 patients conducted by Dr. James Salz and his associates:

- 90% of the patients had 20/40 vision or better from the first year on.
- At the end of the first year *six* patients had lost two or more Snellen lines of best-corrected acuity.
- At the end of two years, only *two* patients still had a loss in best-corrected acuity.
- At the end of three years, *none* of the patients had a loss of best-corrected acuity.[33]

This study confirmed what other researchers have found: Visual acuity stabilizes within the first year, but the quality of vision continues to improve over one to three years.

In another study of 70 patients, two had a loss of best-corrected acuity at the end of a year, but all patients had 20/40 or better uncorrected acuity.[34]

In a third study of 91 patients, only one had a loss of best-corrected acuity at the end of a year and that patient's uncorrected vision was 20/30.[35]

Dr. Stein, who has performed thousands of PRK procedures in Canada, offers additional reassurance: "At one year after PRK, 99% of the patients I have treated have clear corneas and no loss of best-corrected vision."

What Causes Loss of Best-Corrected Acuity?

Corneal haze, irregularities of the epithelium or corneal surface and, less commonly, off-centered treatment are the most common causes of loss of acuity because light can scatter or be unevenly refracted as it passes through the cornea. This can produce a blurred image. Often these problems work themselves out by six months.

Treatments to Improve Acuity

In the early recovery period, haze and irregularities are common and usually disappear as the cornea evens out during the healing process. In the first 2-6 months or so, changing the steroid dosage can help eliminate haze. If haze or irregularities continue to affect vision, the cornea usually can be "repolished" with the laser to improve vision, or the epithelium can be treated to remove irregularities.

Better Vision Than is Physically Possible

"There is a mysterious effect of refractive surgery on vision, "said Dr. Blanton. "It is widely known among ophthalmologists that patients with a certain refractive error after PRK or RK can see better than patients with the same error who didn't have any surgery."

Dr. Blanton described two patients in the Navy study whose final refractive error was -1.00 and -0.50, both of whom had 20/20 uncorrected vision a year after PRK. "Someone who didn't have PRK and was -1.0 might only be able to read the 20/50 line and need glasses to drive," Dr. Blanton said. "There is something about the way the cornea is made a little out of round by the flattening necessary to correct nearsightedness that can give patients better than expected vision with a given refractive error."

REMOTE RISKS

The following two risks are described, not because they are likely (they are extremely unlikely if you have an experienced surgeon), but to reassure you in case you are worried about them.

Off-Centered Treatment

Some decentration of the treatment zone is common and has no negative side effects, as evidenced by the high success rates of PRK. If the treatment isn't centered enough over the pupil, however, PRK can cause glare, halos or astigmatism.

A PATIENT PRESIDENT   When Hawker Siddley Canada Inc. decided to invest in PRK by forming the Beacon Eye Institute, the first patient treated was its president, chairman and CEO, Keith Moore. Since May of 1995 surgeons have performed well over 3,500 PRK procedures in the Beacon Toronto facility. Beacon is expanding into the U.S. and as of February, 1997, had opened fifteen U.S. centers.

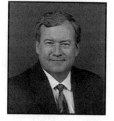

SOME UNLIKELY RISKS
- Off-centered treatment
- Laser malfunction

I can remember the patient information sheet I was given that read: "The procedure takes 20-40 seconds. During this time you will have to focus on a red light. It is extremely important to remain still and focused on the light during this period."

That was all it took to launch me into practice sessions. Every night I would lie in bed with my eyes wide open counting slowly to 40. My eye watered, I had the urge to blink, I swallowed—which I thought caused me to move—and I wondered, "What will happen if I can't do it?"

Let me assure you: the actual experience is nothing like what I was doing to get ready for it. First, you don't have to hold your own eye open. This helps immeasurably. Second, your eye is anesthetized, so you can't feel tears. Third, the sounds and other aspects of the procedure distract you enough to make the time pass very quickly. Finally, the light is easy to see and positioned where you would naturally look anyway, so focusing on it isn't an effort. Even though my treatment involved multiple passes with the laser (which isn't approved yet in the U.S.), I had no trouble fixating on the light for the entire procedure. In fact, it was almost impossible *not* to look at the light!

There are two other reassurances I can offer:

1) A small amount of eye movement will not interfere with the procedure, and

2) If your doctor is a corneal/refractive specialist, he or she has performed dozens, if not hundreds or even thousands of surgeries in which the patient has to "maintain fixation." Doctors learn to tell when a patient's eye is about to move.

"I tell my patients to try as hard as they can," said Dr. Lin, "but if they can't hold the fixation, the good thing is, I'm faster than they are. The second I see a movement begin, I stop the laser. This gives the patient time to refixate and then the laser picks up exactly where it left off. Studies show that an experienced doctor can catch the patient just before he moves," Dr. Lin said.

As a last resort, the doctor can hold the eye in place mechanically with a suction ring, but this is rarely required and isn't necessarily more effective. At least one study has shown that patients can do a better job of holding their eyes still than a machine can.[36]

Since my PRK, laser manufacturers have made fixation easier by adding a flashing light and newer lasers now in clinical trials will automatically track the patient's pupil, making decentered treatment a risk of the past. For now, having a highly experienced corneal surgeon is the best prevention.

Treating Decentration Effects

It's important to keep in mind that if you have glare and halo it doesn't mean your treatment was excessively decentered—these are normal temporary side effects which should subside gradually. If they persist, your doctor will want to determine the cause.

Before and after PRK your doctor should create a colored corneal topography "map" of your cornea (as described in Chapter 8). The computer software can also produce a third image which compares the results of the two tests to show the "after PRK" effect of the treatment. Any decentration will be clearly visible (Figure 11.1). Retreatment of decentration on a still-nearsighted eye might involve repeating PRK or using Astigmatic PRK (see Chapter 16). If the eye is overcorrected—has become farsighted—retreatment with Hyperopic PRK (described in Chapter 18) might be an option.

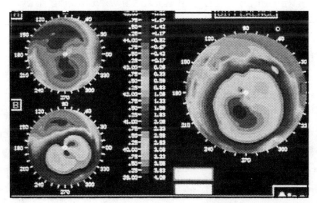

COURTESY OF VISX, INCORPORATED

FIGURE 11.1   These topography maps show the effects of a PRK treatment. The top left shows the cornea before PRK. The bottom shows the cornea after, and the large "difference" image shows the effect of the treatment. The steep and flat areas are apparent in the color printout, but impossible to see in a black-and-white reproduction.

Malfunctioning Equipment

What if the computer program breaks down and tells the laser to correct the wrong amount? What if the laser burns right through the eye? These and other worries are natural, but unrealistic to impossible.

Mark Logan, CEO of VISX said, "The computer controls and the software, plus the fact that the excimer beam can take off only a quarter of a micron in a single pass, are what make PRK such a precise, consistently accurate procedure. If you have a good refraction, the rest is done by the equipment. And it can't make a mistake. It will shut down before it makes a mistake."

With the VISX laser, the operator goes through a number of system checks each day before starting surgeries. Then before each procedure the doctor tests the laser by ablating a -4.0 correction into a piece of polymer plastic. The doctor checks the amount of plastic removed by the laser under a lensometer and if the correction reads -4.0, knows that the laser beam is aligned correctly. "If it says -4.1 or -3.8, the doctor simply punches the lensometer result into the computer and the laser automatically recalibrates itself," Mr. Logan said.

Michael Barra, director of marketing for Summit Technology, agrees: "All the physician has to do is tell the laser what degree of correction is needed. The excimer does the rest."

WEIGHING THE RISKS AND REWARDS

There's little we can do in life that doesn't involve taking risks. Both getting out of bed and staying in bed have risks, as many have pointed out. With PRK, study after study has shown that the potential for risk is minimal relative to the rewards experienced by almost all of the patients.

How High Is the Risk?

There has never been a reported case of blindness or serious infection after PRK and there have been no significant losses of best-corrected acuity.

For 95-98% of patients, the only downsides to PRK are some short-term discomfort, the inconvenience of using eyedrops and making regular office visits, and a few optical effects at night. For most of the rest, the biggest risk is having to undergo a second treatment to fine-tune their correction or clear up residual haze and/or needing glasses to read or see clearly at night. A few PRK patients (less than 1%) end up needing to wear lenses for normal distance vision.

It's important to note that patients who previously have had RK (radial keratotomy) to correct their vision have a higher risk of all side effects and

TWO FULLY INFORMED PATIENTS   How confident are laser manufacturers in their own equipment? Two VISX executives, who should know as
much as anyone about their company's laser, have both had PRK for high
myopia. Katrina Church has been General Counsel for VISX since the clinical trials began and would see any lawsuits filed against the company.
Terrance Clapham, VP of research and development, was co-developer of
the world's first laser for PRK and a VISX founder. VISX is one of the two
laser manufacturers approved for PRK in the U.S.

---

complications when they have PRK to correct residual myopia (see Chapter 14).
Some of even the happiest campers will find themselves needing reading glasses
after PRK when before PRK they were able to take their glasses off to read or
they were wearing slightly undercorrected contacts which allowed them to
see both far and near. That's the only problem with good natural vision, as we
saw in Chapter 5.

How Great is the Reward?

All the patients I talked to said they would have PRK again and urge others to
have it. As Part One described, good natural vision is a life-changing force
that can affect much more than what you do with your eyes.

Without exception, all the doctors I talked with—even ones who hadn't yet
learned to perform PRK—believed it to be a better, safer, more predictable
alternative than any other procedure available for moderate nearsightedness.
For mild nearsightedness, they felt it was a terrific alternative to RK (see Chapter
14).

"I love the procedure," said Dr. Vance Thompson. "I tell my patients that
whether I was a -1.0 or a -10.0, I would have PRK. I think it's the best thing in
the world, but it's still not perfect and I'm not about to tell everyone it is.
Because a very small percentage will have some problems and they won't feel
very good if I didn't give them all their options ahead of time."

Do You *Need* to Feel Lucky?

With an intelligent choice in eye surgeon and pre- and post-care specialist,
the Odds Gods clearly are on your side: If you are -1.0 to -7.0 myopic, the
chances are overwhelming that your experience with PRK will be even better
than my own and your results as good as the other patients' in this chapter.

POSSIBLE COMPLICATIONS OF PRK   Table 11.3

Complication	Typical Description	Possible Treatment(s)
Undercorrection	Less than desired correction. Normal during first 6 months. Could persist.	Retreatment with PRK once vision is stable.
Regression	Patient loses some degree of achieved correction as healing continues.	Doctor might increase steroid drops for a short period. Retreatment is possible if vision stabilizes at lower correction than desired.
Overcorrection	More than desired correction resulting in hyperopia (far-sightedness)	Doctor might reduce dosage of steroid drops to control, or retreat epithelium. If results are problematic for the patient, hyperopic treatments are options (Chapter 18).
PRK-induced Astigmatism	In rare cases, the PRK treatment causes the cornea to become aspherical enough to distort vision.	AK or Astigmatic PRK (Chapter 16) or continued used of corrective lenses.
Loss of best-corrected acuity	After PRK about 1% of patients can't see better than 20/25, 20/30 or 20/40 on Snellen Chart with glasses or contacts, usually as a result of persistent haze or corneal scarring.	Uncorrected acuity might be good enough so that this isn't a problem. Retreatment with PRK is possible if cause is haze, astigmatism or central islands.
Decentered Treatment	The treatment isn't centered over the pupil. Can cause poor acuity, blurring.	Retreatment with PRK is possible or patient can continue to wear corrective lenses.

A CASE OF DRY EYES AND IGNORANCE

My visual results were terrific but I was off the curve with problems the first week. No one realized it, but I was allergic to one of the drops I was using so my eyes burned and watered from the beginning. I also have very dry eyes, so the bandage lens didn't float as easily on my eye as it does on others. This caused more irritation—probably because newly formed epithelial cells were being scratched off every time I blinked. As a result, the first night I couldn't sleep. That's why I made my first mistake:

Marathon Reading

In order to pass the time, since I was in discomfort (not pain) and alone in a hotel room at night, I read most of the night with my treated eye closed. I didn't realize it, but the PRK eye was tracking back and forth just as if it were reading, too. This was like sanding the eye with my eyelid—which increased the irritation and made it even harder to sleep, so I continued to read to distract myself.

The next morning was cool and drizzling. I walked to my doctor's office for a checkup and then took off on foot for five hours—with no glasses— while I waited for my appointment to have my right eye done. I felt much better. The dampness relieved the dryness of the lens. My eyes were open, so I wasn't irritating the eye with my eyelid, and I was entertaining myself by reading billboards and street signs with my "new" left eye. Most important, my mind was occupied by *seeing* rather than *feeling*, so I felt very little discomfort.

The right eye was easier from the start. Even though the drops still burned, I had asked for a sleeping pill and I was able to sleep eight hours. The right bandage lens was removed three days post-op—but the left eye still hadn't healed and continued to burn and tear.

Self-Diagnosis

I made my second mistake six days after my left eye was done. On Sunday morning I woke up at 5:00 A.M. after a fitful night and my vision was very cloudy in the left eye. I went to the mirror and it seemed like the eye had swollen around the contact (but I wasn't certain because my near vision was still hazy). As a veteran self-help enthusiast, I diagnosed my problem as Tight Lens syndrome and decided to treat it by removing the lens and putting in some antibiotic drops.

That was like dropping a match on kerosene. My eye instantly felt like it was on fire and the fire felt like a rocket streaking into my brain—I actually heard the roar! I managed to find and call my local doctor's number, but he was out playing tennis and couldn't return my call until 8:30. Then my husband had to drive me to his office—about 1 1/2 hours away. You've heard the expression "crying your eyes out?" Well, that was what I was trying to do.

By the time I arrived at my doctor's office, I had been in a silent scream for four hours and I couldn't detach my forehead from my knees to get out of the car. Even worse, I couldn't make my eyelid open so the doctor could put in anesthetic drops. When he finally got the drops in, the pain stopped immediately, as if it had never been there. He put a new bandage lens on the eye and sent his shaking wreck of a patient home.

I took Vicodin every four hours just on principle (I wasn't chancing a single jangled nerve) and the next day returned to the doctor. I was relieved to hear that the epithelium had completely healed. He removed the lens and that was the end of all my problems. I had 20/25 and 20/30 vision that day which improved to 20/20 and 20/25 by the end of six months. All optical side effects were gone by that time, too, and my vision has continued to sharpen and brighten ever since. I wish they had an Olympic event for clarity of vision. I'd enter and win!

THE MORAL OF THE STORY

1) If you experience burning every time you put in your eyedrops, tell the doctor,
2) Don't read with your treated eye closed, and
3) **Don't** remove your bandage lens for any reason. If it falls out, call your doctor and refer to the section called "What to Do If You Lose the Bandage Lens" in the previous chapter.

The Cost of PRK

As with every other technology, medical treatments like PRK get better and cheaper nearly every year. So the decision to invest in them requires weighing the benefits you can obtain today against the financial or other benefits of waiting. If you wait a year to buy a computer, for example, you'll get a better, faster one for less money, but what will waiting the year cost you in terms of lost productivity or the opportunity to tour the world via the Internet?

That's impossible to calculate, of course, but weighing the cost of PRK against the costs of the alternatives is easier.

COMPARING THE ALTERNATIVES

First, let's talk about the cost of glasses and contacts. If you wear the second, you probably also need the first. And you need enzyme cleaners, saline, disinfectant, wetting drops, cases, and a whole wardrobe of prescription and nonprescription glasses—for indoors and out. Estimates have it that over $14 *billion*

HOW MUCH WOULD YOU PAY?   Gary Jonas, President of 20/20 Laser Centers believes that "because PRK is elective, most patients will select a doctor based on high levels of service and individualized attention, rather than price." In a survey conducted by *Review of Ophthalmology* only 8% of the prospective patients said that they would pay $1,500 per eye for PRK but not $2,000. The rest would have the procedure even at the higher price.[1] Today PRK costs about $2,000 per eye.

---

a year is spent worldwide just keeping people in vision apparel. How much did *you* spend last year? How much of that did your health insurance cover?

Glasses Aren't Free

I don't know about your experience, but my glasses were costing more every time I bought a pair. As my myopia worsened, the lenses got heavier, so I opted for lighter frames in deference to my nose. This necessitated more expensive "high-index" lenses. But since my eyes were rapidly disappearing behind the stronger (demagnifying) prescriptions, I also bought anti-reflective coatings to maximize the little that was left of what people could see. Then there was the cost of UV protection and scratch resistance and, for prescription sunglasses, polarization. Throw in some designer frames (after all, I wore the things night and day!) and a few leather cases, and I was easily up to $500 a year for a pair of regular and outdoor glasses, plus the cost of eye exams. My vision insurance covered less than a fifth of this.

...And Contacts Aren't Forever

As for contacts...well, I went through at least 40 different pairs of soft lenses in the ten years prior to my PRK—each an effort to solve my dry-eye problem. And added to the exam and lens costs were the costs of all the cleaning aids: boiling units, whirlpool "disk" baths, enzyme solutions and even a couple of ultrasonic cleaners that worked a week or two before breaking. Since I was a protein builder of Olympic proportions, I had to drop off my lenses regularly for a deep clean, and when seasonal pollens embedded themselves, it was time to for a new pair. I tore lenses, washed them down the drain, dropped them between car seats and even drank one from a hotel glass. I estimate I spent, easily, $3000 on soft contacts and supplies *before* I went to a series of gas permeables. I called those my "red-eye specials" because they made me look like a close cousin of the Easter Bunny.

Life Is Different Out Here

In addition to saving all that money on glasses and contacts, I no longer spend time trying to get contacts clean or making frequent eye doctor visits. I don't have a gallon jug of distilled water under my sink and I don't have dozens of little bottles in every bathroom cabinet. I don't lug a 15-pound handbag filled with multiple pairs of glasses and squirt bottles of contact solutions. And I don't apply Revlon's entire inventory of eye-enhancing makeup every time I want to leave the house. Finally, I don't have headaches and nausea from bifocals and I don't have reading glasses stashed in every room of my house.

What I *do* have is good, natural vision (20/25), a $30 pair of department store sunglasses (UV protected) and a $4.95 pair of drugstore readers next to the bed (for reading in dim light when my husband is sleeping). I misplaced my sunglasses on a recent ski trip and picked up another pair for $20—I'll use them for windsurfing this summer. I can see in steam rooms, snowstorms, the shower *and* when I'm draining spaghetti.

Cheap at Half the Price

All these benefits cost me $6000 ($3000 per eye) in January of 1995. They will cost you about $1500-2200—an average of $2000 per eye in most cities—in the next year or so and this price range should remain fairly stable until competing lasers are approved by the FDA—probably in 1998.

WHAT'S INCLUDED IN THE PRICE?

$2000 per eye is a lot of money, but it might cost even more if your doctor tacks on extra charges. Here's what's usually included in the price:

- The pre-screening exam, which normally is free: You fill out a questionnaire about your health and the doctor does a quick check of your prescription.
- The initial vision testing and all follow-up exams. Many doctors charge a nominal $50-$100 fee for the initial tests which they credit toward any procedure you decide to have. This is fair because the initial exams are staff- and equipment-intensive.
- A tranquilizer right before the procedure, if needed.
- The PRK procedure and everything it requires.
- Treatment of astigmatism. As Chapter 16 explains, doctors currently use AK unless they are in Canada or participating in clinical trials.
- Eyedrops before, during, and the week after PRK.
- Pain medication and/or sleeping pills for the first day or two.
- Antibiotics, if required.
- Wraparound "designer" sunglasses (designed by an optician who was more concerned about the health of your eyes than how you look when you wear them). These really help out the first few days.
- Emergency care *by the doctor* during the first week, if necessary. If you have to go to another doctor or emergency room, most likely you'll be responsible for the charges (but your insurance might cover at least part of the cost—see below.)
- Any "fine-tuning" treatments needed during the first year.

Costs usually *not* included in the price:

- Prescription eyedrops after the first week. Steroid drops are the most commonly prescribed and are quite expensive (the FML I was taking was $45 a bottle and I needed two and a half bottles). Fewer doctors are prescribing steroids right out the gate, however, so this cost might be minimal or nonexistent. Your doctor might be able to provide samples to help you out if money is tight, or your health insurance might pay for it (see below).
- Emergency care outside the doctor's office.
- Polarized sunglasses if you need them.
- Additional prescription pain medication.
- Transportation, lodging and meals if you travel for treatment.

Hospital Costs?

If your treatment is being performed at a hospital or surgery center, be sure you understand what the total costs will be. Often the doctor charges a fee for his time and then the hospital bills the patient separately for facility, equipment and ancillary costs. You need to know the "package" price.

WHY DOES PRK COST SO MUCH?

Compared to RK, PRK is pretty pricey—$200 to $700 more per eye in many cases. Chapter 14 will help you decide whether the extra cost is worth it, but here's why doctors are charging their current fees:

Equipment purchase: The excimer laser is expensive to own: The lasers now approved for PRK cost about $500,000. There are other lasers being used all over the world, but they are *not* the ones that produced the results reported in the FDA studies.

Supplies, gas and maintenance: The two gases used by the laser are expensive and the doctor has to maintain his equipment under a service agreement with the manufacturer. This can run $50,000-100,000 per year, depending on how many procedures are performed. "Solid-state" lasers currently are being tested for PRK in FDA trials and in Canada. If they can do the job, these lasers will be less expensive to operate because they don't require gas.

Equipment and treatment supplies: In addition to the laser, all the vision exam equipment and computer hardware and software must be purchased and maintained. Consumable supplies such as medications and bandage lenses must be kept in inventory.

Staff: In addition to reception and patient-care personnel, doctors need at least one technician to help maintain the laser and assist with the procedures.

Per-procedure royalties: When technical advances are shared as fast as they are discovered, the path back to ownership sometimes gets pretty muddy. Early on VISX and Summit decided to settle most of their patent disputes before they both went broke paying legal fees. The result was a unique partnership called Pillar Point Partners which receives $250 every time a PRK procedure is performed in the U.S. The doctor pays the fee when she purchases keycards to make the laser work. The royalties are divided between the two companies (see "A Royalty Pain"). In Canada and other countries doctors pay royalties through other arrangements.

Training: The classroom and lab training costs the doctor about $800. In addition, the excellent surgeons regularly upgrade their skills by traveling to learn new procedures, and stay current with studies and techniques reported by doctors all over the world.

Marketing: To get a PRK practice started, the doctor has to buy or print informational literature, advertise and to set up personnel to handle inquiries and appointments. Some larger partnerships also send out direct mail, rent hotel rooms for seminars, and run infomercials.

SEVEN WAYS YOU MIGHT SAVE ON PRK

Two for the Price of One?
As laser costs decline, royalty payments decrease or disappear, PRK becomes a generally accepted option, and newer competing technologies become approved, the price of the procedure will diminish. In five years it might be possible to have two eyes done for the price of doing one today.

IS MED-TECH TOO COSTLY? The cost of procedures like PRK raises difficult questions. Will medical technology continue to advance if companies are not rewarded for their investment in R&D and clinical trials? How much reward is enough? Who should pay for technology that is life saving if patient's can't? And how do we motivate doctors and manufacturers to find treatments for conditions that don't affect large populations?

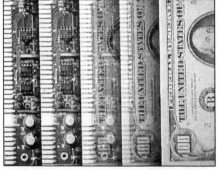

COURTESY OF TERADYNE, INC.

A ROYALTY PAIN

The Pillar Point royalty fees for PRK are unique in the medical world and the subject of much controversy. But the companies needed some way to recover the millions of dollars they had invested in research, engineering and FDA trials. If they hadn't settled their patent disputes this way, they might have gone out of business before they ever obtained FDA approval and everyone—patients, doctors and the manufacturers—would have lost out.

On the other hand, it's not hard to understand why doctors who have invested a half-million dollars in a piece of equipment might feel they should be able to use the laser whenever they want. Imagine how you would feel if you had to pay a fee every time you started up your car! One of the reasons some surgeons are using "gray-market" lasers (see Chapter 13) is to avoid these per-procedure royalties.

From the consumer's standpoint it might have been more beneficial for the manufacturers to work out a way to build their joint patent compensation into the purchase price of the lasers. This might decrease the number of doctors who could afford the technology at the outset and favor large institutions, but that wouldn't necessarily be a bad thing for patients. In addition, doctors with higher patient volume would be able to offer lower prices once their laser was paid off. But price isn't the only reason consumers would benefit from an open market: The royalty fees add to the financial incentive for U.S. doctors to use outdated or unapproved lasers (as described in Chapter 13).

See Now, Pay Later

Many surgeon groups and laser centers have arranged to provide patients with financing plans that allow them to pay for their procedure over a period of time—many as long as three years. Most require a downpayment of at least 10% and monthly payments are based on the total financed plus an interest rate. Most of the plans I've seen result in payments of about $60 a month when the procedure is financed over two years.

Smart patients will not allow the availability of credit to become the most important consideration in choosing a physician.

Good consumers will compare the interest rate and the total cost over time offered by the surgical credit plan to financing available through low-interest credit cards, credit unions, home equity loans and other sources. It might be less expensive to borrow money—or get a cash advance—from another source and pay the doctor in cash.

Pay Now, Save Now

Some doctors offer a discount for cash or credit card payment—I've seen discounts of 10% advertised recently. This could save $200 per eye. If you paid for the procedure with a low-interest-rate credit card, or one that awards mileage or other benefits, you could be money ahead.

Again, and I hate to sound like a broken record, a few hundred dollars in savings would be small compensation for a poorly performed procedure, so take advantage of incentives if they are offered, but don't let them influence your choice of doctor.

Take a Tax Deduction?

In 1996 the Internal Revenue Service ruled that RK was not a cosmetic procedure and allowed the cost to be deducted as a medical expense (IRS ruling #9625049), so there's no reason PRK shouldn't receive the same consideration. At this time, however, medical expenses has to add up to a substantial portion of your taxable income before it can be deducted.

Hand the Bill to Someone Else?

This ruling should pave the way for patients to make the case to their insurance companies that vision correction should be reimbursable like any other medical procedure. As of this writing, however, vision correction is not covered by most health insurance companies if the patient's vision is correctable to 20/40 or better with glasses or contacts. That might not stand in the way of getting all or part of your expenses covered:

- Patients whose job required excellent acuity *and* for whom wearing glasses or contacts on the job could endanger their sight, have succeeded in obtaining insurance reimbursement for refractive surgery as a necessary medical procedure. Example: A firefighter or an ironworker who works in intensely hot environments might need glasses to see, but glasses could be broken on the job and put the worker in danger. Contacts, on the other hand could melt on the eye. Consult with your doctor if you believe you have an employment-related reason for PRK and let his staff go to bat for you.
- Patients with corneal scars or other irregularities that interfere with sight might be able to have them treated with PTK—a procedure described in Chapter 19 which usually is covered by insurance and Medicare—and the doctor might be able to slip in PRK for myopia at the same time for a small extra charge. PTK is so new, however, that the doctor might

have to put the charges in another treatment code to obtain reimbursement. Again, these are possibilities to discuss with your doctor.

- Emergency care following PRK not covered by the cost of the procedure might be covered by your insurance if it is billed as "corneal edema" or some other medical diagnosis. There's nothing untruthful about this—if you need medical care for Tight Lens syndrome, an infection, or pain from swelling (all highly unlikely), your health insurance should cover the cost.

- Prescription eyedrops and medications *might* be covered. Check with your doctor before the procedure and let his staff work with your pharmacist and insurance company.

- If you have a vision plan that reimburses you for annual refractive exams and glasses or contacts, you might be able to make a case that part of the PRK procedure should be amortized out over the period during which you are insured. For example, if your coverage allows $100 a year for exams, lenses and frames, you might be able to be reimbursed $100 a year up to the amount you paid for the PRK procedure, because the procedure is saving the insurance company (and therefore your employer) money it would otherwise spend on vision aids for you.

Two-Eye Discount?

Doctors are going to wish I didn't suggest this, but I believe that patients who have both eyes treated at about the same time should be charged substantially less than patients whose eyes are treated in totally different time periods. There are two reasons:

1) If both eyes are treated in the same session, staff time is minimized and laser time is maximized—both of which reduce the doctor's costs.

2) If both eyes are treated within a day or so of each other, all the follow-up visits cover two eyes instead of one. While it is a little extra work to examine the second eye, it is nothing like two separate series of 6-7 office visits.

As discussed in Chapter 8, having both eyes treated simultaneously has advantages and drawbacks, and is not recommended by the FDA, but if the patient chooses to do it, the fee should be less.

Bargains for Americans?

At this writing, the currency exchange rate between the U.S. and Canada favors Americans. Most Canadian doctors were charging U.S. patients about $1,600/eye ($U.S.) at this writing. Of course, any travel and lodging costs would be additional, and your local doctor might add on her own fee for any pretesting and follow-up care. The exchange rates could reverse themselves at any time, however, and you Canadians might find yourselves steaming South for treatment.

Join a Clinical Trial?

TheResource Guide in Chapter 7 lists a number of clinical trial sites in the U.S., and the Canadian doctors are all conducting trials for various laser manufacturers. These trials need patients wanting to make a contribution and willing to commit to long-term follow-up. If you can qualify for a trial you could save as much as 50% of the cost of the treatment—even more if you are part of an early phase. Read the comparison of treatment centers in Chapter 7 to find out the advantages and drawbacks of being part of trials and remember: the early trials for any piece of equipment or procedure are inherently riskier than the later stages. Be sure you understand the risks before you sign up.

Too Good to be True?

In the next two years if you find a real deal on PRKoutside clinical trials—which often offer lower-cost treatment—take a long, hard look at who's offering the low price and why. There's little to no price competition right now on PRK, because of the fixed costs mentioned above. If someone is able to offer a much lower price, it's probably because he or she is using an unapproved laser. See Chapter 13 for more information about the dangers of "gray-market" lasers and how to find out if your doctor's laser is FDA approved.

Comparing Costs

The PRK Consumer's Checklist will help you compare the costs of treatment at different facilities.

THE PRK CONSUMER'S CHECKLIST

This form can help you gather information, create a budget and compare costs between treatment facilities or doctors. Feel free to make copies.

How Priced?

Item	Included in Package?	Additional?	Total Fee
Initial exam	$_____	$_____	$_____
PRK procedure	$_____	$_____	$_____
Astigmatism treatment, if needed	$_____	$_____	$_____
Eyedrops through first seven days	$_____	$_____	$_____
Pain/sleeping medication	$_____	$_____	$_____
Pre-procedure tranquilizer	$_____	$_____	$_____
Post-op sunglasses	$_____	$_____	$_____
Emergency care by doctor	$_____	$_____	$_____
Retreatments the first year	$_____	$_____	$_____
Steroid drops	$_____	$_____	$_____
Other _____	$_____	$_____	$_____

Hospital Fees, If Any

	Included	Additional	Total
_____	$_____	$_____	$_____
_____	$_____	$_____	$_____
_____	$_____	$_____	$_____

If Treatment Isn't Local

Item	Included	Additional	Total
Local pretesting and follow-up care	$_____	$_____	$_____
Travel to and from treatment	$_____	$_____	$_____
Meals and lodging	$_____	$_____	$_____
Emergency care if needed	$_____	$_____	$_____

Discount for cash, if any   ($_____)

TOTAL ESTIMATED COST $_____

Credit Costs

Interest rate   _____%

# of months to pay $_____

Monthly payment $_____

Total cost over life of loan (# of pymts x # of months:) $_____

from *BEYOND GLASSES! The Consumer's Guide to Laser Vision Correction*, UC Books

PRK and the FDA:
In the USA, It's a Matter of Time

*I*n October 1995, after ten years of development, including six years of clinical trials, the FDA's ophthalmic devices advisory panel approved Summit Technology's excimer laser for use in correcting nearsightedness. A second laser, developed by VISX Corporation, had been marching on the same long path and was given approval in March of 1996.

"This was the first time the FDA had critically assessed safety and effectiveness data of any device for refractive surgery," said Dr. Emma Knight, a medical reviewer with the FDA's Center for Devices and Radiological Health.[1]

The Health Protection Branch of the Canadian Ministry of Health and Welfare no longer considers PRK for myopia below -6.0 to be "investigational."

What Has to Go Through the FDA
The Medical Devices Act of 1976 required that all medical equipment sold in the U.S. be tested in defined clinical trials. Those that were already in existence, such as other lasers used for eye surgery, heart pacemakers, and kidney dialysis machines, were "grandfathered" into approval.

A MAJOR ACHIEVEMENT FDA approval isn't handed out to laser manufacturers every year. In fact, no medical device has ever had to prove itself in such rigorous trials. The approvals for the VISX and Summit excimer lasers were based on safety and effectiveness data on more than 3000 eyes followed for up to three years.

In other words, most of the types of devices currently being used in doctors' offices and hospitals in the U.S. have *never* gone through clinical trials to obtain FDA approval. Furthermore, the FDA does not become involved in surgical procedures *unless* they involve a new medical device, so other treatments for nearsightedness, such as RK and ALK, have never been FDA-approved.

By contrast, the excimer laser for PRK and PTK have had to prove themselves in the world's most stringent tests for safety, predictability and effectiveness: the FDA clinical trials. In addition to FDA scrutiny, all lasers are regulated under the Radiation Control for Health and Safety Act which governs the way lasers are manufactured and labeled and how defects are reported. Some states also monitor the quality and safety of laser manufacturing.

THE FDA APPROVAL PROCESS

A few months ago whenever I heard that some drug or device "has not been approved by the FDA," I was under the impression that there was something wrong with it. As it turns out, that's not necessarily so. When it comes to the FDA, there are only three conditions that count:

1) *Under investigation*: the device is currently being tested in clinical trials.
2) *Approved*: a panel of medical doctors (not employees of the FDA) has reviewed the clinical trial data and is satisfied that the device is both safe and effective when used under the conditions tested in the clinical trials. The panel has recommended approval and the FDA has accepted its recommendation.
3) *Denied Approval*: this speaks for itself.

When you hear that something hasn't been approved, it can mean that it is still in clinical trials, it has never entered clinical trials, it has been removed from clinical trials, or that it has already been denied approval.

While PRK was going through trials in the U.S., both manufacturers were selling their equipment throughout the world and doctors worldwide were performing PRK, reporting on their results and working with the manufacturers

---

CANADA'S PEER-GOVERNED METHOD   "Once a laser is sold in this country, it's up to the surgeon to use it ethically," said Dr. Howard Gimbel of Calgary. "Doctors are monitored by their peers, not the government. The Health Protection Branch looks at the manufacturer's data and requires the manufacturers to continue supplying new data.

to refine the software as well as the laser itself. A number of U.S. surgeons have told me that one of the reasons they became involved with PRK early on was because of the good results that were being reported in other countries.

Still Under Investigation
As of this writing, the following procedures are still *under investigation* in the United States and Canada.

- PRK for nearsightedness over -7.0
- PRK for treatment of astigmatism
- LASIK (see Chapter 15) for nearsightedness or farsightedness
- PRK and other laser treatments for farsightedness (see Chapter 18)
- Laser treatments for the focusing problems that come with age
- Reversible procedures such as the intrastromal ring and implantable contact lens (see Chapter 14).

Who are the Clinical Trial Doctors?
Another common misperception is that the FDA conducts clinical trials. Not true. The trials are conducted by manufacturers with the cooperation of physicians and their patients.

In the case of PRK and PTK, much more than cooperation had to be obtained: each trial site had to purchase a $500,000 laser, hire someone to operate and maintain it and provide the staff and resources to handle the patients as well as collect data.

In addition to the financial and staff commitment, the trial sites are strictly limited in the number of patients they can treat, and patients are often charged little or nothing. Most doctors who work only in private practice cannot afford to participate in clinical trials of expensive equipment. That's one reason clinical trials nearly always are conducted at hospitals and teaching universities.

"The universities and hospitals get involved because they want to maintain their leadership role," said Dr. Richard Abbott, a clinical trial doctor who is one of the five voting members of the FDA's Ophthalmic Devices Panel. "The patients do it because they hope to benefit. And the doctors do it to learn about new technology. If the money can be found, the process can work for everyone."

Phase I: The Blind Eye Study

Prior to Phase I, both manufacturers had conducted several years of animal and laboratory experiments to test the effects of the device on animal eyes and then on human donor corneas. The Phase I study was designed to prove at one location that the lasers could create predictable corrections on living human eyes. The FDA guidelines stated:

"It should be stressed that [PRK is] proposed to correct an essentially benign nondiseased state. It is essential that the procedure performed with the excimer laser be predictable. Predictability is assessed by comparing the refraction achieved after treatment to that targeted before treatment.[2]

In the Blind Eye Study for PRK, conducted by Dr. Marguerite McDonald at Louisiana State University, 10 patients volunteered to allow the laser to be used on their eyes. In some cases, the eyes were blind. In others, the eyes were about to be removed as a result of disease. Dr. McDonald told me that most of these patients, who valued vision perhaps more than any sighted person could imagine, made this gesture out of the hope that their generosity would help others to see.

While the actual procedures took only a few days to complete, the patients were examined over a period of six months. Then data had to collected, analyzed and presented to the FDA.

Morris Waxler Ph.D., research psychologist with the Diagnostic and Surgical Devices Branch of the FDA, said "What we learned is that below -7.0 diopters there are no major safety problems with PRK, so there's no need for future manufacturers to go through a step that doesn't provide any additional information. The only reason we would require data from nonfunctional eyes anymore is if someone came in with another kind of laser, or something that had different output power or different pulsing characteristics. Otherwise there are no real safety concerns that would require another Blind Eye Study for other uses of PRK."

THE AMAZING DOUBLE-BLIND STUDY

The standard scientific method for testing the effectiveness of a drug is a double-blind study wherein neither the patient nor the doctor knows whether the treatment is real or a placebo (harmless substitute). With PRK and other surgeries, of course, double-blind studies are impossible because the effect of the treatment is apparent to everyone.

It came as a shock to the ophthalmic community, therefore, when doctors learned that one of the patients in the PRK Blind Eye Study received a double-blind treatment, of sorts. Dr. Marguerite McDonald, who performed the procedure, tells the story.

"During our Blind Eye Study for the FDA trial, one of the ten patients was a 27-year-old woman who had been diagnosed as blind in one eye at several famous hospitals. She had two causes of blindness, actually: first she had a detached retina, and the operation to cure that made the eye - 4.50. Then she had a brain tumor, which also required surgery. Before both operations, the doctors warned her she probably would continue to be blind in her "bad" eye. Her other eye was 20/20.

"The Blind Eye Study was designed to test the effectiveness of the laser on human eyes: Could we aim for a certain refractive result and achieve it? Since the patients couldn't see, we did whatever corrections we wanted: low, high and in between—just to see what the laser could do.

"When it came time to do this patient, I thought, "What the heck, it'll be easier to measure if we just try for the correction her eye calls for," and so I did a -4.50 correction.

"Seven weeks later, the patient called and said, 'I can see perfectly out of my blind eye!' Well, I thought she was crazy, but I asked her to come in, we taped up her good eye—almost in a neurological headwrap— and she was seeing 20/20 out of the "blind" eye without correction!

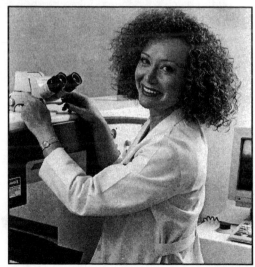

Dr. Marguerite McDonald at the microscope of a modern excimer laser.

"You can imagine how we all felt. At first we were elated and the patient was so excited. But then I began to worry about how I was going to explain this to the FDA! I wrote up the case for a medical journal and luckily had proof that the patient had previously been diagnosed as blind by other reputable doctors.

"It turned out that hers was a case of psychological blindness. Both causes of her blindness had been repaired with surgery, but because she had been told she wouldn't be able to see, she couldn't. When she believed her eye had been corrected, suddenly she could see. This "hysterical blindness" is incredibly rare—the only case I have seen in my life—and stranger still that it ended up in our Blind Eye Study."

As a result, Dr. McDonald can take credit for performing PRK on the first human blind eyes *and* the first human sighted eye—both in the Blind Eye Study.

The Patient's Side of the Story

Carolyn Henry had lost sight in one eye in 1985. By 1987 she was desperate to regain it, so when she heard about Dr. McDonald's experiment, she immediately applied. "I was hoping and praying they would pick me," she said. "I couldn't see anything out of that eye—it was all cloudy— so I was willing to take a chance."

"After the surgery, they put a pressure patch on my eye and I had quite a bit of pain the first day. But after that, I felt nothing. I put my normal eye patch back on and just went in for checkups. When the doctor would take off the patch everything looked blurry just like it had before, so I figured the experiment didn't take.

"One day I was having a party for my two-year old's birthday and I decided to take the patch off. After a few minutes I noticed I could see the birthday cake much better. I went into the bathroom and flushed out my bad eye and then covered my good eye. I could see!"

Today Ms. Henry is a mother of three and a volunteer in the Head Start program. Her vision is 20/20 in both eyes.

Phase IIa: Is It Safe on Normal Eyes?

This Phase was designed to rule out major safety risks. Manufacturers were allowed to test their lasers on 25 patients with nearsighted eyes at five different sites with a six-month follow-up.

"The principle was to give the manufacturers the opportunity to prove that there were no safety problems with their procedures," Dr. Waxler explained. "This phase demonstrated that PRK would not harm. It also gave them a chance to work with their equipment and software and make major modifications before exposing too many patients in a larger trial," Dr. Waxler explained.

Phase IIb: One Last Chance to Make Changes
Once the manufacturers proved in Phase IIa that PRK results were stable and had caused no significant negative reactions, the FDA allowed them to expand their study to at least 75 patients in five sites with a six-month follow-up. This Phase gave the laser makers a chance to see the effects of their procedures on a wider range of patients and finetune them before treating a much larger number in Phase III.

Phase III: Two-Year Trials to Prove Safety and Predictability
When the FDA recognized the Phase IIb data, each manufacturer had to present "protocols" for two-year Phase III trials. These protocols specified exactly how the procedures would be conducted, what medications (such as anesthetics) would be used, how the eye would be treated after surgery, and the timing and content of follow-up exams.

Phase III required treatment of 700 new patients, per manufacturer, at up to 10 sites each with a minimum follow-up of two years. Each test site was allowed to enroll 30 additional patients per year and follow them, as well. Both manufacturers conducted Phase III trials for PTK as well as PRK.

Follow-up exams were required at one week, one month, three months, six months, one year and two years. Patients were allowed to have their second eyes treated after a six-month wait, and data had to be collected on those eyes, too.

In commenting on the size of the Phase III trials, Dr. Waxler said, "700 patients was a very large number; probably too large. There is vigorous discussion going on to reduce that number to significantly fewer patients. Future studies most likely will have lower numbers of participants. Typically each site will have 50-60 patients for that trial. The trial is designed to gather scientific data—not to give the site permission to treat patients. We arrived at the number by calculating what kinds of visual outcomes the manufacturer is looking
for, and how many patients have to be treated, to make the statistics meaningful."-

Because of the size of the studies and the complexity of the data, it took several years from the end of Phase III to final market approval. During this time, doctors at the clinical sites were allowed to continue treating patients. "If the process becomes more efficient," said Dr. Waxler, "there won't be such a delay between submission of the trial data and final approval, and we won't need to give that kind of permission during the review period."

There's also good news for future FDA trial participants. "At the beginning of the trials there was concern over the affects medication might have, but those issues have been resolved. We know we need to allow the physician to make some clinical judgments about what's best for the patient. We don't want to intrude in that so we've decided it's up to the surgeon to determine if one way of dealing with the pain is better than another."

Training Doctors is Part of the Package
Approval involved much more than just giving the manufacturers permission to market their equipment in the States. Both Summit and VISX had to develop extensive physician training materials, courses and credentialing programs before marketing could begin. The FDA minimum training requirements for doctors wanting to learn PRK are:

- A one-day classroom seminar on the procedure and equipment
- A 4-hour hands-on laboratory, usually using animal eyes
- One supervised procedure.

If this doesn't sound like much, it's because it isn't. That's why I wrote Chapter 7.

WHAT FDA APPROVAL MEANS

Once a device is approved, the FDA monitors manufacturing quality and responds to consumer complaints. The companies must report "adverse" events and cannot market a product for other than approved uses.

The FDA has the power to enforce compliance and can halt production, prevent shipping, and fine companies. Individuals can be criminally prosecuted for violating FDA regulations.

The FDA does not go out into doctors' offices and watch procedures, however, so individual doctors can do what they want with their lasers unless someone complains.

"Off-Label" Procedures

In the U.S. PRK is approved only for the treatment of myopia between -1.0 and -7.0 diopters with up to 1.5 diopters of astigmatism. Any treatments not specified in the labeling of the product are not approved.

This presents an interesting dilemma for doctors who, for example, has a highly myopic patient who wants LASIK. The doctor might have a laser, might have the microkeratome and might have years of experience using both. Does this mean he could be jailed if he puts the two together and treats his patient with LASIK? Or, could the doctor do three -7.0 PRK treatments on a -21.0 patient to get him down to 20/20? The International Society of Refractive Surgery believes that the decision should be made by the surgeon based on what's best for the patient.[3]

Other "off-label uses" include using PRK for treatment of astigmatism and farsightedness except as part of clinical trials. These procedures have been performed for years outside the U.S. PRK for the treatment of farsightedness is still quite experimental everywhere.

Many doctors are doing them, however, either as part of defined clinical trials, in addition to them, or on their own. "If the doctor wants to take on that extra legal liability, that's up to him or her," Dr. Waxler said. "As long as the doctor isn't advertising and promoting the products for that use, we're not likely to be getting involved. If the doctor feels a patient would be better served by LASIK, we certainly don't want to get in the middle of that patient/ doctor decision unless some serious public health problems occur."

WHAT ON EARTH IS LASIK?   LASIK, as you will learn in Chapter 15, combines PRK with an instrument that first slices a flap off the cornea.

In other words, the FDA regulates the advertising and the marketing of drugs and equipment, but not the use of them.

"No one can promote LASIK in the U.S. and people don't have the comfort of knowing that it has been proven safe and effective," he added. "We're aware that some doctors are doing off-label procedures. I think it probably would be better if they waited until the studies are complete because we don't know if there are any negative side effects."

"Gray-Market" Lasers

"Gray-market" lasers are ones that are not approved by the FDA for use in the U.S. They could also be called "black-market" lasers. Black markets tend to flourish whenever goods become expensive or in short supply. In the U.S. excimer lasers are expensive, and the ongoing use of them is expensive, if people follow the rules. And, since there are only two manufacturers approved in the U.S., there's little price competition. As a result four types of "gray" lasers have cropped up:

- Lasers made by VISX and Summit and sold outside the U.S. which have been reimported by doctors wanting to avoid Pillar Point Partner royalty fees (Chapter 12). The problem for patients is that these lasers most likely are out-of-date, might have been damaged or knocked out of alignment during shipment, and cannot be tested or maintained using manufacturer parts or service. Since the outcome of the procedure depends, in great part, on the machine's doing its job, a bad laser could mean a bad job.

    "Reimported lasers don't have all the safety features of the lasers that are approved, and they might not have been well maintained," Dr. Waxler added. "It is perfectly fine for a manufacturer to reimport some of its own lasers and refurbish them so they meet the specifications of the lasers that are approved for sale in the U.S."

- Industrial excimer lasers that are adapted to PRK in a doctor's back office or by some third party. I recently found an ad on the World Wide Web for industrial excimers under $25,000—so there's a major cost incentive. Since Summit and VISX invested millions over a period of years in R&D and software design, it's difficult to imagine someone else coming up with the equivalent using raw parts. Nonetheless, as Dr. Waxler said, "there's some of this going on here, which is a problem. All of these lasers are noncompliant.'

- VISX and Summit lasers that have been revised in some way by a doctor wanting to perform procedures not designed into the current products.

Astigmatic or hyperopic PRK are two possible examples of this. There are many great surgeons in the U.S. and Canada who have stretched the PRK technology by reprogramming their lasers and have trained others to do it. Regardless, consumers should be aware that these physician-altered lasers have had no standard testing, and their manufacturers probably won't stand behind the results.

- There are a number of other U.S. and international manufacturers who have developed lasers for PRK, but none have yet completed their clinical trials. Use of these lasers outside clinical trials is against the law in the U.S..

Dr. Abbott, who is working with the FDA's compliance department on the Gray Laser investigations said, "There aren't that many. If everybody did these things, we'd be looking at some real disasters, but we haven't seen many problems." In July, 1997, the FDA panel met and issued guidelines to owners of grey lasers, offering them a short period of time to bring their lasers into compliance or risk penalties, including seizue.

What You Can Do to Protect Yourself
In response to concerns about gray-market lasers, the laser manufacturers have agreed to help readers who might be worried about this problem. If you have any doubts about whether your doctor is using an approved laser, you can call one of the manufacturers and ask if that doctor's site is an approved site. (A tip-off could be that the doctor is offering PRK at a much lower cost, or for a wider range of treatments than her competitors). The phone numbers in the U.S. are:

COMPANY	LOCATION	APPROVED LASER	TELEPHONE
Summit Technology	Massachusetts	Apex	800-880-4582
VISX, Incorporated	California	Star	800-246-8479

What's Under Investigation Right Now?
Mark Logan, President of VISX, said, "Outside the U.S., the VISX system is routinely used to correct astigmatism and higher degrees of myopia. The company has also begun to treat hyperopia, or farsightedness, outside the U.S." The Summit 1995 Annual Report stated that the company is "actively engaged in worldwide clinical trials for the treatment of astigmatism and farsightedness."

According to Dr. Waxler, "Just about every refractive indication is being studied by somebody. There's fairly fierce competition going on in studies of LASIK, astigmatism, hyperopia and other treatments for high myopia."

Are the FDA Trials Too Strict?

Medical devices in the U.S. are more stringently regulated than in any other country in the world. For this reason, said Dr. Abbott, the whole world is interested in what the FDA will do.

The lengthy, very expensive trials required by the FDA have both positive and negative effects on U.S. consumers.

The benefit is clear: by the time a device has received FDA approval, consumers can be fairly confident that it won't cause them major harm and it is likely to be effective. This is a powerful benefit.

The disadvantages were described by a number of the doctors who participated in the PRK trials:

- The trials are a major reason that the PRK procedure is so expensive: American manufacturers have to recoup about $100 million in R&D and clinical trial expenses. "Until receiving FDA approval," said Michael Barra, director of marketing for Summit Technology, "Our regulatory and clinical affairs department was the largest group in the company." Ed Beloze, Summit's product manager added, "It cost more to go through the FDA trials than it did to develop the laser."
- The cost and time involved in clinical trials is a disincentive for manufacturers to invest in new technologies that will serve small populations of people. In order to afford to go through the FDA process, the target audience has to be large enough to warrant the investment.
- The process of approval favors large companies with substantial resources. Small companies might not survive the years it takes to win approval after they have finally developed their product. For Summit and VISX, both start-up companies founded specifically to develop excimer lasers for PRK, it took nearly ten years to obtain FDA approval.
- Because of the rigid protocols necessary to "compare apples with apples" from one clinical trial site to another, patients who participate in the trials can be subjected to more discomfort or risk than is necessary. The fact that bandage contact lenses and anti-inflammatory drugs were not used during the trials is an example of this. The protocol developers felt that adding these variables would make it hard to discern whether side effects or healing responses could be attributed to the procedure or to the lens/drug.

In addition, companies are penalized by the system if they attempt to go back and revise their protocols based on evidence that arises during clinical trials: They essentially have to go back to the start of Phase II or III and begin again. "We have to balance our need for good information with our desire for the best procedures and the mandate not to harm the patients," Dr. Abbott said.

In a sense, the FDA is learning how to evaluate medical devices from the experience it gained at the expense of the excimer laser manufacturers. When trials first began on PRK, the Agency simply took its model for testing medical drugs and applied it to the excimer laser. According to Dr. Waxler, the Agency has learned that this model has its limitations when it comes to investigating devices, and steps are being taken to make the trials easier on the patients who participate in them.

THE GOLD STANDARD: "SAFE AND EFFECTIVE"

All FDA trials are designed to prove, over as few patients as possible, that a device is *both* safe and effective. This not only means that the device or drug won't harm you, but that it offers potential benefits sufficient to compensate for any risks you assume by using it. Using a blowtorch or muriatic acid to remove calluses, for example, might be effective, but it would hardly be safe. On the other hand, many over-the-counter remedies won't hurt you but they might not help much, either. Safe *and* effective is the standard.

"The manufacturers and doctors have been upset by how long it's taken to get approval for PRK," Dr. Waxler said, "but there's another way of looking at all this: Laser vision treatments are not urgent. They don't save lives, for example, like some cancer treatment might. People can see pretty well with glasses and contacts."

That's true, I told him, but I wasn't getting any younger, so why should I have to wait, or go to Canada, when doctors right in my state were trained in the procedure?

"There are people who feel a compelling need to go ahead and get it done even if they have to leave the country to do it. The question is, how much risk do you want to take, given what the information is? If people are reasonably informed about it, then I think that's a personal risk they ought to be able to take. They should ask, 'how risky is it, and how do I know?'"

I admitted that I was a person who wanted my vision fixed strongly enough to take risks even though I didn't understand them.

"Who should take the risk is an interesting issue," Dr. Waxler said. "Should it be the approving officials, or should it be the people who are getting their eyes operated on?"

I asked him whether he had considered having PRK.

"No, I haven't, and I'm not terribly motivated to get it done," he said. "I've worn glasses for some time and I'm perfectly happy with my visual correction. But there are times I'm irritated: I go swimming and I can't see a darn thing. I look at the huge clock across the pool and I can't see what time it is. I can barely see the wall!

"So, maybe I'll change my mind. As I say, people have different motivations and different kinds of work environments. It all depends on how great you expect the rewards to be relative to the possible risks."

Looking at
Your Options

*"But the bravest are surely those
who have the clearest vision of what is before them,
glory and danger alike,
and danger notwithstanding, go out to meet it."*

THUCYDIDES
~420 BC

14

Other Treatments for Low and Moderate Nearsightedness

*G*lasses and contacts remain a viable alternative for correcting nearly any refractive vision problem, but when you take them off, you're left with the problem. For at least a hundred years doctors have been experimenting with permanent cures for myopia.

Except for eye exercises and other "visual therapies," all of the methods have been invasive: They involved some form of cutting into the cornea or, at least, putting stitches in the eye. The fact that so many patients have been willing to undergo these procedures, even when they were highly experimental, is a comment on how driven many of us are to achieve vision without visual aids.

In parallel with surgical techniques, contact lens development followed its own high-tech route to better, cheaper, even disposable, materials and cleaning methods. Anyone who wore contacts in the '60s can attest to the fact that the modern relations bear little family resemblance to the thick plastic lenses some people were able to tolerate back then. Glasses have also improved

---

DO YOU HAVE LOW OR MODERATE MYOPIA?   If your prescription is from -0.5 to about -3.5, you are mildly myopic. Moderate myopia goes up to about -7.0. If your myopia is worse than -7.0, you can benefit from reading the section on RK and other alternatives below as a foundation for understanding the options presented in the next chapter.

---

with high-index lenses that offer stronger corrections with less weight, special coatings to protect against glare and sunlight and graduated multi-vision lenses.

From the early '70s through the '80s refractive surgery took huge leaps forward in a number of directions—spurred, no doubt, by the tremendous size of the potential audience. Corneas were removed, flashfrozen, reshaped on a lathe, then sewn back in place. "Living contact lenses" were created out of freeze-dried donor corneas, (one doctor said they looked like little potato chips), then rehydrated and sewn onto the patients' own corneas. Sections of corneas were sliced off, a tiny divot made in them, and then put back on. And "radial" incisions were cut into corneas.

Of all these techniques, only the last two are still performed with any frequency in the U.S. In Canada and Europe, where PRK has been in wide use for years, RK and ALK have fallen out of use.

ALK (Automated Lamellar Keratoplasty)
In ALK, the front of the cornea is sliced off and the correction is carved into the remaining cornea. ALK is the predecessor to LASIK and both are described in detail in the next chapter. Every doctor I spoke with considered the use of ALK for low-to-moderate myopia to be too risky compared to the other options.

RK (Radial Keratotomy)
In RK, cuts are made in a spoke-shaped pattern around the pupil. Hundreds of thousands of RKs have been performed in the U.S. since the mid-1970s but, as discussed below, doctors now feel it is useful only in the lower levels of myopia. At this point RK is the only widely used alternative to PRK for patients under -7.0.

The differences between PRK and RK are fundamental:
- RK is manual and success depends on the surgeon's skill and experience. PRK is computer-controlled; success depends on the accuracy of the initial exams, the maintenance of the equipment, and the knowledge of the doctor in adjusting medications to control healing.
- RK is "invasive" in that incisions are made into the cornea with a surgical knife. PRK removes a microscopic amount of tissue from the surface of the cornea and involves no incisions. (Figure 14.1)

THE RK OPTION

"Most people agree there is more skill required to perform RK than PRK but I'm not sure that's such a big issue," said Dr. Christopher Blanton. "It's free-hand, like writing with a pencil, but we have markers to guide the incisions. The blade is preset to cut only to a given depth."

Many of the doctors who were clinical investigators in the FDA trials for PRK still perform "mini-RK" procedures (described below) in a small subset of their mildly nearsighted patients and give their patients a choice of that or PRK. Others firmly believe that the long-term risks of RK vastly outweigh any short-term benefits and urge all their patients to have PRK.

Of course, if a doctor isn't trained in PRK, he or she will not be able to offer you both options. Nearly every ophthalmologist can offer RK.

RK and the FDA

It is interesting to me that, during the eight years two U.S. companies struggled to obtain FDA approval for PRK, RK procedures were being performed by the thousands without ever having had to go through the FDA.

"FDA does not regulate radial keratotomy because it is a medical procedure, not a medical device," said Emma Knight, an ophthalmologist and medical reviewer with the FDA's Center for Devices and Radiological Health. "The knife used in RK has been cleared by the Agency for general corneal surgery."[1]

In other words, any ophthalmologist with a diamond blade knife can do it. There are no training requirements or certification programs for RK, as the FDA requires for PRK. A further irony is that there were rare but catastrophic outcomes from RK right from the start and more became evident as patients were followed from one year to the next. During the same period, PRK results were being reported from countries all over the world and there were no catastrophes reported, ever.

Nonetheless, RK is still offered in the U.S. and you might be given this option. Having made the decision to have PRK rather than RK, I have already demonstrated my own bias, but my choice was instinctive: I didn't want any knives close to *my* eyes. *Your* choice should be better informed, so I spent a great deal of time investigating RK and learning what the top surgeons think about it as an option for today's myope. I was surprised to find out that many leading surgeons still offer RK as an option for treating low levels of near-sightedness.

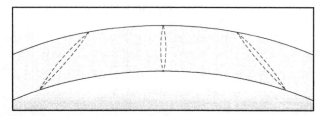

FIGURE 14.1   RK cuts penetrate 85-95% of the depth of the cornea. The length and number of incisions is determined by the patient's age and degree of nearsightedness.

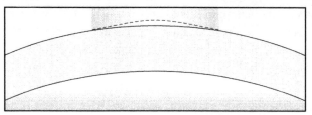

COURTESY OF BEACON EYE INSTITUTE

FIGURE 14.2   PRK removes less than a hairbreadth of tissue from the surface of the cornea. The amount of tissue removed is determined by the amount of correction desired.

How RK Works

RK is performed in a doctor's office under anesthetic eyedrops, just like PRK. The surgeon uses a diamond-blade knife which is preset for depth of cut and angle of incision. Following a pattern transferred to the cornea as a guide, the surgeon makes a series of cuts around the pupil of the eye that radiate out toward the edge of the cornea like spokes in a wheel. The cuts penetrate 85-95% of the depth of the cornea.

When the cornea is weakened by the incisions, the natural pressure inside the eye causes the perimeter of the cornea to bulge out, flattening the center. The degree of bulge, and therefore the amount of vision correction, is determined largely by the number and length of the incisions.

The Number and Length of Incisions

For the first 25 years RK was performed, the number of incisions tended to be 8 or 16 and the incisions extended from a 3-millimeter diameter circle around the pupil almost, in many cases, to the white part of the eye.

This type of RK, which is necessary to correct more than 2-3 diopters of nearsightedness in young people, or 4-5 diopters in older people, is considered "aggressive" today, and is not recommended by any of the surgeons I spoke with.

One of the advantages of RK is that the central optical zone—the "window" over the pupil through which you look—is left untouched by today's more conservative procedures. Unlike PRK, which treats the central visual area, RK begins at the outer edges of the pupil and extends outward from that point.

A New Approach: Mini-RK

In 1990 Dr. Richard Lindstrom, one of the nine PERK surgeons (see sidebar) and a clinical investigator for PRK, came to believe that a "minimal RK" with fewer, shorter cuts would reduce many of the side effects of RK and prevent some of the more serious complications. He also widened the central "clear" zone over the pupil to eliminate or reduce haze and other visual side effects.

Dr. Lindstrom found that 8 incisions that were only 2 millimeters long would produce 92% of the effect of 4-millimeter incisions. After following 100 patients who had mini-RK, he found that 94% achieved 20/40 or better uncorrected acuity with no significant complications.[3]

"Mini-RK turns out to be a way of reducing the invasiveness of RK without sacrificing its effectiveness in treating low-to-moderate myopia," said Dr. Lindstrom, "but I don't recommend it for more than 4 diopters of nearsightedness."

Dr. Christopher Blanton adds: "Compared to the older method, mini-RK may be better for patients at risk of blunt trauma because the cornea is less likely to rupture."

THE "PERK" STUDY   To find out whether RK was safe, in 1984 nine surgeons sponsored by the National Eye Institute began a ten-year Prospective Evaluation of Radial Keratotomy (PERK) on 793 eyes that were all treated using the RK method of the time. All patients were myopes between -2.0 and -8.0. In 1994 the results were summarized:

- 70% did not wear glasses or contacts for distance.
- 53% had 20/20 Uncorrected acuity.
- 85% had 20/40 or better Uncorrected acuity.
- 3% lost two lines or more of Best-corrected acuity.[2]

The researchers concluded, "RK is reasonably safe and effective with serious complications being rare."

Dr. Julius Shulman, author of a book on RK, *No More Glasses* (Simon & Schuster, 1987), and a surgeon in private practice in Manhattan, said, "Mini-RK is good for younger patients with 2 to 4 diopters of myopia or older patients with up to 5 to 6 diopters. I'm very conservative about when I use RK and I bend over backwards to do mini-RK."

Today mini-RKs with two to eight cuts are the most commonly performed with incisions at least a third shorter than in the earlier procedures and with a wider clear zone around the pupil. This is one reason it is hard to use the PERK study data to predict current outcomes: Since modern procedures generally are done more conservatively on less nearsighted people, the results tend to be better.

WHY CHOOSE RK?   Patients choose RK for a variety of reasons including:

- Faster visual recovery
- Less discomfort
- Little or no steroid eyedrops needed
- Lower cost than PRK
- Research results over many years

Mini-RK Minimizes Downsides

All the doctors I spoke with acknowledged that, compared to PRK, there are benefits for those who can qualify for a conservative mini-RK:

- Faster visual recovery: Vision is often 20/40 or better the next day and patients tend to have stable vision after a week or two.
- Less discomfort: Because the epithelium isn't removed during RK, the nerves of the cornea remain protected. Most patients report only a "scratchiness" or feeling like they have an eyelash in their eye. Symptoms usually disappear within a day or two.
- Little or no steroids: In many cases steroid drops are required to control healing and minimize haze after PRK, but after RK there is no significant risk of haze, so steroid drops are only necessary for the week or so it takes the RK incisions to heal. As a result, there is less risk of steroid-related side effects such as infection and elevated internal eye pressure, Dr. Shulman explained.
- 25 years of history: The PERK studies and others allow us to see what happens to patients many years after RK, whereas we don't know what

happens to patients ten years after PRK or other new techniques. On the other hand, RK has evolved over time, so results from earlier studies might not be reflective of, and probably are not as good as, the results doctors are obtaining today. In addition, with RK the patient's outcome is nearly 100% determined by his own doctor's skill and experience, so it will be impossible to predict outcomes from any research that isn't based on your own doctor's experience.

Are You A Candidate for RK?

According to the American Academy of Ophthalmology, RK results are best in patients with low-to-moderate nearsightedness and RK is not recommended for nearsightedness over -5.0 diopters.[4]

Age Matters

Dr. Thompson is not sure he would go as far as the Academy's recommendations: "RK has been around a long time and I know patients who are very happy with their results. But I'm very conservative on who I recommend consider it."

Dr. Thompson would divide your age by 10 to determine the *maximum* amount of correction you should attempt to achieve with RK. So if you are 45 you could have RK to correct up to 4.5 diopters of myopia. But if you're 25, you should only try to correct up to 2.5. He explains the rationale behind this formula.

"In order for RK to work, the incisions have to relax the collagen inside the cornea. 25-year-olds have tight collagen—that's why they don't have any skin wrinkles; 60-year-olds have more relaxed collagen. Therefore, younger patients require longer incisions to correct the same amount of nearsightedness. The longer the incision, and the closer it gets to the pupil, the greater the likelihood that glare will affect vision."

Of the two variables that determine a patient's candidacy for RK—age and level of myopia—age is by far the most important, according to Dr. Thompson. "I can do a 50 year-old's 4-diopter RK in a very conservative fashion, using a 4-incision procedure with the incisions a nice distance from the pupil. If I try to treat 4 diopters with RK on a 25-year-old, that's a maximal RK and all the incisions are going to go into the pupil. I don't want to do that."

"So I divide their age by 10," he summarized, "and below that level I give patients a choice of RK or PRK. Between that level and -7.0, I give them a choice of PRK or nothing. I would rather do nothing than do an aggressive RK. If they're over -7.0 they have the option being in my high-myopia PRK or LASIK studies."

SHOULD YOU HAVE RK?   Divide your age by 10, says Dr. Vance Thompson, and that is the *most* nearsighted you can be and achieve 20/40 or better with RK. A 30-year-old who is -4.0 would *not* qualify under this guideline because 30/10=3, a maximum correction of only three diopters of nearsightedness.

Gender Matters

Whether you are male or female makes a difference too, believe it or not. "A 21-year-old girl will end up undercorrected even if I try for only 2 diopters of correction. Women are classic under-responders," Dr. Thompson said with a perfectly straight face, "because they have tighter collagen than men of the same age."

Health Matters

The same conditions that would rule out PRK tend to rule out RK (see Chapter 3).

Astigmatism Matters

In the U.S., PRK to treat astigmatism is just short of FDA approval, but it is used almost exclusively to treat astigmatism in Canada. Nearly every surgeon in the U.S. I interviewed enthusiastically supports a procedure called AK (Astigmatic Keratectomy) to correct astigmatism during RK or after PRK. Dr. Schulman says that AK works fine, but "the less astigmatism you have, the better your results with RK will be. Additional surgery for astigmatism makes RK more complex and less predictable." AK and laser treatments for astigmatism are described in detail in Chapter 16.

Lifestyle Matters

Dr. Louis Grodin said that one of the chief advantages of RK is the very rapid visual recovery. "With PRK it can take several weeks to get to 20/40 or better and months before their best acuity is achieved. With RK, patients see very well the next day." As a result, patients who can't tolerate much vision downtime, such as truck drivers, often opt for RK.

Dr. Bruce Jackson thinks this is shortsighted, literally: "My PRK patients usually get to 20/25 in a week, and they achieve better, more predictable results over the long term."

What the patient does for a living or recreation also matters: if you spend 24 hours or more at high altitude in short bursts of time, such as ski vacations or mountain climbing, RK might not be the best procedure for you (see "High Altitude" below). Any job or sport that puts you at risk of being struck in the eye would also caution against RK.

Dr. Grodin said, "There's a place for RK in low myopia, but if the patient is into karate or boxing, or any activity that could result in a blow to the eye, PRK is the only option."

Money Matters

A benefit of RK is its relatively low cost. Compared to PRK which involves a $500,000 laser and over $50,000 a year in maintenance costs, RK involves about $15-20,000 worth of equipment. As a result, RK procedures currently cost $500-$1,000 less *per eye* than PRK. For this reason, RK remains popular in less developed countries.

RK SIDE EFFECTS

Some of the side effects of RK are similar to those of PRK and other refractive surgical procedures. Others are unique. Understanding the likelihood and severity of side effects and complications is key to making the right decision.

Pain after RK?

Most doctors described the immediate post-op period for RK in much the same way patients have described PRK with the bandage lens: For 1-2 days most patients experience a sensation of "something in the eye," burning or tearing, light sensitivity, and other irritation. Anti-inflammatory drops have been shown to be effective at reducing or removing most of the post-op discomfort.

In a study of 65 patients, those who were given anti-inflammatory drops reported peak discomfort at three hours after RK and about half of them took some form of prescription pain medication for the first day.[5]

THESE RK SIDE EFFECTS USUALLY ARE TEMPORARY

- Discomfort
- Need for extra caution with the eye
- Optical illusions

The Need for Caution During Recovery

Because of the incisions, there's a longer period of after-care needed to protect against the possibility of infection than after PRK. Patients are advised to be extremely careful with soap, water, swimming, makeup and other possible irritants for a much longer period than the 3-7 days required with PRK. Even rubbing the eyes can cause problems because the incisions seal rather than heal: The cornea always remains unstable.

Optical Side Effects

The very early RKs cut as close as 2.5 millimeters into the central optical zone. Then doctors began using a 3-millimeter zone. "We now know that even a 3-millimeter zone results in greater side effects such as glare and vision fluctuation," said Dr. Shulman. "3.5 millimeters is now the accepted minimum optical center, which reduces optical effects."

Glare

Both RK and PRK patients can experience glare for the first couple of months after surgery. With PRK the cause is slight corneal haze which creates the "dirty windshield" effect of scattering light. With RK, glare is caused by scarring at the incision sites.[6]

Dr. Blanton said that the risk and degree of glare depends on the size of the patient's pupil. If it enlarges at night into the area cut by RK, glare will occur.

Starbursts

Because RK involves incisions that never fully heal, the surface of the cornea can become uneven at the incision sites, causing the tear film to refract light unevenly. This can result in a starburst effect in bright light during the day or night. In some patients the effect is temporary; in others it might subside but never really disappear. In a few, starbursts actively interfere with vision.

"Generally glare and starburst get better over the first few months," said Dr. Lindstrom, "just like glare and halos do with PRK."

Haze Not a Problem

Because the central vision zone of the cornea is not treated, haze, which can cause a short-term loss (and, rarely, a longer-term loss) of best-corrected acuity after PRK, is not a problem with RK.

RK COMPLICATIONS

The list of complications, both short- and long-term, is longer for RK than PRK. Most doctors feel that the risks of complication are much lower today with more conservative RKs, but there are no long-term studies to prove one case or the other. As with PRK, there's no way of knowing in advance who will have complications.

Undercorrection and Regression

As with PRK, RK is not a perfect science in that the degree to which the cornea flattens is dependent to a large extent on the individual patient's eye. As we learned above, age can be a factor, but some people "age" slower than others because of firmer collagen, and this can cause the cornea to under-respond to the RK surgery or to regress gradually after surgery.

Add to this the fact that most doctors go out of their way to do the most conservative possible RK, and you end up with a 10-30% possibility of undercorrection.

Undercorrection can be treated with another RK or with PRK, but there are greater risks in both cases than if the patient had just had one RK and stopped.

No Contact Lenses After RK?

If an RK patient ends up undercorrected and chooses not to be retreated, chances are he will end up wearing glasses. The PERK study surgeons reported that "many patients have difficulty wearing contact lenses if they are required after RK." [7]

Most likely this is because there are "bumps" in the epithelium over the incisions which make it harder for the tear film to float the lens. As a result the lenses cause irritation and are less comfortable.

POSSIBLE RK COMPLICATIONS

- Undercorrection and regression
- Overcorrection
- Fluctuating vision
- Loss of best-corrected acuity
- Progressive hyperopia
- Perforation during surgery
- Infection and ulceration
- Rupture of cornea or eyeball

What If It Doesn't Work the First Time? Repeat RKs

The reason any refractive surgery is repeated is because the results were not as expected. Repeat RKs are called "enhancement procedures." Some doctors place new RK incisions directly over the earlier ones. Others go out of their way to avoid this.

Is Retreatment Likely?

Three factors seem to affect whether a patient will need retreatment: the surgeon's experience, the method of RK used, and the patient's own healing response.

The "Russian method" of performing RK, which involves cutting the incisions from the periphery of the cornea towards the pupil, appears to generate more retreatments: up to 40-60% of the cases. The "American method" retreatment rate is much lower: 10-20% of the cases.[8] The Russian method might also be riskier. Dr. Blanton said he has witnessed cases where an incision accidentally crossed the center of the pupil.

Every surgery requires a learning curve and surgeons new to a technique do not obtain the same results as those with experience. Dr. Blanton, who uses the American method, analyzed his first 100 RK cases and compared the first 50 to the last 50. In the first group of patients, 36% had to be retreated to get to their desired correction. In the last group, only 8% needed a second treatment.

During a seminar I attended (incognito) for patients interested in PRK, I was surprised to find the surgeons actively promoting RK. They said that "enhancement" procedures were necessary in about 20% of cases in order to allow the patient to drive without glasses or contacts. Other studies from very experienced surgeons have shown enhancement rates as high as 32%. But included in these studies were patients who had fairly high myopia. Modern RK procedures limit the amount of correction attempted, which in turn reduces the chance that patients will need an enhancement.

"If the surgeon is skilled and experienced," Dr. Blanton said, "The enhancement rate can drop below 10%."

The need for retreatment is determined by how happy the patient is with his results, and that can be age-related. "Young people want to get to 20/20 if they can, because they can use their focusing abilities to see near," Dr. Blanton said. "Patients over 50 actually enjoy a little undercorrection because they can read without glasses. Most of my patients achieve 20/25 instead of 20/20, but this nearly always makes them happy."

Retreatment Risks

Some doctors place enhancement incisions directly over the original ones, believing that this leaves more of the cornea intact. Others always create a new incision and never go over the old ones.

After performing corneal transplants on six patients who had vision loss from complications after RK, doctors at the Madigan Army Medical Center in Tacoma wrote, "Severe loss of vision was the [reason] for surgery in each case, and was associated with aggressive and repeated incisional attempts to correct astigmatism, hyperopic overcorrection and residual myopia."

The report concluded, "The risk for loss of vision increases with increasing number of incisions, intersecting incisions and very small optical zones." [9]

In other words repeat RKs can be risky. While there are no long-term follow-up studies on the results of repeat PRK procedures, every doctor I interviewed said that the worst outcome from retreatment has been either overcorrection or loss of 20/20 best-corrected acuity.

PRK to Retreat Traditional RK

According to some estimates there are over 200,000 Americans who have had RK in at least one eye. If the PERK studies are any indication, about a third of them still need to wear glasses. Now that PRK is approved, should these patients get a "buff and polish" job to take their vision the rest of the way?

Dr. Lindstrom has performed many PRKs on patients who had undercorrected RKs. "I only do it to correct real problems and I make sure patients understand the risk," he said. "In patients who have PRK over a traditional deep-incision RK, the risk of haze goes from only 1% with straight PRK to 10% for PRK after RK. There is also a greater risk of loss of best-corrected acuity."

How effective is PRK in treating undercorrected RKs? The research offers widely varying results:

- A study of 91 eyes that had PRK performed after RK found that 90% had 20/40 or better at the end of a year.[10]
- A different study found that 93% had 20/40 vision or better at six months after PRK and there was no significant haze after one month.[11]
- In a multi-site one-year study participated in by Drs. Robert Maloney and Roger Steinert of 107 eyes which had PRK to treat uncorrected myopia after RK (and 3 after cataract surgery), 74% had 20/40 or better vision a year after they had PRK to correct RK. Nearly 30% of the patients lost two or more lines of best-corrected vision, however. While the researchers do not recommend using PRK after RK as a planned two-stage

procedure, they concluded it was a "viable option" for treating eyes undercorrected by RK.[12]

- Dr. Marguerite McDonald participated in a study of 25 eyes treated with PRK after RK and found that only 53% of the patients were 20/40 or better after a year and 14% had lost two lines of best-corrected acuity. "For -6.0 myopia and lower, there is a somewhat reduced chance of success for PRK after RK compared to PRK alone," she said.

So, what are you going to do? The odds seem to favor retreatment with PRK rather than repeat RKs. If you have had RK and are not happy with your results, you might consider talking with a doctor who is very experienced in PRK to get an evaluation of the risks and benefits of having your eyes re-treated with PRK to increase your current uncorrected acuity.

About Face: Mini-RKs to Retreat PRKs

Doctors also go the other direction and use mini-RKs to take an undercorrected PRK patient closer to 20/20. While using the laser for retreatment is more common, there are cases where the doctor fears that an enhancement PRK could result in overcorrection.

Dr. Lindstrom said that mini-RKs to enhance PRK have been very effective and produce no higher complication rate. "But we don't plan for it; we try to get there in a single pass with PRK."

Overcorrection

As with PRK, there is the risk of overcorrection (causing farsightedness) with RK. In one published report a patient "in the ideal range for correction by RK" had surgery on both eyes. She ended up being 9 diopters farsighted and lost one line of best-corrected acuity. As the eye healed, the farsightedness pro-gressed.[13]

Fluctuating Vision

Many studies of RK have noted that most patients experience a "diurnal" change in vision: Their vision might start out fine in the morning and decrease to the point that they need distance glasses by late afternoon.

Dr. Shulman speculated that vision fluctuations throughout the day might be caused by the normal rise and fall of the internal pressure of the eye on an already weakened cornea. At night, pressure from the eyelid plus a reduction in oxygen to the eye might cause the eye to flatten back out, producing better vision in the morning. "As the incisions heal, these changes become less sig-nificant until vision stabilizes," he said.

THIRD TIME WAS CHARMED

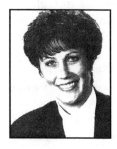

Name
Sandy Richards, 34

Occupation
Executive Assistant,
Michigan

Pre-Op Vision (before RK)
Left eye: -8.75
with 0.50 astigmatism

Right eye: -8.75
with 0.25 astigmatism

Post-RK Vision
Right eye: 20/400
with .75 astigmatism

Left eye: 20/30
with trace astigmatism

After RK enhancement:
Right eye: -3.25
with .75 astigmatism

After PRK retreatment:
Right eye: 20/20
with no astigmatism

PRK Surgeon
Jeffrey Machat, MD

Sandy Richards was a high myope who started wearing contacts in the fourth grade. She also had trouble seeing well enough to drive at night—a common problem with high myopia. At the time she chose to have RK, she didn't know about PRK and it was three years away from FDA approval in the U.S.

"I was outside the recommended range for RK and the doctor shouldn't have performed it on me, but my left eye came out fine, no problems. My right eye didn't—it was about 20/400 after RK, so I still needed glasses. To improve it, three months later the doctor did an 8-cut enhancement RK. Now I had 16 cuts in my right eye and nobody had bothered to tell me this could be a problem.

"After all three RKs it was a good three full days before I lost the sensation of a "lash" in my eye and my eyes watered the entire time. It was not fun. I kept using the numbing drops and when I mentioned it to the doctor he said, 'You're only supposed to use those on the first day.' My reaction was, 'O.K., but why didn't you tell me?'

"Even after all this my right eye still wasn't better than -3.25 and my astigmatism was much worse. The doctor said that he couldn't do any more, thank heaven, and suggested I see a doctor in Canada who was using a laser. So I went to Dr. Machat's former office in Windsor, Ontario. He examined me and told me that he couldn't help me with the laser he had in Windsor and suggested I go to his Toronto center where they had a newer machine that could also correct my astigmatism.

"So in April 1993 I trekked to Toronto on a Thursday, had PRK in about five minutes and slept while my husband drove the five hours home. PRK wasn't nearly as uncomfortable as the RKs—it was much, much easier.

"I went back to see Dr. Machat in Windsor on Friday. My eye was about 90% healed and he removed the bandage contact lens. I asked him how long I should wait before getting back into my aerobics class and he said "You can do it tonight, if you feel like it." I was amazed.

"A week after PRK my vision was still a little blurry, but I could function without glasses. In two weeks it was 20/20. Because that eye had already had RK, however, my vision would shift from morning to night. In the morning I could see 20/15, but by night it wasn't nearly as good. I asked Dr. Machat if he could fix this, but he said he couldn't take away the incisions that were the cause of the problem. Over the last two years, though, I've noticed that my vision has gotten progressively more stable throughout the day, but I still have starbursts from the RK. My night vision in the RK eye has also improved: Up until about nine months ago I wore weak distance glasses when I drove at night, but now I never do.

"I was so excited with my results. At that time Dr. Machat was just starting TLC-The Laser Centers and I decided I wanted to be part of it. He found a place for me, and here I am three years later.

"My big regret is that I didn't do my homework and wait for the laser. I have two small kids and I'm constantly worried I'll get hit in the eye and lose my sight. With PRK there is just so much less to worry about."

In their 11-year results published in early 1996, the PERK study group reported, "The average change in vision from morning to evening was between -0.50 and -1.50. 3% lost best-corrected acuity of two lines and 1% gained two lines."[14]

In other words, after 11 years, patients' vision could degrade from 20/20 in the morning to 20/80 in the afternoon, when they'd need glasses to drive or watch the evening news.

Daily vision fluctuations have not been reported as a side effect of PRK.

Loss of Best-Corrected Acuity

The risk of loss of best-corrected acuity was higher in the PERK study (3% lost at least two or more lines) than in studies following patients who had PRK.[15] Mini-RK techniques probably will demonstrate a better track record.

Progressive Hyperopia

This is one RK side effect that gives every refractive surgeon concern: Over the long term, RK patients have slowly continued to "improve" to the point that they become hyperopic, or farsighted. In the ten-year results of the PERK study, 43% of 693 eyes had shifted into farsightedness by at least 1 diopter at the end of ten years.

Dr. Shulman said there is irony in this, "We used to think that total removal of myopia after RK was the ultimate in a perfect result. Now we know that the closer a patient is to being 20/20 after RK, the more likely, if there is no regression, she will end up farsighted years later."

Dr. Steven Schallhorn believes that this is one complication that ultimately will spell the demise of the practice of RK in North America once PRK becomes more widely available. "The shift toward hyperopia after RK is common and unacceptable given the alternatives available," he said.

Another summary report expressed similar concerns. "The ultimate outcome of RK may never be known in many or even most patients because of a long-term refractive shift toward increased flattening of the cornea. This phenomenon of long-term instability is a major weakness of the RK procedure performed in the 1980s."[16] Dr. Lindstrom believes that hyperopic shift will be proven to be significantly less in eyes treated with mini-RK.

At this writing, the standard treatment for farsightedness (hyperopia) after RK is surgical. Many doctors, including Dr. Lindstrom, use a compression suture, called the Lasso technique, to steepen the cornea temporarily until a better treatment is available.

Perforation

The very word sends chills down most spines. "It happens in 2-10% of the cases," Dr. Blanton acknowledged, "but almost always it means nothing to the patient."

Perforation is the result of the knife going through the cornea into the inner eye. Since corneas vary in depth—most are between 480 and 550 microns deep—and blades can vary by a few microns in length, a long blade and a thin cornea could result in perforation. There are two types of perforations:

Microperforations occur when the surgeon notices that the blade is going too deep, immediately retracts the knife, and the perforation seals itself. "Most patients do very well when this happens," Dr. Blanton said.

Macroperforations occur when the doctor doesn't notice that the blade is penetrating the cornea, it continues to go deeper, and a larger gape, or hole,

HIGH ALTITUDE AND PROGRESSIVE HYPEROPIA

One thing you can say about the military is that it is remarkably thorough when it goes about investigating something. In several Army studies, patients who had RK were sent on a plane ride or placed in a hypobaric (low pressure) chamber for a number of hours to see what would happen. The result of these real or simulated high-altitude jaunts was a trend toward flattening of the cornea—a shift to hyperopia.[17]

This information is important to an organization that might, for example, depend on its members' ability to perform search, rescue or tactical missions in a high mountain region.

Dr. Blanton said that a joint Army/Navy study made similar findings but in some cases the tests were done shortly after RK—before the incisions had any chance to heal—and this could have affected the results. He and Dr. Schallhorn led a Navy expedition to investigate the phenomenon in more depth.

"We took a number of people to the top of Pike's Peak in Colorado [altitude 14,110 feet] and kept them up there over 72 hours. In the group there were 11 RK eyes, 12 PRK eyes and 17 eyes that had never had surgery. During the time they were up top, the RK eyes demonstrated a significant shift to hyperopia, and this didn't happen in any of the other eyes. The effect was greatest in the

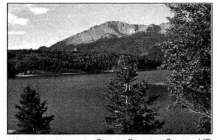

PHOTO BY CHRISTOPHER BLANTON, MD

Pike's Peak as seen by Dr. Blanton during the Army/Navy study.

patients who were only 4 months post-op and least in the ones who were more than two years post-op. When we came back down, all the eyes returned to the state they had been in before the trip."

Dr. Blanton theorizes that hyperopic shift is caused by oxygen deprivation at high altitudes. "The cornea requires oxygen to maintain its normal thickness and clarity. At high altitudes everyone's cornea swells, but the RK patients' vision was affected by the swelling." This is thought to be because the weakened corneas bulged more at the sides, which had the effect of flattening the center, causing farsightedness. Another Army study determined that this effect takes at least six hours to develop,[18] so

PHOTO COURTESY OF CHRISTOPHER BLANTON, MD

Drs. Schallhorn (left) and Blanton set up shop atop Pike's Peak.

RK patients probably won't experience problems during air travel unless they're crossing many time zones.

This could cause trouble people who have to perform at high altitudes over a period of days, though. For them, the potential for hyperopic shift should be factored into a decision about whether to have RK. Exposure to high altitudes for less than 24 hours doesn't seem to cause much of a problem.

---

results. "If left alone, these perforations leak fluid from the inner eye. The doctor nearly always notices the leak, pops in a couple of stitches, and the problem usually is solved," continued Dr. Blanton. "It's usually not a horrible thing, but there are cases where patients with perforations end up getting infections. In those cases there can be serious complications and poor outcomes." The stitches are left in for about six weeks and can be bothersome as well as interfere with vision.

Early-Stage Infection

A pre-existing eye infection can cause complications after RK just as with PRK. But unlike with PRK, after RK there are open incisions to collect bacteria which can cause infection weeks after the procedure. For this reason, mini-RKs seem to generate the same rate of infection as more aggressive RK procedures.

"Infection is very rare," said Dr. Shulman, "but it's a risk factor. The more damage you do to the cornea, the less resistance it has to infection. Antibiotic drops can be used to prevent or treat the problem."

Infection is the main argument against treating both eyes in the same visit. If an infection occurs in one eye, it can spread to the other, putting both eyes at risk.

Late-Stage Infection and Ulceration

If you've ever had a cat who ended up with an abscess after a fight, you'll understand what can happen to RK incisions. With cats, the outer skin heals over the wound (probably because they take such good care of it), trapping bacteria inside which then can abscess.

It appears that the same thing can happen after RK: The surface of the incision closes, but any bacteria trapped deep inside can fester and cause infection or ulceration. For cats, the treatment is to drain the wound, add antibiotics and keep the wound open until it heals from the inside out. This is hard to do with eyes!

Studies have shown that when infection does occur, the bacteria usually is found in the incision, and doctors speculate that the bacteria were placed in the incisions by a contaminated diamond-blade knife and didn't show up until later because they were injected so deeply into the cornea at the time of RK. Because antibiotic drops don't penetrate to the inner part of the cornea, just as they don't when applied to the surface of a cat's wound, the bacteria were able to survive and multiply.[19]

In the PERK study there were no early cases of infection, but there were two cases of infection that occurred after seven months and one at two-and-a-half years.

Another study reported on a 39-year-old man who developed a corneal ulcer in an RK incision site eight years after surgery. Doctors were unable to find any reason for the infection other than his previous RK.[20]

Susceptibility to Blunt Trauma

The worst complication of RK is the extremely rare case in which the eye ruptures after being struck with force (blunt trauma). The rupture can occur along the incision sites and affect only the cornea (and therefore perhaps be solved with a corneal transplant), or it can open the eyeball itself, causing permanent loss of sight.

Out of hundreds of thousands of cases, though, there are only a few reports of rupture and some doctors believe that most of the time an untreated eye would have ruptured under the same circumstances. In at least one report, patients whose eyes would have been expected to rupture did not, despite serious injury. A woman who died in an airplane crash had multiple broken bones in her face. Another man was struck in the eye by a racquetball. In both cases the patients had undergone RK but their eyes remained intact after the trauma.[21]

On the other hand, when rupture occurs it is serious. In one study researchers said, "Several cases of ruptured corneas after blunt trauma in eyes [treated with RK] have been reported, even ten years after the procedure, and in the majority of patients this event is associated with sight-threatening complications."[22] The researchers found that "eyes which have undergone RK require approximately 54% less force to rupture" than unoperated eyes.

The good news in this study, for people interested in RK, is that mini-RK provided much higher resistance to blunt trauma than aggressive RK. The researchers concluded that "Mini-RK may be particularly useful in patients at high occupational risk of subsequent ocular trauma." However, they cautioned

BLUNT-TRAUMA RISK AFTER PRK   There haven't been any reports of corneal or eyeball rupture after PRK—which makes sense because PRK doesn't weaken the cornea. Dr. James Salz reported on two patients who suffered blunt trauma after PRK—one from a fist fight and the other from a karate kick. Both injuries healed the way an untreated cornea would be expected to heal.[25] Of course, there's no way of knowing whether an RK-treated eye would have ruptured under identical conditions.

When eyes treated with RK were compared to eyes treated with a very deep PRK (beyond the level approved in the U.S.), researchers found that eyes treated with a deep PRK (10-diopter correction) are less likely to rupture with blunt trauma than eyes treated with RK.[26] Other researchers studying whether eye-bank eyes would rupture after extreme PRK concluded that PRK "does not weaken the cornea after degrees of ablation commonly used in the clinical setting." [27]

---

that even though mini-RK might protect the cornea from minor trauma, it probably wouldn't protect the eyeball from rupturing after major trauma.

This finding has been supported in other studies. Laboratory experiments attempting to investigate the likelihood of eyes rupturing after RK have found, time after time, that untreated eyes can withstand much more force before rupturing than RK-treated eyes. In addition, eyes treated with RK tend to rupture at the incision sites.[23] This is why most doctors won't perform RK on patients at known risk of being struck in the eye, such as boxers or karate students.

The experiments proving this tendency might be flawed, however, because eyes (such as pig or sheep eyeballs bought from a slaughterhouse) are given RK incisions and then immediately put in a bench press to test them for susceptibility to rupture. Since the eyes aren't in a living being, there's no way to know whether they would have ruptured if they had been able to heal for several months. The studies do show that blunt trauma such as a blow to the eye from a baseball or a car accident in the first few weeks or months after RK can expose the eye to a substantial degree of risk. Reporting on the rupture of an RK eye seven-and-a-half-years after surgery, a researcher concluded, "Our case documents that the weakness of the keratotomy wounds persist up to 91 months after the operation."[24]

Simultaneous RK

Treating both eyes with RK, or any other surgery, during the same visit is controversial and some of the leading eye surgeons disagree on whether this is wise.

The benefits of treating both eyes at the same time are the same as for PRK: less awkwardness between surgeries, faster release from glasses and contacts, less downtime, fewer follow-up visits. Dr. Thompson said, "I'm not a fan of simultaneous eye surgery, but it is appealing to get both eyes done at once."

These benefits have to be balanced against the possibility of an infection that could start in one eye and spread to the other, jeopardizing both. "Much of this risk can be eliminated if the surgeon uses a new blade on each eye," Dr. Maloney said. "Switching from one eye to the other with the same blade is a very poor idea."

Treating one eye at a time allows the doctor to observe an individual's healing response and use that information to finetune the procedure for the second eye, perhaps achieving a better result. "Standard calculations on how many incisions to make for patients at any given age are based on averages," Dr. Salz said. "If the patient heals more aggressively, he can end up overcorrected. If you learn this on one eye, you can take steps to prevent it in the second."

In a study of 20 patients who had both eyes treated with RK at the same time and 71 patients who had their two eyes treated at different times, it was found that the simultaneously treated eyes had more identical vision after surgery. The researchers noted, however, that the risks of infection should be carefully considered before operating on both eyes on the same day.[28]

In another report, researchers concluded after examining four patients with severe infections after simultaneous RK that "Sight-threatening [infections] can occur after radial keratotomy and we believe that simultaneous surgery of any kind should be discouraged."[29]

Dr. Salz agrees. "I go ballistic on simultaneous RKs," he said, "especially now that PRK is approved, because they deprive the patient of an important option. There is no way patients can understand certain side effects of RK until they have experienced them. Starbursts at night don't bother some people, but drive others crazy. If a patient only has one eye treated and has starbursts, we can offer PRK for the other eye. If both eyes are cut, that option disappears."

RK *vs* PRK: MAKING THE DECISION

Having read all of that, how are you going to decide? There are three basic approaches to making the decision: compare research results, compare treatment characteristics, or compare doctor opinions. A fourth method—all of the above—probably makes the most sense. Table 1 summarizes the primary treatment characteristics. Below are some notes on comparing research results and, finally, some considered medical opinions.

In the end it will come down to how much nearsightedness you have, how long you can put up with less-than-perfect vision, and how much faith you have in your doctor's surgical skill.

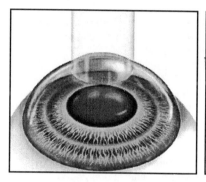 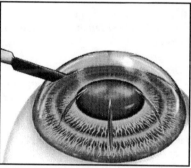

COURTESY OF BEACON EYE INSTITUTE

PRK   **RK**
Which is right for you?

On Comparing Research Results

There are at least five problems with relying on research results to make a decision in this case:

1) Technology and surgical methods didn't stand still while we waited for the PERK ten-year follow-up studies. Between the time the long-range study was begun and when the results were analyzed, the mini-RK method came into being and the older techniques were improved.

2) The patients didn't stand still either. Even with control groups, it's impossible to know for certain if changes in vision occurred because of side effects from surgery or whether they would have occurred in the normal progression of the patients' lives.

3) Likewise, PRK evolved during development and clinical trials, and is continuing to evolve, so even FDA approval data isn't going to give you the results of current methods being used.

COMPARING PRK WITH MINI-RK	Table 14.1

PRK	**MINI-RK**
Who?	
•In U.S. for -1.0 to -7.0 myopes over age 18.	•Myopia to -4.0 or -5.0, depending on degree of nearsightedness
•Widespread use in Canada	•Widespread use in U.S.
•Approved by FDA and Canadian Health	•Not reviewed by either organization
•Requires experienced doctor, well maintained equipment	•Requires surgical skill, experience, and a knife.
How?	
•Procedure planned by computer	•Procedure planned by surgeon
•Laser vaporizes less than 10% of cornea	•Knife penetrates 85-95% of cornea
•Done under anesthetic drops	•Done under anesthetic drops
•Less risk with simultaneous treatment	•More risk with simultaneous treatment
•Nonreversible	•Nonreversible
Where?	
•Done over central optical zone; can cause scarring or loss of best-corrected acuity.	•Done outside central optical zone, so scarring usually is not a visual problem, but there can be risk of loss of best-corrected acuity
Healing	
•More discomfort possible the next day	•Minimal discomfort likely
•Good vision can take a week or two	•Vision better sooner; good the next day
•Outer cornea completely heals in less than a week	•Incisions never fully heal
•Patients can wear contacts after PRK, if necessary	•Might not be able to wear contacts after
•Correction stabilizes in 2-6 months	•Correction stabilizes in 1-2 weeks
Side Effects	
•Haze	•Starbursts
•Glare	•Glare
•Results stable, once attained	•Vision tends to fluctuate during the day and can change over a period of years.
Complications	
•Some short-term risk of overcorrection	•Long-term risk of progressive hyperopia
•Little risk of infection	•Serious infections at the incision sites can occur even years later
•No change to integrity of eyeball	•Eye can rupture more easily
•Repeat treatments safer	•Repeat treatments riskier
Cost	
$1500-2000 per eye plus steroid drops	$600-1500 per eye

4) Since RK is so dependent on individual surgical skills, using data generated by other doctors might be meaningless as a predictor of your own doctor's outcomes. Even a gifted surgeon can have a "bad hand" day every once in awhile.

5) There are no ten-year follow-up studies on PRK patients.

Dr. James Salz conducted his own comparison of RK and PRK in 1995. In a three-year follow-up study of 107 of his PRK treatments and 117 of his RKs, the visual results for the patients were nearly identical. In addition, the side effect rates and the number of serious complications were minimal and also identical.[30] It should be noted, however, that Dr. Salz is one of the world's most experienced corneal surgeons and has performed both procedures since they were first introduced.

Some Expert Opinions

The best available help might be surgeons who have used the older methods and now use or have access to the newer ones. Without exception, all the U.S. investigators for PRK have also performed RK. When you go to your doctor you'll hear his or her views. Here's an opportunity to hear from some of the others. I haven't included Canadian doctors in this summary because none of them perform RK.

Dr. Vance Thompson

"I've been doing both procedures for over six years and I'm still doing them both. I've treated ophthalmologists who chose RK even though they knew about PRK. RK has a few benefits and there are long-term success stories. It's attractive not to have surgery over the visual axis and I like the quickness of the visual recovery. Even though I feel that PRK will become the most commonly performed procedure for correcting vision, I feel it's important to teach patients about all their options.

Dr. Richard Lindstrom

"PRK patients tend to improve over the first 18-24 months and there doesn't seem to be any long-term instability. RK problems tend to get worse with time—corneas lose stability and there's hyperopic shift. That's the reason I'm now much more conservative in using RK. I'm doing less RKs all the time.

"At our center the surgeon has a vote, but so does the patient. If you look around the world at other advanced countries, not that many patients are voting for RK, so I'm not going to push it on the patient. It turns out PRK works fine and it looks like LASIK is getting better and better. Patients will have all those options.

Dr. Christopher Blanton

"We need more than one tool in our toolbox. PRK is not a panacea because all surgery has its risks. For some patients, RK has a better combination of benefits and risks." Dr. Blanton recently completed a review of the last 150 cases treated in his Navy clinic that were more than 18 months post-op. 5% had perforations without negative results, there were no early infections, there was one late-stage infection, and 1-3% lost some best-corrected acuity. The *worst* outcome was 20/25.

"PRK is so new, we don't know how those patients are going to do in ten years. We are now starting to ask: 'What is the incidence of glare and halo problems at night?' All that said, I have referred family members for RK and I would do it for PRK."

Dr. Lewis Grodin

"There's still a place for RK in low myopia where optical zones can stay in the 4-millimeters range. I tell my patients, 'to correct low myopia you've got four options: glasses, contacts, RK and PRK.' The research doesn't come down in favor of one or the other, so I let them make up their own minds."

Dr. Robert Maloney

"I tell patients to take their age, divide it by ten and then have PRK no matter what the result. PRK is more predictable in treating low myopia than RK and is safer in treating higher levels. Whichever category the patient falls into, he's better off with PRK."

Dr. Steven Schallhorn

"PRK, while it's not perfect, might prove to be preferable to RK in young, active people, especially those exposed to a wide variety of conditions. I've seen cases of sudden ulceration of RK eyes, and there have been documented cases of RK eyes rupturing when hit. RK works because it weakens the structure of the eye.

"As for mini-RKs, the risks are lower, but so are the rewards. I wouldn't even consider it for someone under age 40 with more than 3 diopters of myopia. In addition to the risks of infection and rupture, many patients have unstable corneas that change over the years. This is very disturbing because it means that even after several years their corneas are not healed. Deep portions of the cuts might *never* heal.

"By contrast, PRK doesn't weaken the eye and the cornea fully heals afterward, but it *is* performed over the optical center. If there is residual haze or scarring, there could be some loss of vision. In our study of 100 Navy personnel who had PRK, however, nothing even came close to being vision threatening. There are patients who aren't good candidates for PRK, but RK isn't a preferable alternative."

The American Academy of Ophthalmology

A 1993 report by the American Academy of Ophthalmology included the following comments:

> Published data indicate that radial keratotomy (RK) usually achieves partial improvement in uncorrected visual acuity in patients with non-progressive low and moderate amounts of myopia. Undercorrection occurs commonly, and the amount of correction cannot be predicted accurately for an individual patient...The unpredictability of the refractive outcome stems from several factors, including: 1) The biologic variability from one individual to another, 2) Variation in surgical techniques among surgeons, 3) Difficulty in making all incisions uniformly, and 4) Inability to measure and control the biomechanical properties of the cornea.
>
> Improvements in the surgery are occurring...and some series of radial keratotomy cases have reported better uniformity and predictability of outcome. The potential of this procedure to render good visual acuity without glasses or contact lenses must be weighed against its known risks. [31]

WHAT ABOUT LASIK?

I knew you were going to ask. LASIK is a combination of ALK and PRK which was developed to solve some early problems that arose from using PRK to treat high levels of nearsightedness.

In LASIK a flap is cut off the front of the cornea while the eye is under suction, and then PRK is performed to remove tissue from the interior of the cornea. The flap is carefully placed back on, where it seals itself without stitches. LASIK requires a much more skilled and experienced surgeon than PRK. Like RK, LASIK exposes the eye to the risk of infection, but there are some other rare but serious risks as well. Because the procedure is complicated and has the potential to damage the eye, most of the doctors I spoke with do not recommend it for patients under -7.0, since PRK is a proven safe and effective treatment for them.

The next chapter describes LASIK in detail, along with its benefits, risks and complications. If your doctor is urging you to consider it, I hope you'll take the time to read that section, the patient case stories there, and learn

CHOOSING THE BEST-AVAILABLE OPTIONS

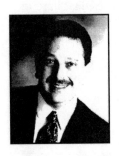

Name
Jeffrey Robin, MD, 40

Occupation
Ophthalmologist, Ohio

Pre-Op Vision
-4.50 with no
astigmatism

Procedures
Right eye, RK
Left eye, PRK

Post-Op Vision
Right eye 20/20
Left eye, 20/20

RK Surgeon
J.Charles Casebeer, MD

PRK Surgeon
James J. Salz, MD

Back in 1991, Dr. Jeffrey Robin was head of refractive surgery for the Illinois Cornea Center. "I had worn glasses since about the fourth grade," he said, "and got contacts right before college. Neither solution was right for me.

"The lenses were uncomfortable and easily torn, and with glasses I always felt I was missing something visually." Having performed several thousand RK procedures on patients, when he turned 35 he decided it was time to get some good natural vision for himself—at least in one eye. PRK was starting to gain momentum in Canada and Europe, but in the U.S. trials had just begun, so he opted for RK.

"I had an 8-incision RK on my right eye with a 3-millimeter optical zone, but that was considered conservative back then. My vision was 20/20 the morning after surgery and I felt only a little uncomfortable."

A year later, PRK was entering Phase III trials in the U.S. and Dr. Robin decided it might be an even better option for his left eye. "I had about the same amount of discomfort after PRK as I had with RK," he said, "but it took longer to get to 20/20—nearly two weeks. The big difference between the two eyes now is that the PRK eye has much more stable vision. There are no fluctuations or starbursts as I have had in the RK eye. I should mention, though, that I experienced both these effects with contacts."

Dr. Robin is 40 now and hasn't worn glasses for five years—not even for reading. Since 1992 he has performed over 650 PRKs as part of the FDA clinical trials plus more than 5000 RKs. "I don't do many RKs any more. Most patients decide that the few benefits—early visual recovery and lower cost—just aren't worth the risks."

Dr. Robin currently is comparing PRK and LASIK (described in Chapter 15) in the FDA trials for a new excimer laser and feels LASIK will one day become the treatment of choice for all levels of myopia. "If I had to have my vision corrected today, I would have LASIK," he said, "but if I had waited, I would have worn glasses five more years."

HAD BOTH, NO REGRETS

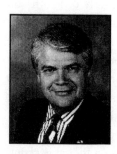

Name
Tom Rodriguez, 49

Occupation
Men's clothing retailer,
California

Pre-Op Vision
-4.50
with no astigmatism

Procedures
PRK and RK

Post-Op Vision
PRK: 20/15
RK: 20/30

Surgeon
Michael Gordon, MD

Tom Rodriguez had PRK back in 1993, as part of the FDA trials, when patients were required to wait six months between eyes. To avoid the wait, Mr. Rodriguez opted to have his second eye treated with RK.

"I wasn't being frivolous— I felt very much off balance because the results were so dramatic with the laser. I waited about two months and then I just felt I couldn't stand it, so Dr. Gordon suggested the RK." Mr. Rodriguez was 46 at the time, so with Dr. Thompson's "age-divided-by-10" formula, a mini-RK could correct his -4.50 vision.

"At the time I was doing a lot of traveling for work and I was president of the Hispanic Chamber of Commerce, which involved public speaking. I had reached the point that I was tired of wearing glasses and had no success with contacts. My niece worked in Dr. Gordon's office and told me about PRK.

"To this day, quite frankly, I've had so much better results with PRK than with RK. But with the RK eye a little nearsighted I've been able to read without glasses even though I'm 49.

"After PRK I had about a day and a half of discomfort, but it wasn't to the point of being painful—I didn't even use the pain medicine they gave me." [This statement surprised me because Mr. Rodriguez was part of the FDA trials and he did *not* have benefit of the bandage contact lens or the anti-inflammatory drops.]

"After RK my eye looked pretty bad because a couple of blood vessels had burst, but there was even less discomfort: I walked in, had the procedure and walked out feeling like I hadn't even had the surgery. The only thing that happened was I had 'dry eye' after the RK for awhile—which made it uncomfortable to open my eye first thing in the morning. I used some eyedrops and that helped. I've also noticed some fluctuation in my vision in that eye.

"I never even needed glasses until after college. Now, 30 years later, not having to wear them has given me a whole new outlook on life."

what the doctors in this book are saying about it. It bears mentioning here that there have been no long-term studies that prove the safety of LASIK and some doctors are concerned it might cause damage to the eye that won't be apparent for a few years. Early reports from a few studies indicate that the visual outcomes of PRK and LASIK are nearly identical, but that LASIK might avoid some of the temporary side effects. On the other hand, there have been cases of lost sight and corneal transplants after LASIK and its predecessor ALK, while in PRK's ten-year history, no patient has had these kinds of problems.

Most of the publicity you hear about LASIK centers on the same claims made for RK: fast recovery and no pain. But as you have learned from reading the patient cases in this book, most PRK patients have only very short periods of discomfort, if any, and some LASIK patients also have a period of discomfort while the epithelium heals around the incision site. Most PRK patients achieve 20/40 vision within the first week or so, as do LASIK patients, but LASIK might get them there a few days sooner. Unfortunately, some doctors are taking advantage of the proven safety of PRK procedure to imply that LASIK has the same track record, just because it uses the same laser. There is no research that shows this is true.

In the hands of a gifted and experienced surgeon LASIK might prove to be fine for the very nearsighted, but we don't know that for sure yet, and we don't know if it's better or worse than PRK. Until we have credible studies following large numbers of patients over several years, LASIK, and its supporters, have a great deal to prove.

WATER-JET SURGERY: THE RK/PRK/LASIK OF THE FUTURE? The wave of the future might well be pressure-washing excess tissue from the cornea instead of removing it by laser. Two companies, Medjet and Surgijet, are developing ways to harness a high-speed stream of purified water so it can make precise cuts or remove tissue with even less harm to the remaining cornea. The devices are relatively inexpensive, handheld and powered by a CO_2 cartridge—which would make the waterjet procedures much lower cost than laser, if FDA trials prove that they can do as good a job predictably and safely.

ON THE HORIZON:
REVERSIBLE/ADJUSTABLE CURES

Just as PRK revolutionized refractive surgery by allowing surgeons to precisely sculpt the cornea right on the patient's eye, three new procedures which are in development and clinical trials could be the seeds of another revolution.

These "reversible" techniques have undeniable appeal because they might allow surgeons to correct vision by implanting a device today, and then later remove or change it if the patient's vision changes or the correction did not go as planned. It will be 1998 or 1999before these treatments complete clinical trials.

One consolation for those of us who go ahead and have RK or PRK now is, if we're not 100% happy with our results, one of these reversible procedures might be the ticket to perfection. And for those of us who achieve 20/20 vision, a reversible procedure might give us bifocal or near vision in one eye to help us avoid reading glasses at a future date (see Chapter 17).

Unlike PRK and RK, where the surgery is over when it's over, these procedures all involve leaving something behind. Long-term safety questions arise whenever a device is implanted into the body, together with the risk of the incisions required for the procedure. In addition, infection can accompany an implant if it is contaminated before being placed in the eye or if bacteria are injected during the implantation process.

Implantable Contact Lens (ICLs)
Doctors currently are investigating an implantable contact lens which is placed inside the eye on top of the lens, but below the iris.

One doctor said, "We make a little incision in the side of the cornea and inject a light, delicate lens under the iris. This is simple to perform and totally reversible. We can insert lenses to correct myopia and astigmatism and deliver instantaneous, next-day perfect results. There doesn't appear to be any instability and, because the lens is designed just like a contact lens, the results are completely predictable. The entire surgical experience takes 1-2 minutes."

Dr. Salz, who is investigating the ICLs said, "I've examined 100 eyes that were treated with the implantable contact lens by Dr. Roberto Zaldevar in Argentina. Patients have instant visual recovery without the usual side effects of RK and PRK and very high-quality results long term."

Wow. Are there any downsides?

Complications include all the risks of any incisional procedure plus glaucoma and problems with swelling at the retina, although none of these had yet appeared in a study conducted by Dr. Salz.[32]

The major reservation many doctors have about ICLs is the possibility that the artificial lens will cause cataracts in the natural lens. "This is not a horrible complication though," said Dr. Salz, "because in that case we simply remove the natural lens and the ICL and replace them with an artificial lens—just as we do for cataract surgery."

Dr. Roger Steinert is not so optimistic. "These procedures are unquestionably aggressive—and the solution to any problems that arise is even more so. They are high risk based on our current level of knowledge."

INTRASTROMAL DEVICES   The *stroma* is the body of the cornea, right under the epithelium. An *intrastromal* device is one placed inside the body of the cornea.

Intrastromal Corneal Ring Segments (ICRS)

Dr. Richard Abbott has been involved with the development of the ICRS for nearly 10 years and is just beginning Phase III trials for the FDA study. Dr. Lindstrom is also participating in the trials.

The intrastromal ring segments are two tiny plastic 150-degree arcs. A special diamond-blade instrument is used to create a very short groove outside the visual area on either side of the pupil and the rings are placed in the cornea. This causes the periphery of the cornea to bulge and the center to flatten. The degree of bulging is determined by the thickness of the segments, although "thick" would hardly be the way to describe them: They range from ¼ to ½ millimeter in thickness.

In the preliminary three-month results of the first 75 cases, which were presented in March of 1996, 92% of the patients had 20/40 or better vision and the rest had 20/50 or better. All the patients were within two lines of best-corrected acuity.

"Since the incisions are only 1.8 millimeters in length, the epithelium is hardly disturbed—so healing is much faster," said Dr. Abbott. "On the first day patients are seeing well, and by the third day they usually are seeing very well with minimal discomfort. When the segments are in place, they're less noticeable than a contact lens. Best of all, we can remove the device if there is a problem later."

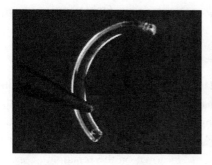 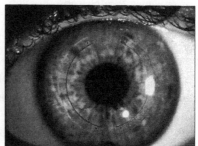

Courtesy of KeraVision, Inc.

A closeup, magnified view of the KeraVision ICRS before it is implanted. The ring is inserted into an incision less than 2 millimeters long.

This is an eye with the ICRS in place. Look closely and you can see a vertical arc to the right and left of the pupil.

Dr. Lindstrom said that the intrastromal ring is less likely to cause halos because it is outside the zone of normal pupil dilation. There's no risk of haze because the central visual area isn't affected. In addition, corneal topographies of the first 75 patients show that the flattening of the cornea is greater around the edges than in the center. This is the opposite of what happens during PRK and is said to produce less glare, and therefore better contrast sensitivity.

Since the procedure is done under suction, like LASIK (see Chapter 15), the same risks apply: Increased eye pressure can damage the retina or the optic nerve and cause permanent loss of sight and the microkeratome cuts can cause damage to the eye. In addition, any surgery that involves incisions and/or insertions brings with it the risk of infection. The groove needed for ICRS penetrates two-thirds of the depth of the cornea. The other drawback for some might be cosmetic: the ICRS can be seen when the eye is viewed closely.

The ICRS currently is being tested on a limited number of patients with up to -5.0 myopia. At this time, no astigmatism or hyperopia is being treated with it, but there's potential for it, Dr. Abbott said.

Dr. Abbott believes the ICRS is at least three years away from being widely available.

Dr. Roger Steinert said, "It isn't apparent to me why any patient would choose such a procedure. It's moderately invasive and doesn't have a demonstrable advantage over the laser." He fears that the effects of the ring could be temporary and that the insertion of foreign material into the eye could cause problems years later. "Only time will tell, but the burden of proof is on those

who implant a foreign substance into patients' corneas. Only years of experience will tell us whether this is safe."

Intrastromal Lens
A hybrid approach, of sorts, is a contact lens inserted into the cornea. This
has the advantage of avoiding the human lens (and therefore diminishing the
risk of cataract formation), and avoiding any major removal of cornea tissue.

The lens is either inserted into a pocket cut into the cornea, or a cap or flap
is sliced off the top of the cornea, the lens set down on the remaining cornea,
and the cap replaced. According to Dr. Raymond Stein, the first method uses a
lens that is less permeable to water and other eye chemicals. The second uses
a more adaptable lens material. But this method requires use of the
microkeratome and suction, which as you'll see in Chapter 15, carries some
substantial risks.

"Historically," Dr. Steinert said, "lenses placed behind the cornea in the
front portion of the eye have been associated with a low-grade inflation inside
the eye that causes severe damage, and can result in the need for a cornea
transplant."

NONSURGICAL ALTERNATIVES

This will be a short section, because there aren't many effective vision-correction alternatives that don't involve some form of surgery.

The obvious alternatives are glasses and contacts, but you know about
those already: They are relatively inexpensive ways to give functional vision
to just about anyone with a refractive vision problem. Below are some other
nonsurgical options.

Visual Therapies
Eye exercises, hypnotherapy, biofeedback, acupressure and meditative "vi-
sualization" exercises have all been used in an attempt to correct refractive vision
problems and presbyopia. You can even buy instructional videos from mail order
catalogs for a few of the methods. These are some of the advantages:
- They are lower cost than surgical alternatives
- They have no direct risks, side effects or loss of best-corrected acuity
- Many are relaxing and reduce stress—something all of us can use!
- They can temporarily reduce eyestrain.
- They can improve vision a little as long as the treatment continues.

But there are a number of disadvantages:
- All require a substantial time commitment
- If they don't work, the money spent is wasted
- The results are not permanent for nearsightedness, farsightedness or astigmatism because they affect the eye's focusing ability, not refractive capability.
- They probably will not eliminate glasses or contacts for people with more than the mildest of vision problems.

Dr. Carl Hirsch says that eye exercises have been shown to work for some patients "if they're very dedicated. It's kind of like doing stomach exercises: The improvement lasts only as long as you keep on doing them."

Orthokeratology: Braces for Your Eyes

This treatment has been around since the early 1960s and is offered by a number of optometrists as a semi-permanent solution to mild nearsightedness and astigmatism.

Called Ortho-K, or Precise Corneal Moulding, the procedure attempts to flatten the center of the cornea and round out any astigmatism by using a series of gas-permeable contact lenses. Patients wear them as much as possible every day, even sleeping in them if they can, and they change to a new lens every two or three weeks. Each new lens is designed to alter the shape of the cornea just a little bit more until, after a few months, it is flattened enough to refract light properly.

After the cornea is reshaped, patients must continue to wear "retainer" lenses at night or for at least four hours each day. "With Ortho-K patients can spend most of their time seeing without glasses or contacts," says Dr. Hirsch, who offers the treatment in his own optometry practice.

I asked him why anyone would want to do this if they could have PRK and never wear contacts again. "Until very recently PRK wasn't an option in the U.S.," Dr. Hirsch reminded me. "Now, cost is the main reason: Ortho-K only costs about $500-$1,200 per eye, depending on the number of lenses needed to reshape the cornea."

THE NON-ALTERNATIVE ALTERNATIVES

Into this group I place the health-food approaches and all the appealing but noneffective kinds of "glasses" that are supposed to fix vision permanently. Rather than trying these, save your money for designer frames the next time you need glasses; the money will be better spent.

Vitamins and Herbs

Drinking quarts of carrot juice will make your skin turn orange, but it won't change the way your eye refracts light. Taking megadoses of Vitamin A (which is necessary in the right amounts for good vision) is downright dangerous. Other herbal and vitamin treatments can improve your overall health and even have an impact on eye diseases such as glaucoma, but they won't fix your vision problem, and that's just a reality.

Pinhole or "Laser" Glasses

You've seen the infomercials. They remind me of those hilarious photos from the fifties where people in a theater are wearing 3-D glasses. Instead, participants are looking through cards or glasses that have small holes pierced in them. The only thing "laser" about these glasses is that the holes might have been cut with a laser diecutting machine.

Pinhole glasses are based on a physical truth: the holes have the effect of reducing pupil size and as the pupil gets smaller, the depth of field increases. That's why squinting can help nearsighted people see a little better. If you're only a little nearsighted, this can be just enough to make light focus right at the back of the eye.

The opposite is also true: When the pupil widens to take in more light, as it does when it's dark, the depth of field decreases as the eye tries to focus. This is called "night-induced myopia" and is why some naval aviators wear glasses when they are flying at night, as Dr. Schallhorn mentioned in Chapter 2.

Staring through a tiny hole in a card has the same effect as reducing pupil size: it cuts down on the amount of light entering the eye. Take the card away and the pupil adjusts to more light by expanding, so the effect is gone. Doing this over and over again can give you eyestrain, but it will not make your pupil narrow permanently. If it did, you would be sorry, because you would have a hard time seeing at night!

So unless you plan on going around with pinhole glasses on (and please don't drive if you do!), my recommendation is to try another method of vision correction or stick with glasses or contacts.

PLOT IDEA FOR LOIS AND CLARK   Clark Kent loses his superpowers and then his glasses! The Daily Planet is burning down, he knows Lois is trapped, but where is she? Remembering what he read in *Beyond Glasses!* the ever-resourceful Kent gropes in his desk for his business cards, stabs some holes in each one with his pencil, and holds them to his eyes. Wait! Is that Lois under a falling beam? He lunges to save her, drops his "glasses" en route, and trips over Lex Luther. Will the evil Lex save Lois? Or is she doomed because her Superguy lost his Supereyes?

Amber-Colored Sunglasses

A recent spate of infomercials claiming that yellow- or brown-tinted sunglasses can improve your vision outdoors takes advantage of another optical reality: screening out short-wave light (blues and greens), makes the viewer feel that she is seeing better. In reality, tinted lenses have not been shown to increase visual acuity, and there's no connection between the advertised lenses and the superior acuity of a hawk, eagle, owl or any animal. If you want amber-colored sunglasses, there are less-expensive ways to get them, with the same results as those advertised on television.

Help for the Very Nearsighted

*H*igh myopia, like high hyperopia, is more than just a worsened degree of the problem. People who are extremely nearsighted and wear glasses have a greatly reduced field of vision, for example. They also have more trouble with night vision, even without surgery, and a greater susceptibility to retinal defects and injury.

For someone who is -10.0 or above and can't wear contact lenses, just getting to 20/100 or 20/150 can be a tremendous improvement. Very high myopes are functionally blind without lenses—and this puts them at risk in emergencies. With a reduction in nearsightedness they can get around with their lenses off, and glasses can be much lighter in weight and less demagnifying.

Ironically, the very people who need vision correction the most have the hardest time getting it. All the available procedures, including PRK, are less predictable at the higher levels of nearsightedness and most aren't approved for use in the U.S. outside clinical trials. Nonetheless, doctors in the U.S. and Canada have had some fantastic successes with even the most severe cases of myopia, so the option of permanent vision correction is worth more than a

---

WHAT IS HIGH MYOPIA?   For the purposes of this book, high myopia is nearsightedness above -7.0, which is the limit for PRK in the U.S. Many doctors break high myopia into two, or even three, groups, such as -7 to -10, -10 to -15, and -16 and up.

---

second look if you have vision worse than -7.0. Chapters 6, 9 and 11 contain background information which will help you better understand some of the options for high myopia.

PRK FOR HIGH MYOPIA

PRK, as approved by the FDA, slightly flattens a 6-millimeter zone on the surface of the cornea with a gradually widening circular beam, in a single pass of the laser (see Figure 15.1). This is called single-zone PRK. The FDA requires doctors to perform the procedure in one step, without stopping, except to recenter the beam if the patient moves. In Canada and other countries, this is only one method of performing PRK. There are others that are used more often, even for the lowest levels of nearsightedness.

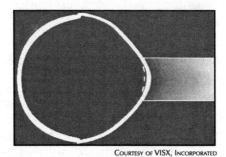

COURTESY OF VISX, INCORPORATED

FIGURE 15.1 As this graphic exaggerates to illustrate, the PRK procedure removes a tiny amount of tissue from the surface of the cornea to create a flatter central cornea.

The Problems with Single-Zone PRK for High Myopia

Single-zone PRK has been used successfully to treat high myopia[1] but there are higher rates of side effects and complications for a number of reasons:

- The more nearsighted the patient is, the more tissue has to be removed from the cornea to correct it. A narrower treatment zone requires less tissue to be removed, but people who are very nearsighted tend to have large pupils. When the pupil dilates past the central, most deeply treated area, halos can result. That's why doctors went to a wider zone in the first place.

- No matter how narrow the treatment zone, single-zone PRK for the higher levels of myopia requires a deeper ablation in the central visual area and this can stimulate a more aggressive healing reaction right in the

SMALL GLASSES AREN'T JUST FOR STYLIN'   Fashion issues aside, people with higher levels of nearsightedness often opt for smaller frames because the lenses can be thinner and therefore lighter in weight. Even with small frames, though, glasses for those over -10.0 tend to be thick and they greatly demagnify the appearance of the eyes to the outside world. Small bifocal and trifocal lenses can pose a problem—especially when they are blended to remove the line—because there's not much room on the lens for each correction.

---

spot where we least want it. The result can be haze severe enough to interfere with vision.

- The need for retreatment is greater in higher myopes because more aggressive healing can cause regression, so vision returns to some level of nearsightedness.[2]
- To compensate for aggressive healing reactions, and prevent regression, high myopes require larger doses of steroid eyedrops over longer periods of time. This increases the risk of steroid-related side effects such as increased eye pressure and cataract formation. Even though the side effects can be treated and steroids stopped, it's an extra problem for the patient.
- Visual recovery (the amount of time it takes to get to 20/40 or better and to regain near focus) is slower at higher levels of myopia because more healing has to take place and because doctors tend to overcorrect to a larger extent to allow for more regression. As a result, patients can experience farsightedness for a month or more. This gradually diminishes over the next two or three months.
- Finally, higher myopes might have a harder time maintaining focus during treatment—perhaps because they can't see the fixation light, or because the time under the laser is longer. This increases the risk of off-centered treatment, which in turn can cause irregular astigmatism and loss of best-corrected acuity.

One Solution: Two-Stage PRKs

One way doctors have dealt with these problems is by breaking treatments for high myopes into two separate stages. The first might take the patient's eye to -2.0 (20/100). Then, six months later when the eye has fully stabilized, a second procedure could very predictably take the patient the rest of the way. As inconvenient as this might be for the patient, it gives the doctor a chance to see what the healing response is, reduces the risk of haze and halos, and gets the patient to a good result without overcorrection, even if it takes longer.

Another Solution: Multizone PRKs

Doctors have developed techniques to reduce the depth of the ablation required, which reduces regression from overhealing, and to create a smoother ablation, which reduces haze. These treatments are called multizone PRKs, and are only available in the U.S. through clinical trials. All the Canadian doctors who contributed to this book have been developing and using these techniques for years.

During the time between treatments the patient can wear glasses or contacts. Dr. David Lin told me about a scientist whose vision was -27.0 before PRK. "Her field of vision was extremely narrow with glasses," he said, "but she worked in a chemical lab and the fumes made wearing contacts during the day impossible. We were able to take her to -1.50 in a single procedure and she was so delighted that she hasn't come back for retreatment. For her, it made all the difference just to be able to see normally with lightweight glasses and have some functional vision without them."

The Theory Behind Multizone Treatments

The thickness of a lens for correcting vision problems is in part determined by the diameter of the lens: Smaller diameter lenses are thinner for any amount of correction. For you math lovers, the formula Dr. Charles Munnerlyn developed to calculate the depth of PRK treatments in its simplified form is: The depth of the treatment zone or thickness of a lens is equal to:

$$\frac{(\text{diameter of lens or treatment zone in millimeters}^2) \ \times \ (\text{\# of diopters of correction})}{3}$$

Dr. Raymond Stein explains, "There's a significant difference in depth between a 3-millimeter treatment zone and a 6-millimeter zone. To correct someone with 10 diopters of nearsightedness with a 3-millimeter zone, we would go a maximum of 30 microns deep in the center. With a 6-millimeter zone we would have to go down 120 microns."

As mentioned above, however, the narrow zone tends to result in halos because the pupil widens past the treated area and light enters through an untreated (still nearsighted) part of the cornea. In addition, the deeper treatment can cause aggressive healing and haze.

One way around these problems is to try for the best of both worlds: the wider zone to prevent halos and a shallower ablation depth to avoid haze.

How Multizone PRK Works

Multizone PRK lets the doctor create two or more distinct zones which are blended smoothly from the deepest central ablation to a shallower ablation at a normal 6-millimeter treatment zone. Newer lasers allow treatment beyond 6 millimeters, tapering the zone out as far as 9 or 10 millimeters.

Multizone can be called "start and stop" PRK, as opposed to the "once you start you shouldn't stop" PRK that has been approved by the FDA to date.

Dr. Steven Schallhorn provides this example. "Let's say that a doctor is treating a -10.0 patient with multizone PRK. The goal is to remove ten diopters of nearsightedness from the eye. The doctor might 'tell' the computer: 'give me a 5-diopter correction in a 5-millimeter zone.' The computer would then open the laser beam at 1 millimeter and gradually widen it to 5 millimeters in a series of pulses that remove tissue 42 microns deep.

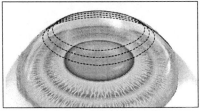

By Beacon Eye Institute/Joseph Schmalenbach

FIGURE 15.2 In multizone PRK, the cornea is treated with several different diameters of treatment zones. The wider shallow zones overlap the smaller, deeper zones to create a smooth ablation.

"Then the doctor might say. "give me 2.5 diopters at the 5.5-millimeter zone." The computer would take the beam from 1mm wide to 5.5 millimeters but the deepest ablation would be only 25 microns deep.

"At this point, 7.5 diopters have been corrected. Now the doctor might repeat the last step but increase the zone width to 6 millimeters. The width of the laser beam would then increase from less than 1 millimeter to 6 millimeters, 30 microns deep. At the end you have a gradually shallower ablation with no abrupt edges between the zones because each larger zone overlaps the smaller ones."

The multizone treatment just described would be 23 microns, or 20%, shallower at the center than a similar single-zone PRK. It should be stressed that neither treatment would result in a dent in the cornea—the cornea will still be convex in shape after the treatment.

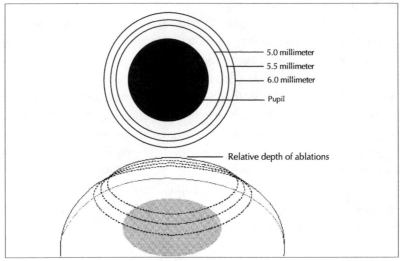

BY JOSEPH SCHMALENBACH

FIGURE 15.3 As these schematics demonstrate, in multizone PRK the treatment zones overlap, with each larger zone tracking over the smaller, to create a smooth ablation.

The Benefits of Multizone PRK

Multizone PRK has two potential benefits:

- It can reduce the amount of regression and/or haze because the shallower ablation incites less of a healing response.
- It can reduce the occurrence of halos or make them less noticeable because the overall treatment zone is larger.

Dr. Donald Johnson said that multizone techniques compensate for the mechanical nature of the laser. "There are microscopic 'stutters' as the aperture opens which can create stair-step-like patterns to the ablation. By going over the area several times with different treatment diameters, we can smooth all this out."

Doctors have speculated that the "rest periods" between zones also might be beneficial in that they allow the tissue to settle down between ablations.

How Well Does Multizone PRK Work?

Dr. Howard Gimbel, who has been using Multizone PRK for several years and is now using newer scanning laser beams to do it, said, "For patients over -8.0 we are seeing clear corneas in 84%, trace haze in 13% and mild haze in 2.5%. There have been no losses in best-corrected acuity.

A study of 14 eyes between -10.0 and -24.0 found that at six months, 10 of the eyes were between 2 and 4 diopters of attempted correction and four needed to be retreated. Three patients lost two or more lines of best-corrected acuity as a result of haze.[3]

A peer-reviewed study of 315 eyes conducted by Dr. Mihai Pop demonstrated that multizone PRK can be safe and effective for all levels of myopia and astigmatism. He used up to seven treatment zones in the higher myopes. About half the eyes were over -6.0 and forty were between -10.0 and -27.0 diopters of nearsightedness. More than half had at least 0.5 diopters of astigmatism. At the end of six months, without further retreatment:

- 89% of the 119 patients who started out under -6.0 had 20/25 acuity or better. One patient lost and one patient gained more than two lines of best-corrected acuity.

- 75% of the 82 patients who started out between -6 to -10 had 20/25 vision or better. Two patients lost and 15 gained more than two lines of best-corrected acuity.

- 25% of the 32 patients who started out between -10.0 to -27.0 had 20/25 or better and 78% had -2.0 [about 20/100] or better. Six patients (19%) lost and 25 gained more than two lines of best-corrected acuity.[4]

"In cases of haze, we used to wait six months to retreat patients. Now I retreat after a month. I don't let the scar form," he said. "In our study there was no loss of 20/40 best-corrected acuity."

In a review of the first 840 eyes treated with two-zone PRKs in Dr. Raymond Stein's private practice, 95% of patients between -1.0 and -6.0 were corrected to 20/40 or better, as were 85% of the patients between -6.0 and -8.0, and 73% of the patients between -8.0 and -22.0. Only 1% lost more than one line ,and one per cent gained more than a line, of best-corrected acuity short term, but there was no loss of best-corrected acuity in 99% of the eyes after two years.[5]

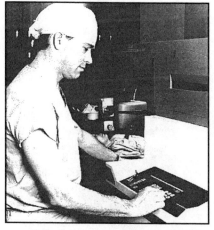

Today's lasers are easily programmed, as Dr. Robert Maloney is doing here. In multizone PRK, the number of zones and the amount of tissue removed in each is dependent on the amount of correction targeted.

BY CHARLIE MARTIN, COURTESY OF JULES STEIN EYE INSTITUTE

Not all reports are this positive, however. Dr. Richard Lindstrom has performed multizone PRK on over 50 patients who were -8.0 and higher. "Personally I've not been impressed with our PRK results for high and extreme myopia with PRK. 10% of the patients from -8 to -15 lost two or more lines of best corrected vision from surface hazing or topographical abnormalities like a central island. In patients worse than -15.0, this number increases to 15%. We had to use a lot of steroids which also can cause problems."

Dr. Schallhorn cautions that we don't yet have enough data to know whether multizone treatments are superior to single-zone PRK or other alternatives such as LASIK (see below). "It might not be a free lunch. The transitions from one zone to the other could cause a reduction in contrast sensitivity which could affect night vision."

In addition, even if certain doctors are getting good results with their own equipment, there is no guarantee other doctors will achieve the same results.

Multizone Side Effects and Complications
All the PRK side effects and complications discussed in Chapter 11 can occur in higher levels of myopia, but their occurrence is diminished by the multizone procedure. Studies indicate, however, that the rate of side effects varies greatly from one surgeon to the next and it's difficult to compare studies because of differences in ranges of myopia, treatment methodologies, and length of follow-up.

Haze and Loss of Best-Corrected Acuity
In Dr. Pop's study, at the end of the first month there was no difference in the amount of haze between the under -6.0 group and the -6.0 to -10.0 group, but it took longer for haze to disappear in the more nearsighted patients. This means their visual recovery was slower. At the end of six months, three of the

---

POTENTIAL MULTIZONE PROBLEMS   Some of the potential problems with single-zone PRK are also possible with multizone. They include:

- Haze and slow visual recovery
- Loss of best-corrected acuity
- Induced astigmatism
- Halos and other optical illusions
- Regression and undercorrection

THE MOUNTIES FINALLY GOT THEIR MAN

Name
Vincent Yeung, 37

Occupation
Pharmacist,
British Columbia

Pre-Op Vision
-11.0

Procedure
Multizone PRK

Post-Op Vision
Right eye: 20/25

Left eye: 20/20
with retreatment

Surgeon
David Lin, MD

Vincent Yeung was a high myope and so it is not unusual that one of his eyes required a second treatment to finetune his vision.

"I had my two eyes treated six months apart and wore a contact on the untreated eye in between procedures. It was a problem because I work around chemicals, I have allergies, and my eyes tend to build up protein deposits on the lenses. I went through three or four lenses that spring.

"My eyes had gotten progressively worse until I was about 29. I looked into RK but it just didn't seem that reliable. By the time I got to Dr. Lin's I had done my research on PRK and I felt pretty calm. Evidently, the worse your myopia is, the longer it takes for the eye to hea. I knew going in I was going to have to wait between eyes because I couldn't be without good vision—at least in one eye.

"The first [right] eye was easy. I drove back to work right after the procedure and never felt any sensation whatsoever. I didn't even take Tylenol. The bandage lens was removed two days later but I could see right away and the eye stabilized at 20/25 fairly quickly.

"The left eye only got to 20/50 after four months, so Dr. Lin did a quick touch-up procedure. Oddly, I had some pain after that procedure for about four hours. It helped to apply pressure to the eye. It's been 3-4 months now and I have 20/20 vision in that eye. I have large pupils, so even though my daytime vision is great, at night I still see some halos and occasionally use drops to close my pupils a little. I don't have any trouble reading, though.

I'm a volunteer Mounty now, something I wouldn't have attempted before, and that gives me a great deal of satisfaction. I've been able to get into scuba diving, and I'm back to swimming and skiing. Badminton and squash are even more fun than they were before. PRK has widened the world for me.

patients (about 1%) had lost more than one line of best-corrected acuity because of haze—a lower percentage than with the single-zone PRK results reported in the FDA trials.

About 20% of the very high myopes in Dr. Pop's study lost two or more lines of best-corrected acuity, most because of haze. 78% gained at least one line.

Dr. Pop said, "All haze disappears after PRK eventually and most never interferes with vision. When it does, we retreat it."

Dr. Johnson added, "I usually don't prescribe steroids at all any more for patients under -7.0 or -8.0. I watch them carefully the first month, and if there's no haze, I don't put them on the drops. With multizone PRK, haze is extremely rare. For higher levels of myopia, the answer isn't certain yet. I use as little as possible and keep close tabs on the patients."

Dr. Stephen Trokel, who initiated the multizone approach back in 1992, believes that multizone treatments have a great deal of potential. "As we learn how to make the ablation smoother, glare and haze should be decreased."

Induced Astigmatism

In Dr. Pop's study, the multizone approach caused mild to moderate astigmatism in nine patients who had no astigmatism before PRK. Residual or induced astigmatism can affect visual acuity but if it does, it might be able to be improved by retreatment.

Other Risks Affecting Acuity

The risks of a decentered treatment are low to zero with multizone PRK because the eye is recentered between zones. Even if one or two zones are slightly off-centered, the others zones take care of the problem.

None of the patients in Dr. Pop's study had central islands at six months—probably because the multiple passes over the central visual area left a smoother surface than with single-zone PRK.

Halos and Other Optical Effects

Two of the 315 patients in Dr. Pop's study reported significant halos at six months and both were retreated. Dr Stein said, "After two years few patients reported marked symptoms, and of those with symptoms, most were satisfied with their visual outcome."

Regression and Undercorrection

The higher the level of myopia a patient starts with, the more likely she will end up needing a second treatment. This can be part of the plan, however, as

◦ GRACEFULLY AGING IN NEW MEXICO

Name
Rosina Yue, 43

Occupation
Registered nurse and
Artist, New Mexico

Pre-Op Vision
-10.0

Procedure
Multizone PRK

Post-Op Vision
20/30

Surgeon
Richard Lindstrom, MD

When it came time to get her vision corrected, Rosina Yue traveled all the way from New Mexico to Minnesota.

"I had read about the laser treatment in the *New York Times* but it wasn't approved yet. When my brother told me about Dr. Lindstrom's trials in Minneapolis, I made an appointment. I was tired of wearing contacts and worried about depending on them in an emergency. Also, I want to age gracefully and this seemed like a good way to make an improvement in my life. My first eye was treated in February of 1995.

"Because I'm a nurse, I like to know everything about what's going to happen to me, but with this procedure I didn't; that made me very nervous. I also didn't realize they would be scraping the epithelium off my eye, so that was scary. There was no pain during the procedure and I didn't have any trouble fixating on the light.

"When I first sat up my vision was foggy—like I was looking through a filmy window. I didn't have any discomfort until the next morning and then my eye started watering and twitching. It felt like something was in it. I didn't take any medication, though. I just kept the eye closed. The epithelium healed within 24 hours.

"As the week progressed, my vision got clearer and clearer and I was so excited, I felt like crying. The results were so dramatic it made me wonder what was happening in my brain to make it adjust to being able to see this well. I kept worrying the effects wouldn't be permanent.

"For the first three months my vision kept on improving, then it declined a little. The period between eyes was a little uncomfortable for me—I felt out of balance.

"Finally, the left eye was treated six months after the first and it took longer under the laser—there was more zapping—but the recovery went about the same. I only need reading glasses now—which I find to be kind of fun—they're an accessory. I also wear very weak distance glasses when I drive at night.

"PRK has simplified my life. I'd do it again in a minute. It has been a morale-boost at a very deep level."

EVOLUTION OF A MULTIZONE OUTCOME

	Refraction	Acuity
Pre-op:	-10.0	20/400
1 day post-op:	+1.0	20/100
1 month post-op:	+1.0	20/30
3 months post-op:	-0.75	20/25
6 months post-op:	-1.25	20/40
1 year post-op:	-1.75	20/30

The table above shows how Rosina Yue's uncorrected acuity in her first eye evolved from just prior to treatment through the first year. She had 20/30 vision at the end of the first year, even though her refraction had regressed a little. This is typical of patients after vision-correction surgery—their functional vision is better than their refractions would indicate. Also typical is a progression from slight farsightedness right after PRK to slight nearsightedness after the cornea is fully healed.

in two-stage PRKs, to prevent an overly aggressive healing response. There was less regression in the multizone patients treated in Dr. Pop's study than in other studies of single-zone PRK. Generally regression can be retreated if it results in less than 20/40 acuity.

What Other Canadian Doctors Say About Multizone PRK

Dr. Johnson has been developing multizone procedures for years. "Doing high levels of correction with single-zone PRK can leave the patient with irregular astigmatism—which is very difficult to treat. I will treat patients who are -15.0 or higher in four zones: 3-millimeter, 4-millimeter, 5-millimeter, and 6-millimeter. Then I'll do a double pass on the 5- and 6-millimeter zones. This gives a deep ablation at the very center but a very smooth transition to the outer edges. "

Dr. Bruce Jackson said, "We've treated up to -22.0 with multizone PRK and obtained extremely good results, but I'm more comfortable treating patients whose vision is -15.0 or better. For higher myopes we break their correction into two treatments spaced a month or two apart. This tends to produce less regression and haze."

Where to Go to Have It Done

In the U.S. multizone PRK hasn't yet completed FDA trials: so for highly near-sighted Americans, the alternatives are to be treated in Canada, at a clinical trial site in the U.S. (see Chapter 7), have single-zone PRK or one of the other options described below, or wait.

The Cost of Multizone PRK

Multizone PRK is performed by the doctors who do it when they feel it's appropriate. They don't charge extra for this technique, which is nice of them because multizone takes quite a bit longer than single-zone PRK. Prices are the same as for single-zone PRK: $1,500-$2,000 per eye, at this writing.

INCISIONAL APPROACHES TO HIGH MYOPIA

As briefly described in Chapter 14, a wide variety of methods for treating nearsightedness have been adopted and abandoned. One, called *automated lamellar keratoplasty* (ALK), is falling out of use today, but is the big sister of a new technique called *LASIK*.

First Some Background: ALK

ALK is a method for correcting nearsightedness (and farsightedness, see Chapter 18) which uses an instrument called an *automated microkeratome* to slice off a cap about a third the depth of the cornea. Then the doctor uses a surgical knife to carve a small lens-shaped amount of corneal tissue out of either the cap or the remaining cornea. The cap is replaced and the natural pressure of the eye creates suction to hold it in place. Newer methods of ALK don't slice the cap all the way off, so a "flap" is created instead and the treatment is done in the underlying cornea. Generally, no stitches are used.

The advantages of ALK, when it succeeded, were little discomfort for the patient and fast visual recovery because the epithelium wasn't disturbed. Temporary drawbacks included halos and night vision problems.

The big problem with ALK is its difficulty and imprecision: not only does it require an extremely skilled and experienced surgeon, but even the best surgeons have a hard time knowing exactly how much tissue to remove. In addition, the microkeratome can fail, and the incision is subject to problems.

As a result, there have been some disastrous outcomes with ALK, including the need for corneal transplants and even permanent loss of the eye and/or vision. With PRK and RK as available alternatives, none of the surgeons I spoke with recommended ALK for patients other than high myopes. It just isn't worth the risk.

Dr. Vance Thompson has used ALK to treat myopia as high as -30.0 but he warns, "It requires *very* experienced hands. ALK survives in the states because of the regulatory atmosphere. It has been used successfully by skilled sur-

---

WHAT IS LASIK?   LASIK is an acronym for **LAS**er-assisted **I**n-situ **K**eratomileusis. LASIK is a combination of ALK and PRK.

---

geons to treat high myopia when they use ALK for most of the correction and then plan to take the patient the rest of the way with mini-RK at a later date, but ALK shouldn't be used a second time on the same eye."

128 eyes with high myopia or residual myopia after RK were treated with ALK and followed for a year. 86% gained 20/40 or better uncorrected vision and 6% lost two or more lines of best-corrected vision.[6]

When PRK became widely used and research showed it was safe, researchers began to wonder if the benefits of ALK could be combined with the safety and predictability of PRK. The result was the birth of a combination technique called LASIK.

How LASIK Works

LASIK combines the microkeratome used for cutting the flap in ALK with the laser used for performing the correction in PRK.

The Microkeratome

A microkeratome is an instrument which applies suction to the eye to flatten it. It contains a blade that is preset by the surgeon to cut a defined depth and width. The depth of the cut is controlled by a plate.

Once it's started, the instrument automatically moves the blade across thecornea, like a cheese cutter. It is preset to stop at a point just short of cutting the cap completely off. The resulting flap is about 160 microns thick

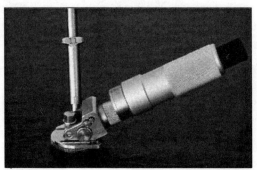

This microkeratome is a $50,000 instrument designed to shave sections from the cornea within several microns of accuracy. It uses disposable steel blades to reduce the risk of infection.

COURTESY OF CHIRON VISION CORPORATION

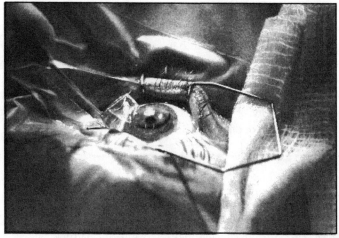

PHOTO BY NICK LAMMERT

FIGURE 15.4 In LASIK, the eyelids are propped open, suction is applied, and a flap is cut from the front of the cornea. Then the doctor very carefully pulls back the flap to ready the eye for PRK.

(one third the depth of the cornea) and about 9 millimeters in diameter—much wider than even large pupils (see Figure 15.4).

Flap and Zap

Once the flap is created, the doctor removes the microkeratome, carefully folds the flap back, wipes the cornea dry, and then positions the laser beam over the eye where it pulses enough times to create the desired correction (see Figure 15.5). Then he carefully puts the flap back in place and patches the eye. The patient goes home with a mild "something in the eye" feeling, comes back the next day to have the patch removed, and might have excellent vision right then. Other than antibiotic eyedrops, usually no other medications are required.

FIGURE 15.5 During the laser step of LASIK, the interior of the cornea is treated just as with surface PRK. The flap is folded back down and it seals without stitches.

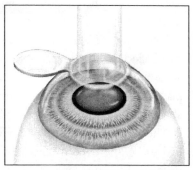

COURTESY OF BEACON EYE INSTITUTE

FLIP and ZAP   In an earlier version of LASIK, the doctor removed the cap altogether, flipped it over, took it to the laser, programmed the laser to pulse the underside of the cap enough times to make the correction, carried it back to the patient, and then very carefully tried to put it back in its original position. This technique eliminated the risk to the interior of the cornea but increased the difficulty of getting the cap back on the eye correctly without causing astigmatism or other visual impairments.

Goodbye ALK?

LASIK offers much greater precision than ALK in the correction of myopia because the surgeon doesn't manually cut into the cornea—the laser is programmed to remove exactly the right amount of corneal tissue.

Dr. Thompson said, "If I had high myopia, I'd be in the study for LASIK or wait until we get the outcomes of the study. I feel that LASIK will be approved in a couple of years and ALK will be history.

"ALK is doomed," agrees Dr. Michael Gordon, "but we'll keep the flap, because LASIK is here to stay."

And Dr. Lindstrom predicts, "By the end of 1996, I expect all my ALK cases will become LASIKs."

Not OK'd by the FDA

The FDA has *not* approved LASIK. Emma Knight, an ophthalmologist with the FDA said, "From FDA's standpoint, we want to know not just if LASIK is as good or better than PRK... we must also be sure there are not any greater risks than with standard PRK. So we've asked people to do randomized studies." [7]

Outside the clinical trials, LASIK is being performed by a few doctors in Canada, a few doctors in the U.S. who have filed for investigative status with the FDA, and "off-label" by other doctors in the U.S. who have access to lasers for PRK (see Chapter 13). In mid-1996 a group of 30 U.S. doctors began the Clinical Evaluation of LASIK study in which each will submit the results of 50 LASIK cases to a central data collection site for analysis and then to the FDA. A chief goal of the study, in addition to analyzing the effectiveness of LASIK in treating various levels of myopia, is to help standardize the procedure among surgeons and educate others about the benefits or drawbacks of various techniques.

The microkeratome used for LASIK was invented before medical devices had to be approved by the FDA, so it, as well as all the newer models, has never had to go through FDA trials for safety and effectiveness.

The Benefits of LASIK over PRK

Doctors who perform LASIK are enthusiastic about its benefits:

- Fast visual recovery: Patients can see very well as soon as the eye is unpatched the next day, so there's little vision downtime.
- Little or no discomfort because the epithelium is hardly disrupted. A bandage contact lens isn't even necessary, but the eye must be patched for the first 24 hours to protect the flap.
- Lower risk of haze formation because the cells under the epithelium (called "Bowman's layer") aren't disturbed.
- Less regression because less of a healing response is stimulated.
- Fewer incidents of glare and halos because the affected portion of the epithelium is outside the central visual area.
- Reduced need for steroid eye drops, so there's less risk of side effects from drops.
- Astigmatism can be easily corrected at the same time as myopia—if the doctor has the software to do it.

Dr. Jeffrey Robin, whose eyes were treated with RK and PRK several years ago (his story is in Chapter 14), performs LASIK now, even for moderate levels of myopia, as part of an investigation. "I would have LASIK today if I still needed vision correction. I had to take 10 days off work after PRK. I wouldn't have to take any time off with LASIK."

How Well Does LASIK Work?

A review by Dr. Marguerite McDonald reported on the results of the few published studies available on LASIK in late '95. Only one had more than a year of follow-up data and that was only on seven eyes:[8]

- In 10 eyes from -10.0 to -25.0, 66% had 20/40 vision or better after a year and there was no loss of more than one line of best-corrected acuity.
- In 150 cases of LASIK, 85% of the eyes had 20/40 or better after three months.
- In multicenter FDA trials of LASIK begun in 1991, of 57 eyes with pre-op vision between -6.0 and -25.0, 66% had 20/40 or better and 34% had 20/25 or better after six months. 79% were within one line of pre-op best-corrected acuity, 15% lost two lines and 6% lost more than two lines of their previous best corrected acuity. 12% had trace haze at 6 months and 5% had mild haze—higher percentages than with the FDA trial results for PRK.[9] Dr. McDonald commented, "If this is the best-case scenario, LASIK may not pass the FDA guidelines for excimer surgery, which requires less than five percent incidence of loss of two lines or more of best-corrected vision."

MARKETING THE REFRACTIVE HIGH

Is fast visual recovery important? It depends on who benefits. "Faster visual recovery has tremendous appeal from a marketing standpoint," Dr. Schallhorn said, "because euphoric patients are the best source of referrals. Patients who take a few weeks to get to good vision aren't nearly as effective at selling the procedure as ones who have 20/20 vision the next day.

"One of the crucial missing pieces of information is, what are the functional outcomes of refractive surgery? We do a great deal of testing of the eye, but no one has yet studied the effect of the surgery on how well the patient functions in daily life—reading, driving, occupational tasks."

Dr. Richard Abbott added, "There is a refractive high that people get after vision-correction surgery. After the refractive euphoria ends, some aren't as happy as others. We're just now beginning to study the actual lifestyle and performance benefits of procedures like PRK." Dr. Abbott is beginning a National Institutes of Health study of patients who have had PRK matched against patients who have kept on wearing glasses and contacts."

In evaluating how important speed of visual recovery is to you, be sure to remember that with whatever procedure you choose, you'll have an immediate improvement in vision—even if the images you see aren't crisp for a day or two. Getting to 20/40 or better appears to be faster with LASIK than it is with PRK, in many cases, but the importance of fast visual recovery must be weighed against the relative risks of the two procedures.

- In a subset of the above study, and the only two-year study available at that time, out of seven eyes, 71% had 20/25 or better. All had best-corrected acuity of 20/25 or better.

Another study that followed five extremely myopic eyes for a year after LASIK found no loss of best-corrected acuity in four of the eyes. One eye had some persistent vision problems and another had astigmatism as a result of the surgery. The average refraction pre-op was -21.0 and the average post-op was -1.50.[10]

In early 1996, doctors in Saudi Arabia reported results of LASIK on 88 eyes that ranged in nearsightedness from -2.0 to -20.00. Five months post-op 71% of the eyes had 20/40 or better vision with results best in the lower myopes. Three (3.4%) had lost two or more lines of best-corrected acuity, but there were no sight-threatening complications. The researchers concluded that LASIK could be effective but that modifications needed to be made in the laser programming to make the results more predictable.[11]

A study published in early 1996 out of Spain reported the six-month results of 43 eyes with pre-op vision of -7.0 to -18.5 that were treated with LASIK.

Researchers said that none of the eyes ended up overcorrected or with "visually significant" haze and that patients experienced rapid visual recovery. They noted that predictability of results was more accurate for the patients whose vision was below -12.0.[12]

Another 1996 study in Egypt compared 40 eyes treated with LASIK to 40 treated with Single-zone PRK. All eyes started out between -6.0 and -10.0. At one year post-op, the LASIK eyes had 10% better success at obtaining 20/20 vision. None of the LASIK eyes developed haze, but 90% of the PRK eyes had experienced it.[13]

Side Effects and Complications

The LASIK technique has been evolving all over the world since the early '90s. Some doctors have serious reservations about it, while others support it wholeheartedly. However, nearly all the patients I spoke with described the LASIK experience much the way people describe PRK: a period of brief discomfort followed by a time of visual adjustment. "Discomfort after LASIK is not uncommon," Dr. Salz said, "usually because of epithelial abrasion." One journalist told me that she had an extreme "something in the eye" sensation for ten days after LASIK. "It made me regret having done it, but now I'm thrilled," she said.

"LASIK could blow PRK off the map in the U.S.," Dr. Jeffrey Robin predicted. "It might not be perfect, but it's looking like it's best we have right now." In late 1995, Dr. Robin began using LASIK to treat low-to-moderate myopia (below -6.0).

"I love LASIK," Dr. Thompson said. "It's fun to perform and doctors like to do it. But nobody wants to talk about the risks of flap surgery. It's the riskiest form of refractive surgery. There are no monitored studies that are over a year old to tell us what the long-term effects are. PRK, on the other hand, has gone through the trials, we know what the downsides are and it has never caused a case of blindness, or the need for a corneal transplant."

POTENTIAL LASIK PROBLEMS   Doctors worry about these complications:

- Loss of the eye
- Loss of blood supply to the optic nerve
- Loss of the cornea
- Retinal tears or deterioration
- Perforation of the eye or the flap
- Infection
- Loss of best-corrected acuity

Dr. Schallhorn agreed, "We have to be wary of any new procedure that's being hyped before we have data from long-term, multicenter trials. Rather than offering the best of ALK and PRK, LASIK could prove to combine the worst of both. We just don't know."

Problems with Applying Suction to the Eye

In order to raise the cornea up so the flap can be cut, during the LASIK procedure a suction ring is applied around the cornea and pressure inside the eye is raised to 60 millimeters of mercury. The resulting increase in intraocular pressure shuts off the blood supply to the eye, so for about 20 seconds the eye "goes dark." This can be dangerous to the retina, the blood vessels and the optic nerve. Under normal conditions, the flap is cut and suction is released immediately without a problem.

Dr. Pop said, "The big problem for all myopes over -10 is that their retinas are more fragile. If you pump up the eye pressure to 60 millimeters of mercury and then suddenly release it, the vessels in the macula can be damaged. The question is, will we see more detached retinas and more hemorrhages in patients 5-7 years after they've had LASIK?"

Cutting off blood supply to the eye is similar to cutting it off to the heart. "There are reported cases of infarction caused by the microkeratome," Dr. Thompson said. "This is like an 'eye attack' and when it happens, it's lights out forever." He was quick to add that this is extremely rare, "but just think about how eager everyone is to embrace LASIK. What happens when a patient comes in to get his nearsightedness corrected and now he's needing a corneal transplant or loses his sight altogether?"

Dr. Jeffrey Robin pointed out that thousands of LASIK cases have been performed with no reported problems. "In young, healthy eyes, there's little concern about damage to the retina."

LOOSE LIPS ON SLIPS   Dr. Steinert said, "Some doctors are guilty of selective recollection of their own bad results. A very vocal LASIK enthusiast stated at an American Academy of Ophthalmology meeting that he had performed several hundred LASIKs 'with no complications and no loss of best-corrected vision.' A few months later in a social conversation the same doctor regaled us with his 'wouldn't you know it' story of how his worst LASIK disaster was when the microkeratome jammed in the middle of a procedure on a very wealthy individual and left the patient needing a corneal transplant—and the surgeon needing a lawyer."

Problems with the Microkeratome

As I write this, doctors are expecting to see new, improved microkeratomes. Today's models use steel blades, rather than diamond ones, so they can create an uneven cut which might make it difficult to reposition the flap. An analysis of three brands of microkeratomes stated that all "produced irregular surfaces with chatter lines." [14]

In addition, microkeratomes require the doctor to set a plate which limits the depth of the cut. If the doctor forgets to set the plate, or sets it at the wrong level, the eye can be cut open by the microkeratome. In fact, the documentation for one of the microkeratomes has a bold warning:

WARNING   Failure to use the appropriate plate or set the plate could result in permanent damage to the cornea and possible perforation into the [front] chamber of the eye.

New "fixed-plate" models which are not yet widely available should make it impossible for this to happen, but other dangers remain.

Dr. Pop said, "I personally know of three cases where the natural lens had to be removed after it was cut into by the microkeratome because the suction brought the lens right up to the front of the eye."

Dr. Schallhorn said that he has observed ALK surgeries in which suction suddenly released while the blade was cutting and the blade ended up going through the cornea at an angle.

Dr. Robin said, "I don't know of any eyes lost from LASIK in North America. There are reports out of South America and Europe of doctors forgetting to set the plate and incising the eye. The new microkeratomes will make it impossible to forget to set the plate and will enable doctors to make a more uniform cut each time."

Dr. Robert Maloney, who performs LASIKs as part of the randomized PRK/LASIK FDA trials, cautioned, "Improvements in microkeratomes will make these surgeries safer, but even a perfect microkeratome won't make LASIK perfectly safe, because there's no way to make a*ny* surgery 100% safe."

Dr. Maloney continued, "Eyes have been lost from a faulty microkeratome or an inexperienced surgeon, but I've never personally witnessed one of these cases. When suction is lost during the cutting of the flap, the blade can enter the cornea at an angle. This can be a minor problem or a major one. The worst case would be cutting into the eye. The second worst case would be cutting the cornea to the point that the patient needs a transplant."

In addition to the placement of the cut, the depth of the cut is difficult to control precisely. A recent study showed that most LASIK cuts were 20% too deep, on average.[15] This can pose a problem in patients with thinner-than-average corneas who have high myopia, because the pulses could penetrate the very inner layer of the cornea (the "endothelium"). Unless the doctor stops and does a special measurement during the surgery—which isn't part of the procedure—he has no way of knowing exactly how deep the cut was.

Dr. Steinert said, "I have performed a corneal transplant on a patient who had flap surgery right here in New England, and there aren't even that many patients here who have had flap surgery. In the thousands of PRK procedures done in the U.S. since 1989, not one single patient has even remotely come close to needing a corneal transplant."

In a preliminary report, researchers in the FDA LASIK trials, while concluding that LASIK "appeared to be an ideal technique to correct myopia up to -20.0," also said that "the outcome of the procedures is most affected by the accuracy and ease of the microkeratome cut. When an even, smooth cut is achieved, the best and most predictable results are obtained."[16]

Problems with the Flap

Another potential problem is loss of, or damage to, the flap—either at the time of surgery or later. The flap can be cut all the way off accidentally, which requires the doctor to reposition it exactly where it was—not an easy task. If the edges don't match up with the underlying cornea, scarring and irregular astigmatism can result in loss of best-corrected acuity.

Dr. Bruce Jackson said, "The flap can wrinkle when it's set back down or the doctor might have a hard time getting it back in exactly the right position. As an indication of how fragile the flap is, you can retreat the patient at a later date simply by lifting the flap back up and adding more pulses—the flap only seals around the edges."

This fact caused several doctors to worry that the patient might rub the flap off during the night, even many months after treatment. Dr. Robert Maloney said, "I'm told it can happen, but I've done more than 600 ALKs and LASIKs and I've never had a patient rub the cap off."

A study of 12 cases of cap problems after ALK noted that three "fell off" (one after six months, the other two after one month)." The rest were intentionally removed because of irregular astigmatism (6), dislocation (2), fragmentation (1) and haze (1).[18]

COMPLICATIONS WITH MICROKERATOMES   In May of 1996, the American Academy of Ophthalmology listed twelve reported problems with automated microkeratomes, including the following. The word "flap" can be used interchangeably with "cap."

- Decentered ablations
- Holes in caps
- Large over- or undercorrections
- Problems getting the cap to readhere
- Infection
- Scarring at the edges of the cap.[17]

In the study of 57 eyes mentioned above, two patients had perforated flaps during the surgery. One had to have a corneal graft five days after the procedure, which did not work, and "the patient remains highly myopic." One eye had mild wrinkling of the cell layer beneath the epithelium. At the end of six months, results from only 24 eyes were reported on and 7 of these had vision worse than 20/40. At the end of a year, 14 eyes were reported on and eight had vision less than 20/40.[19]

In the study of 128 eyes treated with ALK, one eye lost the cap, five eyes developed irregular astigmatism and five others had an increase in astigmatism.

Problems with the Zap

The biggest unanswered question about LASIK is what happens to the cornea long term after laser pulses remove tissue inside it, rather from the surface of it. Most doctors feel that the inner 150-200 microns of the cornea shouldn't be disturbed because a buffer zone is needed to protect the endothelium—a single-cell layer at the back of the cornea that is vital to keeping the cornea clear. Unless the endothelium does its job of pumping water out of the tissue, the cornea turns hazy and then white, like the normally white part of the eye. A damaged endothelium can result in the need for a corneal transplant because the endothelium does not regenerate.

In 1995 doctors in Switzerland reported that performing LASIK on pig eyes appeared to have no effect on the endothelium, but all their measurements were taken within six hours of the surgery.[20]

Dr. Thompson said, "There are no studies that tell us whether lifting up a third of the cornea and zapping the rest of it with a laser will have a long-term negative effect. It is possible that shock waves from the laser pulses could damage the endothelium."

Sadly, those who could benefit most from LASIK are at the highest risk of endothelial damage: If the flap is cut at 160-200 microns in a 500-micron cornea, this leaves only about 100 microns for treatment—which might not be enough room to correct a patient greater than -10.0 all the way to 20/40 or better with a sufficiently wide treatment zone without endangering the endothelium.

Problems with the Epithelium

A known side effect of flap surgery is overactive regrowth of the epithelium. Instead of growing back over the surface of the cut, it grows down into it and under the flap.

"Epithelial regrowth under the flap is fairly common," Dr. Maloney said, "and because the epithelium is pearly white, it can interfere with vision. In about 5% of the cases we have to lift the flap with an instrument and wipe away the epithelium. Then we set the flap back down. It doesn't cause a terrible problem."

In the study of 57 eyes, 12% had trace and one eye had "mild" epithelial regrowth.[21]

Problems with Infection

Any time the cornea is cut into, there is danger of infection and inflammation. Since the flap never fully heals, this danger never really ends.

Dr. Lin, who began performing LASIK for high myopia in mid-1995, said, "Infection at the interface of the flap and cornea could be worse than a surface infection after PRK, but the likelihood of infection might be reduced because the epithelium isn't removed."

Dr. Steinert said, "There's a growing awareness of a problem with inflammation around the edge of the flap which can occur years after the procedure."

Problems with Inexperienced Doctors

Dr. Jackson said that even in the few studies available on LASIK, the results are from top-notch surgeons who do very high numbers of cases. "What will the results be for the average doctor who only does a case a month?"

At least one study showed that the predictability of the depth of the flap was dependent on surgeon skill.[22]

Dr. Steinert agrees and wonders whether this has anything to do with how enthusiastic some are about it. "The blunt reality is that PRK can be learned by many reasonably competent doctors and is becoming widely available. LASIK is very surgeon-dependent and restricts the market to far fewer surgeons."

Problems with Off-Centered Treatment
Just as with single-zone surface PRK, the LASIK ablation can be off-centered. Multizone ablations beneath the flap could reduce or eliminate this risk.

Optical Side Effects
The incidence of glare, flare and halo appear to be lower after LASIK than after PRK. In the study of 57 eyes, only one patient reported "marked" halos and one reported mild "ghosting" [flare].[23]

Simultaneous LASIK?
Doctors who are opposed to simultaneous eye surgery make no exceptions for LASIK, but others think the risk might be exaggerated.

Dr. Jeffrey Robin said, "I'm planning to treat both eyes simultaneously and correct astigmatism at the same time so patients can get as much correction as possible in one visit."

Dr. Maloney added, "I think doing both eyes at the same time is fine, as long as the surgeon uses a different microkeratome on the second eye. Just as with RK, the risk of transferring infection from one eye to the other is much higher if you use the same instrument on both eyes."

COMPARING PRK TO LASIK

There have been very few studies comparing PRK results to those of LASIK, and none with long-term follow-up. In a rare study conducted in Eygpt, 40 eyes between -6.0 and -10.0 were treated with PRK and then the same surgeon treated 40 eyes with the same refractions with LASIK. About half of the PRK eyes ended up with 20/20 vision at the end of a year, but 60% of the LASIK eyes achieved that goal. The researchers added that none of the LASIK eyes developed haze.[24]

In the U.S., trials are just beginning in which patients will be randomly treated with LASIK or PRK and then followed for a year or more. This will provide good comparisons of the results of the types of treatments studied but will give little guidance on new techniques that emerge while the trials are in progress. The studies should begin to tell us what the incidence of certain side effects and complications are, at least as performed by very highly skilled surgeons.

"LIKE *ALMOST* WINNING THE LOTTERY"

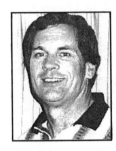

Name
Richard Lilja, 46

Occupation
Technical writer,
California

Pre-Op Vision
Left eye: -6.75
Right eye: -7.75 with
 mild astigmatism

Procedure
LASIK

Post-Op Vision
20/40

Surgeon
Michael Gordon, MD

I spoke with Mr. Lilja three weeks after his first eye was treated with LASIK. Before we began talking he wanted to make one thing clear: "If you're going to tell me anything about LASIK, I don't want to hear it until my other eye is done." I said he had a deal. The next time I spoke with him was two weeks after his second eye was treated, and we checked in several times thereafter.

"About a year or so ago I looked into RK. I went to a few seminars but nobody would commit to any results. Worse than that, they all said I probably wouldn't be able to wear contacts if the RK didn't work.

"So, I pretty much put the whole thing on hold until recently. Then I went to Hawaii and one day I fell off the board when I was out windsurfing. A wave washed out one of the contacts and there was such a difference between my two eyes, I knew that if I lost the other contact I could end up on Molokai. It brought back memories of when I used to go to the beach and I'd come out of the water and not be able to find my towel."

"When I got home I went straight to Dr. Gordon's. He said I was a candidate for his LASIK study, so I skipped the seminar and just set the date for February 27, 1996.

"The night before my first procedure I started getting the flu. Between that and the Valium, pain pills and eyedrops, I was just out of it. The whole thing took about ten minutes and there was zero pain. I couldn't see anything except the focusing light. The laser part lasted about five seconds, then Dr. Gordon taped a plastic shield on my eye and I was done. I felt like I was like looking through Vaseline, but that was just the shield.

"On the way home I felt a little cheated. It was like, 'I paid all this money for five minutes?!!' But then I looked out the side of the plastic shield and it was unbelievable. The feeling was, 'This is good! This is great!'

"I felt absolutely nothing for 24 hours and I slept all that night. A day later I started to have a feeling like there was dirt under a contact lens. This lasted a few days and the eye was a little hazy compared to the eye I was still wearing a contact lens on. When I went in to be checked my vision was 20/30.

"Even though I've been through it once, I'm still concerned about Eye Two. I can't wait to get it over with."

The Right Eye   Two weeks after his second LASIK, Mr. Lilja and I spoke again.

"This eye was a completely different experience. For one thing, the procedure took a lot longer and Dr. Gordon seemed to spend a lot more time putting the flap back in place. I was pretty uncomfortable during the procedure. I felt the suction on my eyeball and the laser seemed to take five minutes—even though I knew if was only taking a few seconds. Maybe it was because I was more aware this time—I didn't have the flu.

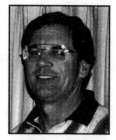

Before his first LASIK

"I didn't see as well right away, up close or far, and I felt some irritation afterward. The eye was only about 20/100 the next day and I still can't read the newspaper. It has been two weeks and the eye is still red and a little swollen.

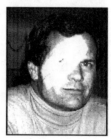

After his first LASIK

Three Weeks Later   "The redness went away right after I talked to you. But I have to say I'm a little disappointed in the second eye and I'm still not seeing very well out of it. I might have to have AK to correct some astigmatism. It seems like my two eyes aren't working together quite well enough and I see worse with both eyes together than I do with my left eye alone.

"I had some trouble with night vision for a little while—it was kind of like starbursts—but that's getting better. I have to say that if my eyes never get any better than this, it's still fantastic. The trouble is, it's so good, I just want it to be perfect. It's a little frustrating—like *almost* winning the lottery!"

Two Months Later   "I just went in for a check-up and my overall vision is about 20/40. I still can't read with my right eye, so I just use my left eye, and I'm having trouble seeing my computer screen.

"My distance vision is acceptable, but I know it's not perfect. I can't read the freeway signs very well, for example. There's a big wall map in my office and I can't read any of the words on it. On the positive side, my last job assignment was outdoors and it was very dusty. I loved not having to wear contacts. All in all, I guess I'm pretty satisfied, but I think I'm going to have to have a touch-up procedure."

UPDATE   Mr. Lilja had an Astigmatic Keratotomy on his right eye to remove the astigmatism (see Chapter 16 for information about AK) and now has monovision: he uses his left eye for reading and his right eye for distance. "It works great. I can read anything, but when I look into the distance, I notice my left eye isn't perfect. I could have AK in it, but then I might lose my reading vision. I'm not complaining: my vision is really terrific."

Another problem with comparing treatments is that the more involved the procedure, the more it is dependent on the individual doctor's skill—and so the harder it will be for patients to use research data produced by other doctors to predict their own outcome.

Dr. Mihai Pop said, "If a doctor performs only LASIK and is very good at it, patients probably are safe in having it. If the doctor has done surface PRK for a thousand cases, go with that. Excimer laser surgery is like any other: Experience is what counts."

The Cost
Right now LASIK costs about $300-400 more *per eye* than PRK. There is more surgical skill and equipment involved and the procedure takes a little longer.

What the Experts Say About LASIK *vs* PRK

Dr. Vance Thompson
"I'm not doing LASIK outside my clinical trials. I think one of the beauties of PRK is that it has gone through the trials and survived very intensive scrutiny. LASIK hasn't come through that. I can tell patients that LASIK has less discomfort and you see faster, but I can't tell you what its safety and predictability is over the long term.

"Even though there are doctors other places who have done thousands of cases, they're not doing studies. In fact, there are no peer-reviewed studies of the kind the FDA would require for approval. That's why the whole world sits on the edge of their seats over what happens in the U.S. with the FDA."

"I tell people this: For -6.0 and under, there's no doubt in my mind that PRK is the way to go. For -10.0 and above, I'm becoming confident, but not yet totally convinced, that LASIK's the way. For -7.0 to -10.0, I tell them that I don't know which is best for them and if they need me to tell them, I tell them to wait. If they can make a decision based on the facts as I can present them, then I'll do what they choose.

Dr. Richard Lindstrom
"About 50,000 LASIKs have been done worldwide with very few reported problems. At this time we've abandoned PRK for -8.0 and up. For extreme myopes you need to do a multizone LASIK or you cut too much tissue out of cornea. Right now I use ALK to get the first 15 or 20 diopters and then I use the laser to get the rest. By end of the year we probably will only be doing LASIK, even on extreme myopes (-27 and -28)."

NO MORE LINES

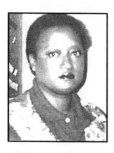

Name
Deby Hammond, 41

Occupation
Legal word processor
California

Pre-Op Vision
Right eye: -7.0 with .75 astigmatism
Left eye: -8.25 with .25 astimatism

Procedure
Right eye: PRK
Left eye: LASIK

Post-Op Vision
Right eye at 6 months: 20/50
Left eye at 3 months: 20/40

Surgeon
Michael Gordon, MD

Deby Hammond had her right eye treated with PRK only a few weeks after it was approved in the U.S. Three months later she had her left eye treated with LASIK. I spoke with her a month after the second eye was done.

"Before I went through all this, my vision was about 20/1600. Now it's been a month since my left eye was done and I'm seeing 20/30 overall.

"I was wearing contacts but by evening my eyes would get very dry and they were a pain in the neck. Glasses hurt my nose and it was a hassle to carry around prescription sunglasses, regular sunglasses, all that stuff.

"Last year I had to go into bifocals and I thought, 'Oh, no, I don't want that line.' By the time you pay $50 to get the line removed and then more for the ultra-light lenses, and a tint... and then there were only certain frames I could choose because my lenses were so thick...it was expensive!

"A friend at work was fed up with her lenses too, and she did all the legwork to research doctors. I made an appointment with Dr. Gordon and asked a trillion questions. I was most concerned about what would happen to my vision as I get older.

"Right after PRK my eye looked great—no one could tell I had anything done. I could still wear a contact in my left eye and see perfectly for distance. I had a little trouble using the computer for about a week, then it was fine. The only problem was when I was getting ready to have the second eye done and I had to stop wearing my contacts a week ahead of time.

"The day after I had LASIK just happened to be three months after my PRK, so Dr. Gordon checked both eyes. My first eye was 20/30 and my brand-new eye was already 20/25! I didn't have any discomfort to speak of after either procedure. And now, of course, I don't wear glasses or contacts at all. Sometimes you finally do something and then you just stand back and say 'Why did I wait so long?'"

UPDATE At this writing Ms. Hammond was six and three months post-op, her vision had regressed a little and she was planning to have both eyes retreated with PRK.

Dr. Donald Johnson

"Multizone PRK strongly competes with LASIK for high levels of myopia without the risks of cutting into the cornea. I do it on the highest myopes to ensure the smoothest possible surface and I've treated up to -25.0 in a single procedure. LASIK is surgery for the surgeon. PRK is surgery for the patient."

Dr. Marguerite McDonald

"There's nothing better than a good LASIK and nothing worse than a bad one. Third-generation technology is giving us extremely good PRK results with rapid return of best-corrected acuity. This may allow us to treat a wider range of myopic corrections than we first predicted."

Dr. Roger Steinert

"We're in the middle of a PRK trial on -6.0 to -12.0 myopia and are getting spectacularly good results, even though patients are randomized between single-zone and multizone PRK. So far the healing responses are indistinguishable from those of PRK in the lower levels of myopia. Until we follow large numbers of patients for several years, we can't say we've solved the problems of PRK for high myopia, but the results look encouraging.

"We are simultaneously running trials on LASIK. It appears that LASIK patients do better optically in the first month, but after that PRK patients do better, with better uncorrected vision and minimal loss of best-corrected vision."

Dr. James Salz

"We're going by the book and not doing LASIK, because I refuse to use a gray-market laser and the currently approved lasers aren't programmed for LASIK. We need multi-site studies that show whether LASIK beats PRK and we don't have them yet. In a year we'll have a much better idea of which is best for which degrees of nearsightedness.

"Patients need to be aware that doctors can't do hundreds of microkeratome procedures without complications. Even the inventor of LASIK will not perform it on patients lower than -6.0; for them he uses surface PRK. Only 1% of all myopes are worse than -10.0; for them we might find that implantable contacts are a better solution."

Dr. Robert Maloney

"I prefer PRK for low to moderate myopia, because haze is so rare. For high myopia I prefer LASIK, because it eliminates the risk of haze and vision recovers quickly."

Dr. Howard Gimbel

"I've performed 300 LASIKs in the last year and I'm doing more all the time. However, the results I can get with PRK are so good, LASIK might be unnecessary. Doctors who are really pushing the benefits of LASIK are comparing it to older PRK treatment results. With newer methods such as multizone PRK, and with the new types of laser treatments which create a smoother surface, the results I'm seeing with PRK match those of LASIK.

"To make the risks of LASIK acceptable, the results have to be superior to those of PRK. We don't know if they are."

Dr. David Lin

"Surface PRK results are so good for -6.0 and under, why add a more invasive step to the procedure if you don't have to? The gray zone is from -6.0 to -10.0; Only time will tell. Faster visual recovery, less discomfort, fewer eyedrops— they're all great if the results are equal. For high myopes the results are fractionally better with LASIK and the recovery is faster."

Dr. Michael Gordon

"I think LASIK is an excellent procedure but we don't know for which types of cases the risks of LASIK begin to outweigh the benefits. It will be one or two years before we begin to have the answers to this question. People who are using LASIK for very low myopia are out to lunch in my opinion, because the proven results of PRK are so good at the lower levels."

Dr. Bruce Jackson

"I don't do LASIK right now because I'm not really happy with any of the microkeratomes that are available and there are no LASIK studies with results as good as the results that have been shown for PRK. LASIK is very popular in the U.S. but people aren't as crazy about it here in Canada. I don't think it will be the solution over the long term—slicing the cornea isn't something you want to do if you can avoid it. The reason ALK never took off is the same reason LASIK will fall by the wayside: there are too many risks."

Dr. Jeffrey Robin

"Canada is the only country in the world, besides the U.S., that isn't LASIK-crazy, but surgical techniques like ALK and RK have never taken hold there. When you start to look at what's happening in all the unregulated societies of the world, PRK is getting to be a tough sell. They're all going to LASIK."

Dr. Mibai Pop

"We'll always have specialists trying new procedures and getting good success rates, but we have to match the doctor to the procedure. The best technique is the one the average doctor can do without ruining the eye.

"LASIK might turn out to be better than multizone PRK, but we don't know yet. We hear that there's fast visual recovery, but we don't know what the quality of vision is in 3-6 months.

"We know the complications of PRK and we know we can treat them fairly easily. We don't know all the risks of LASIK and many can't be solved short of a cornea or lens transplant. The bottom line is, I favor surface PRK. I think we can perfect it even more with the new scanning lasers that are in clinical trials right now. Because PRK is much less dependent on an individual doctor's skill, I think it's going to become the procedure of choice for all levels of nearsightedness."

THE DOCTOR WHO IS WAITING TO SEE

When Dr. Marguerite McDonald was five, she could hardly see. "Even though my dad was a surgeon, no one knew I needed glasses. I never squinted, I just ran around seeing color blocks: A block of green was the front grass, a block of blue was the sky. If I got close enough to my mother, I could see a piece of her face—like her nostril or part of her lip. But I thought that was how it was for everybody.

"So one day when I was five my mom took me with some other kids to a new shopping mall. We were told to go play in the park while she and the other mother went shopping. I went running full-tilt right into a little manmade lake that I didn't see because it was covered with green scum— it matched the grass. I'm in the pond, my legs are trapped around the bottom of an old wooden bridge and I'm drowning. A 12-year-old dove in and rescued me and my mother ran over screaming, 'Marguerite! Why did you jump in that lake?'

"Of course, I said that I didn't see the lake. She said, 'We've been letting you cross the street for a year. How did you do it?' I told her I did it like everyone else—I stood on the curb and listened for cars!

"When I got my glasses, I saw faces for the first time: my mother's, my father's, my sisters'. I made them tie those glasses on me and I would not let anyone take them off for at least three weeks. My mother had to wash my face around them. I said to myself, 'Seeing is the best thing on earth and someday I won't need to wear these things.'

Sweet Fifteen

"There was an old law in Illinois that you had to be 15 in order to wear contact lenses. So guess where I was on my 15th birthday? I left the doctor's office with these horribly thick, uncomfortable lenses—they felt like rocks, but I was smiling— and I went to see my girlfriend. My eyes were bright red and dripping wet. Her older brother opened the door and said 'Marguerite, is that you? Where are your glasses?' Then he said, 'Do you want to go to the movies tonight?' I thought, 'That's it; this is the key to social success.'

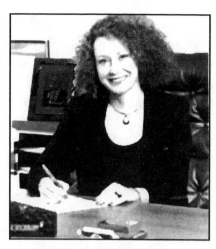

Marguerite McDonald, MD

"But contacts were so uncomfortable, I vowed that some day I would be free of all this. Someday I would *help* other people be free. No one should have to be an optical cripple. That was the start of everything and the motivation behind everything I have done."

Dr. McDonald is one of the three doctors in the world who can be credited with developing the PRK procedure (see Chapter 6). She performed the first 10 PRK procedures in the FDA Phase I trial in June of 1987. She was also one of the nine surgeons who were part of the National Institutes of Health 10-year PERK study on RK, and, with Dr. Herbert Kauffman, developed the "living contact lens," technique (epikeratophakia) for high myopia.

After all of this, Dr. McDonald, whose vision is -12.0, still wears contacts. I asked her why. "I'm waiting to see 3-year follow-up data on LASIK before deciding if I want that or PRK. So far there's only one LASIK study on seven eyes that is more than a year in duration. The very latest Multizone PRK data looks like it might even outperform LASIK in my case, and it could be that LASIK will be reserved only for the super-high myopes. All that is being studied right now and the jury is still out."

"I've waited this long, I'll wait another year. Then I'll see."

ON THE HORIZON

In parallel with developing PRK and LASIK, doctors are beginning to investigate new techniques, new instruments and new types of lasers for the very nearsighted. Some are in clinical trials in the U.S. and are being tested in Canada. If you are interested in one of the following treatments, see the resource list in Chapter 7 for possible treatment centers near you.

Clear Lens Extraction (CLE)

This technique is identical to the lens replacement done during cataract surgeries, except that a normal lens is replaced by an artificial lens. The new lens is designed to correct myopia and/or astigmatism. It is held in place by the same membrane that holds the natural lens.

In a study of 31 highly myopic eyes treated with CLE, 77% achieved 20/40 or better. Five eyes were later retreated with RK or AK to finetune the correction. In one case the eye had to be reopened and the artificial lens replaced to achieve good vision for the patient. After an average follow-up period of 20 months, the major problem was clouding of the membrane that held the lenses. There were no retinal or macular problems.[25]

Dr. Salz is investigating the use of CLE for high hyperopia but said, "I don't think we're going to find that CLE for high myopia is the answer. High myopes have a much higher risk of retinal detachment without surgery. Eye surgery increases this risk. While a detached retina can be solved with yet another surgery, who wants to have their eye cut into twice? Implantable contacts might be the way to go."

Reversible Treatments

The implantable contact lens and the intrastromal corneal ring segments are two methods which share the benefit of being reversible or easily adjusted. They are described in more detail at the end of Chapter 14.

VISION ALERT! Ever wonder why we're told to wear protective eye shields when we play racketball or squash? In 1996 German doctors reported on 26 cases of retinal detachment after young patients were struck in the eye with a ball while playing squash. Doctors were able to reattach the retina in 22 of the eyes but only 42% ended up with 20/40 or better *best-corrected* vision. [26]

Dr. Jackson said, "The early results on these are interesting but I still think PRK is going to end up being better, even for high myopia. The less you have to cut into the eye, the better off the patient will be."

"I think implantable lenses and intrastromal ring segments have a lot of possibilities for treating high myopia," Dr. Gimbel said. "For low-to-moderate nearsightedness, PRK works so well that there's no reason to risk incisions of any type."

Scanning Laser PRK

Some of the doctors involved in this book are currently testing lasers such as ones made by Novatec, Nidek and Autonomous, which use narrow beams that move back and forth (scan) across the surface of the eye in a computer-controlled pattern. "The scanning technique distributes the energy more evenly to create a much smoother surface than we can obtain with a stationary beam that simply widens," Dr. Gimbel said. Another feature of the new lasers is automatic eyetracking to enable on-centered ablations even if the patient's eye moves a little.

The new lasers don't require the use of gases, which reduces their size (and therefore the amount of space that must be dedicated to them) as well as the cost of operating them. This should, ultimately, result in lower prices for PRK and LASIK.

Mark Hamilton of Novatec said that their LightBlade laser system has the potential for treating high myopia, hyperopia, and both regular and irregular astigmatism. The laser is in FDA Phase II clinical trials and being tested in Canada by some of the doctors who contributed to this book.

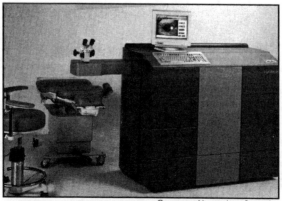

COURTESY OF NOVATEC LASER SYSTEMS INC.

The new "solid-state" lasers, such as this one from Novatec, could offer smoother surface PRK treatments at lower cost.

Intrastromal Lasers: LASIK without the Flap?

What if you could get all the benefits of LASIK without cutting a flap? Novatec is working on a module for its LightBlade laser which is designed to bypass the epithelium and go straight through to the cornea, where it would scan back and forth to perform PRK, or create incisions like those used in RK or AK. The wavelengths are said to be almost as short as those used for PRK, so it should emit cool light and do little damage to surrounding tissue. This module is not yet in clinical trials, but preliminary animal research looks promising.

Water-Jet PRK and LASIK?

The wave of the future might well be pressure washing excess tissue from the cornea instead of removing it by laser, or using a high-speed stream of purified water to cut the LASIK flap. Two companies, Medjet and Surgijet, have developed instruments which might be able to cut or remove tissue with even less harm to the remaining cornea than a laser, and with less risk than a microkeratome. This could be good news for the highly nearsighted because less disturbance to the cornea would mean less risk of haze and faster healing.

Medjet's "hydrokeratome," which received a patent in September of 1996, has created LASIK flaps on cadaver corneas which are perfectly spherical and clean-edged, according to observers. The hydrokeratome is much simpler than a laser—it consists of a hand-held instrument and tubing attached to a footpedal, all powered by a CO_2 cartridge—and much less expensive to maintain and operate. As a result, hydrokeratome procedures not involving a laser will be lower in cost than laser alternatives. Medjet was entering clinical trials in the Fall of 1996 for removing the epithelium prior to PRK and other surgeries as a first step to proving its technology.

THANKS ARE IN ORDER   I'd like to extend my thanks to Dr. Gordon for enabling me to interview two of his patients while they were in the middle of the vision-correction process. He could have referred me to any of hundreds of his cases where the patient outcome was already known, but instead, as a contribution to this book, made it possible for me to capture the experiences of Deby Hammond and Richard Lilja as they unfolded.

16

What If You Have Astigmatism?

*I*f you are nearsighted or farsighted, chances are better than even that you are also astigmatic, and there are those who wear contacts and glasses *only* to correct their astigmatism. If you have it, whether and how to treat it should be part of your total decision about correcting your vision.

Who Has Astigmatism?
Dr. Donald Johnson said that about two thirds of his nearsighted patients have more than 0.25 diopters of astigmatism. Dr. Raymond Stein pinpoints it further: 35% have astigmatism over one diopter and most of these have over 1.5 diopters of astigmatism.

What Happens If You Don't Correct It?
The initial FDA approvals of PRK stated that PRK could be used for treating myopia in patients who have up to 1.5 diopters of astigmatism—but not for treating the astigmatism itself. This could lead patients to the incorrect conclusion that treating the astigmatism is not necessary.

QUICK REVIEW   As detailed in Chapter 5, astigmatism is an irregularity in the shape of the cornea which causes the cornea to be steeper in one dimension than in the other (Figure 16.1). As a result, light is focused at two points in the eye, instead of one. That, in turn, causes blurred vision.

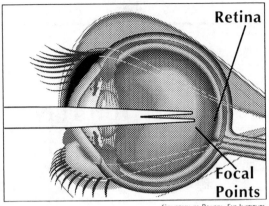

FIGURE 16.1   With astigmatism, light comes to two focal points inside the eye, instead of just one, and the brain "sees" a blurred or double image. This graphic shows an astigmatic nearsighted eye.

If your glasses or contacts correct your astigmatism, you probably aren't aware of its effect on your vision. And without lenses, your myopia or hyperopia most likely causes enough blurring to mask the effects of any astigmatism.

If you have your nearsightedness or farsightedness corrected, however, the astigmatism will become all too apparent unless it is positioned outside the central visual area. It might be noticeable only in your near vision (as mine is) or only the distance, or both.

Mark Logan, CEO of VISX Corporation said that allowing patients with myopia to be treated with PRK *without* treating the astigmatism gives patients bad results. The VISX application to the FDA requested a limit of 1 diopter of astigmatism, which was approved. "The ultimate solution is to treat the astigmatism at the same time we treat the myopia, like doctors do in Canada."

Dr. Vance Thompson agrees. "If a doctor ignores astigmatism while treating myopia, chances are the patient won't be happy unless the astigmatism is very mild."

Dr. Roger Steinert said that some patients see very well with up to 1.5 diopters of astigmatism and others need treatment. "After about 1.5 diopters, there's a marked drop-off in vision and most patients need the astigmatism corrected."

Dr. Bruce Jackson sets a lower limit: "If you don't treat astigmatism, patients have slower visual recovery and they never see as well. If you leave 1 diopter of astigmatism, the patient will not get to 20/20."

Dr. Donald Johnson said, "I always treat any degree of astigmatism over 0.25 diopters. Anyone who is left with a half diopter of astigmatism is not going to be very satisfied no matter how wonderfully their PRK turns out."

And Dr. David Lin added: "If a patient has any degree of astigmatism, PRK by itself is not the treatment of choice. You need to treat the astigmatism too."

Astigmatism and the FDA

Since 1992, PRK has been used extensively and successfully outside the U.S. for the treatment of astigmatism. Because the FDA trials were so long and expensive for PRK, the manufacturers decided to postpone simultaneous studies for Astigmatic PRK (APRK), which had been started. As a result, until recently the only option for treating astigmatism in the U.S. has been AK, described below. Canadian PRK patients generally receive APRK or Astigmatic LASIK (see Chapter 15) as part of their treatment if they have astigmatism.

On October 15, 1996 the FDA acknowledged the need to include astigmatism as part of any treatment for nearsightedness by expediting their review of VISX's application for treating 0.75—4.50 diopters of astigmatism with their laser. VISX has held a long track record for safe, effective APRK treatments in countries outside of the U.S.

According to a release issued that day, the VISX application was granted expedited review status because "no legally marketed device is available for the safe treatment of astigmatism ... and the alternative treatments being employed entail substantial risk of morbidity for the patient." By "morbidity" they mean damage or death to the eye, not the person.

WHERE TO GO IF YOU HAVE ASTIGMATISM If you are considering laser vision correction and have more than 0.50 diopter of astigmatism, your options for the near term are likely to be:

a) Treatment in Canada
b) Treatment with a VISX laser
c) PRK plus AK (see below)
d) Having your PRK treatment in a center that is conducting a clinical trial for APRK (see Chapter 4 for some locations).

The good news is that upgrading a VISX laser for APRK is simply a matter of overnighting new software to the doctors; so patients will be able to take advantage of APRK approvals almost as soon as they are announced.

Full approval for the VISX APRK treatment was expected in early 1997. But does this mean every PRK patient can then receive astigmatism treatment if she needs it? No—because Summit lasers and others still in clinical trials have not yet obtained these approvals.

What Kind of Astigmatism Do You Have?

There are two types of astigmatism: regular and irregular. Regular astigmatism can be treated with APRK or AK, as described below. Irregular astigmatism *might* be treatable. The reason doctors require you to stop wearing contact lenses before your initial exam for vision correction is so they can determine how much and what kind of astigmatism you have, if any.

Regular Astigmatism

Regular astigmatism (see Figure 16.2) is distributed nearly evenly on either side of the center of the pupil in a "bow-tie" or "figure eight" shape. For this reason it's also called "symmetrical" astigmatism. The astigmatism can occur in any orientation (axis). For those of us who have it, regular astigmatism is natural—it occurred at birth or in the development of our eyes during childhood.

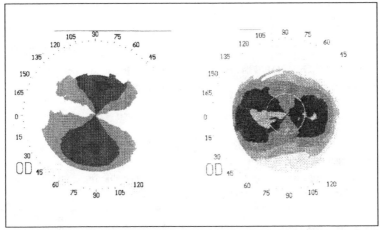

FIGURE 16.2   Regular astigmatism in different orientations are shown on these topography maps of two different eyes. You can see the bow-tie shapes of the corneas.

Irregular Astigmatism

Irregular, or asymmetric, astigmatism tends to congregate mostly in one section of the cornea (see Figure 16.3). While it is relatively rare in the total population, it tends to occur more frequently in people who want their vision fixed—because this type of astigmatism interferes with vision and can make wearing contact lenses more difficult.

Irregular astigmatism is more likely to be caused by trauma to the eye. Wearing contact lenses, particularly rigid ones, can cause corneal "warpage" which can lead to irregular astigmatism. This usually disappears when the patient stops wearing lenses for a few weeks. If it remains, your doctor will want to analyze the cause.

Accidents which affect the surface of the eye, previous incisions to correct vision, and corneal surgery, such as transplants, all can cause irregular astigmatism. Some forms of irregular astigmatism cannot be treated, or fully treated, with APRK or AK.

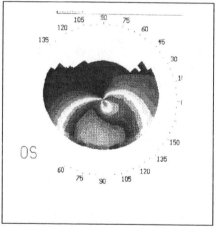

COURTESY OF PACIFIC LASER EYE CENTRE

FIGURE 16.3 In this eye with irregular astigmatism, the corneal topography shows that the steepest (lightest) surface primarily is in one quadrant of the cornea.

Keratoconus: A Special Case

Keratoconus is a type of irregular astigmatism that is caused by a progressively thinning cornea. As the cornea gets thinner on one side, the pressure inside the eye causes it to bulge out—forming a cone shape. The tendency toward keratoconus is inherited and, at this time, there is no cure. In most cases the condition can be managed with rigid contacts which help retain the cornea in a proper curve.

Every piece of literature I read from laser manufacturers, laser center operators and doctors in private practice cautioned that keratoconus should not be treated with PRK. The fear is that removing even a small amount of tissue would further weaken an already thin cornea.

On the brighter side, Dr. Donald Johnson said that he has treated cases of keratoconus successfully, and two doctors in Sweden used PRK to treat five eyes in which keratoconus had progressed to the point that cornea transplants were necessary (and therefore they had little to lose by trying PRK). At the end of the first year, keratoconus was reduced in four of the five eyes and their visual acuity was improved. The eyes did not have any unusual healing problems and there was no sign that PRK caused accelerated corneal thinning. These doctors concluded that the fear of using PRK to treat keratoconus is "speculative" and might be exaggerated.[1]

The Importance of Being Tested

To treat astigmatism properly the doctor needs to know not only how much you have (the refractive error in diopters) but which type it is and where it is located on the cornea. That's where videokeratography comes in. As described in Chapter 8, this test provides a topographical "map" of the surface of the cornea, which pinpoints any irregularities.

After doctors reviewed corneal topography maps of 106 eyes of people who consulted the University of Texas for vision correction, 35 of the corneas were found to be abnormal in some way and 32 of these eyes had irregular astigmatism. After examining the patients, the doctors believed most of this was caused by "warpage" from wearing contact lenses, and the effect was more severe in rigid lens wearers. Three of the patients were diagnosed with keratoconus. The doctors believed that all of these conditions would have escaped diagnosis if only a visual examination had been conducted.[2]

The message here is, you can't have the right treatment unless you begin with the right diagnosis. Stop wearing your contacts before the initial exam, and don't skip a corneal topography exam even if astigmatism isn't evident in your refractive exam.

OPTIONS FOR TREATING ASTIGMATISM

If you have your PRK procedure in Canada and have astigmatism, most likely it will be treated at the same time as your nearsightedness or farsightedness. Those who are treated in the U.S. have different options:

As mentioned above, clinical trials for APRK are underway at this time, and since PRK has already been approved, APRK approval should be more rapid—perhaps by the time you read this. When it is, doctors will be able to add a software program to systems approved for APRK systems purchasing new equipment. Until then, doctors outside clinical trials can't buy the software in the United States.

Astigmatic PRK (APRK)

As described in Chapter 6, PRK can be used to treat astigmatism at the same time other vision correction is done. It is performed as a separate step right after the epithelium is removed.

The surgeon programs the laser for APRK, performs the procedure, which rounds up the shape of the cornea in just a few seconds, and then reprograms the laser for myopic or hyperopic PRK to change the steepness of the cornea. APRK can also be used to treat astigmatism in patients who are not myopic or hyperopic.

How APRK Works

The VISX method of APRK involves a computer-controlled aperture of the excimer laser which opens in a gradually widening slit oriented to match the position of the astigmatism on the patient's eye. As it opens, the laser beam removes tissue in an elliptical pattern, (Figure 16.4) which has the same effect

---

APRK IN CANADA Dr. Howard Gimbel began using the VISX laser to treat astigmatism way back in 1992. "Even then we had no problems with the procedure," he said. "If anything, patients tended to be undercorrected rather than overcorrected—and that was something we could fix by retreatment." Dr. Johnson added that most of the PRK treatments in Canada also include APRK. "Very few doctors use incisions to treat astigmatism here." Dr. Raymond Stein says that 90% of the patients at the Beacon Eye Institute have APRK as part of their PRK treatments.

as a "toric" (astigmatic) contact lens. The number of pulses of the laser determines how much irregularity is removed—1/4 micron is vaporized with each pulse. Instead of an aperture slit, other systems use a mask which controls the position of the treatment.

Irregular astigmatism might be treated differently, with the aperture set to open in a gradually widening circle, as it does with myopic PRK. Drs. Johnson and Mihai Pop have both reported success using this method.

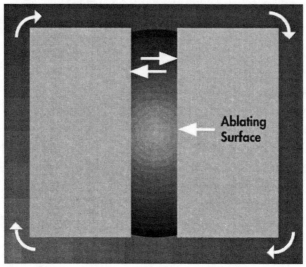

Courtesy of VISX, Incorporated

FIGURE 16.4 A rectangular aperture controls the effect of the cylindrical laser beam, creating an elliptically shaped ablation.

How Well Does APRK Work?

Results from studies in other countries and early clinical trials in the U.S. indicate that APRK combined with PRK has about the same success rates as PRK for myopia alone. In other words, the patient gets the bonus of the extra treatment without giving up many, if any, of the benefits of PRK. There should be no extra cost if it is done in the same visit.

• A group of doctors in Australia performed APRK and PRK procedures on 150 eyes—some with myopia as high as -15.0. At the one-year follow-up period, 77% of all the patients had 20/40 vision or better. 6% lost two or more lines of best-corrected acuity, but 9% *gained* two or more lines. Only 8% reported "adverse reactions" in the post-op period—none vision-threatening.[3]

- A U.S. study of 70 patients treated with APRK and PRK reported that 71% had 20/40 or better vision at six months. At the end of a year, of the 12 patients available for follow-up, 83% had 20/40 or better and there was no "significant" loss of best-corrected acuity.[4]
- Another U.S. study of eight eyes that were part of FDA Phase IIa trials were treated with APRK and PRK and then followed for 18 months. In six of the eyes astigmatism was improved, and the position of the residual astigmatism had shifted. two had 20/20 or better, five had 20/40 or better and all had 20/50 or better. One eye had an increase in best-corrected acuity from 20/20 to 20/15. For two eyes it decreased from 20/20 to 20/25.[5]

Side Effects of APRK

All the potential side effects of PRK also can be caused by, or increased by, APRK. If astigmatism is treated alone, side effects are likely to be greatly reduced, if they appear at all, because less tissue is removed from the central visual area. Because doctors are careful about how much tissue they remove during APRK, to ensure that they don't overcorrect the patient's vision, quite often some astigmatism remains after the treatment (as it did in my case). The remaining astigmatism might be in a different position (axis) than it was before surgery. Mine went from 80 degrees in both eyes to 20 and 135 degrees. If residual astigmatism interferes with vision, it usually can be removed in a subsequent treatment.

APRK also has the potential to create irregular astigmatism if it doesn't remove all the astigmatism in the first attempt. In most cases, if these results create vision problems they also can be solved by retreatment.

In the U.S., until APRK is approved, astigmatic patients who have PRK will only have the option of AK unless they are part of a clinical trial or they go to Canada.

Astigmatic Keratotomy (AK)

AK is a descendant of RK (radial keratotomy). With RK, the incisions are made in a spoke pattern around the pupil. With AK, the surgeon makes two short incisions either in an arc or, (less commonly) in straight lines, around the pupil. "The incisions aren't quite as deep as with RK," Dr. Robert Maloney said, "and they average about 2-to-3 millimeters in length. Whether one or two incisions are made depends on the amount of astigmatism."

AK is based on the same principle as RK: the incisions weaken the cornea, allowing the internal pressure of the eye to cause it to bulge—making the cornea more evenly spherical to compensate for the astigmatism. Unlike APRK, AK does not physically remove tissue from the cornea.

AK is permanent and, unlike RK, does not appear to be subject to progressive change. AK is used to correct regular astigmatism only. "The incisions do not treat irregular astigmatism," Dr. Maloney said. "In fact, they make it worse."

Where and When Can You Have AK?

Many RK patients have had AK to treat either their natural astigmatism or astigmatism that was caused by the RK, so eye surgeons who do (or did) a high volume of RK procedures usually are very experienced with AK. Doctors new to incisional refractive surgery might not be qualified to perform this technique.

AK can be done before, during, or after PRK. Dr. Richard Lindstrom said he performs AK routinely for up to 5 diopters of astigmatism. "80-90% of patients can have their astigmatism and myopia treated in one visit. We do the AK first and then 30 seconds later we perform PRK. It's easier on most patients to try to get the whole job done at once and have a retreatment only when it's necessary. If you plan for a two-stage procedure, then it's guaranteed you will have to have two separate surgeries, two separate recovery periods."

How Well Does AK Work?

All the U.S. doctors I spoke with who had experience with RK and AK said that AK is effective in correcting mild-to-moderate levels of astigmatism. Four studies confirm this:

- A multi-center study of 160 eyes with 1-6 diopters of astigmatism treated with arc-shaped incisions concluded that the greater the number and length of the incisions and the older the patient, the more effect AK would have on the eye. Male eyes responded more to the treatment than female eyes.[6]
- A study of AK in 26 eyes (including 6 with early forms of keratoconus) concluded that AK is more effective in milder degrees of astigmatism. In the entire group AK reduced astigmatism by about 50%.[7]
- In a study of 11 eyes, nearsighted people with astigmatism were treated with AK followed a month later by PRK. Results showed that astigmatism had been reduced from an average of 3.14 diopters to about 0.10 diopters.[8]
- A study of 173 eyes which had T-shaped AK incisions to correct astigmatism as high as 5.5 diopters, found that there was no loss of more than two lines of best-corrected acuity, and that age had no effect on the success of the treatment. 16% of the eyes required a second treatment.[9]

Side Effects of AK

The incisions are placed at the 5, 6- or 7-millimeter zone. That is wider than most pupils, so any optical effects from them usually occur when the pupil is very dilated—at night. However, people with naturally large pupils can experience glare, starbursts and loss of best-corrected acuity.

It is possible that AK can result in overcorrection, causing hyperopia. In a report of 15 cases in which this happened, 13 were successfully treated by resewing the AK incisions.[10] Dr. Schallhorn cautioned that AK after PRK can result in overcorrection if the patient's uncorrected vision is close to 20/20 when the AK is performed. However, a 1996 study of 40 mildly astigmatic eyes that were treated by AK in a 5-millimeter treatment zone found that only two eyes ended up overcorrected. The researchers concluded that further investigation of the effect of the smaller treatment zone on glare and contrast sensitivity was needed and was underway.[11]

Dr. Christopher Blanton said that the risks for infection and perforation with AK are about the same as for RK (see Chapter 14). Dr. Julius Shulman said that AK was unlikely to expose the eye to greater risk from blunt trauma. "The two small incisions don't affect the stability of the cornea much."

Retreatments after AK

If AK doesn't remove all the astigmatism, the option is to retreat the eye with AK, adding more incisions to the eye, or wait for APRK. There is a limit (probably very low) to how many incisions a patient should allow to be made in his eye, but Dr. Maloney said, "Four or fewer incisions is not a problem and probably no more risk than APRK."

WHAT COULD GO WRONG, DID   A doctor in North Carolina wrote about the case of a 30-year-old who had keratoconus in his right eye. Two AK incisions were performed to treat it, but some astigmatism remained. An additional two AK incisions were made. Even though this smoothed out the asymmetry of his astigmatism, a corneal ulcer developed in the eye, bacteria formed in the incisions and the cornea became even thinner. As a result, his vision began to regress at about two months after the last procedure.[12]

Advocates in the States

Many doctors in the U.S. no longer recommend RK for patients with over 3 or 4 diopters of myopia, but will perform AK, at least until APRK is available on the lasers they use.

Even though Dr. Louis Catania adamantly opposes RK, he reluctantly recommends AK with PRK for cases of severe astigmatism. "In the U.S. there's no other way to get a good visual result right now, unless you're part of an FDA study." He cautions that AK shouldn't be used to completely eliminate high degrees of astigmatism, "A reasonable amount of surgery would be a 2- to 3-millimenter incision way outside the optical zone, but if I had my way, I would prefer to do it all with PRK."

"In experienced hands, AK is safe, very effective, and easy on the patient," Dr. Maloney said. "Like RK, there's a learning curve and more experienced doctors get the best results."

"We probably will always be doing some AKs for enhancement after PRK," Dr. Lindstrom said. "Most of the time this just means one small incision under local anesthetic and you're done."

Dr. Vance Thompson performs AK on the patients who want it. "Some people say 'At all costs I don't want a knife in my eye.' For them, they can be in an APRK study, or go to Canada, or wait."

What About ALK for Astigmatism?

I attended a seminar not too long ago in which doctors were promoting ALK for the treatment of astigmatism. "We just remove the cap, cut a little elliptical disk out of the center of the cornea, and drop the cap back on." (See Chapter 15 for a more complete description of ALK.)

I ran this idea past a number of my experts and they all agreed that ALK for astigmatism isn't predictable, it exposes the patient to more risk than is necessary, and it usually doesn't work. "ALK is *not* a treatment for astigmatism," Dr. Lindstrom said with finality, summing up the feelings of the group.

A Word on Astigmatic LASIK

For doctors who support LASIK for myopia and hyperopia (see Chapter 15), using the laser to remove astigmatism is a natural progression, if they have the software on their lasers to do it. Again, LASIK is highly dependent on the skills of the individual doctor and there are no long-term studies of its predictability, effectiveness or safety in treating any form of vision problem. All the known risks of LASIK apply as well as the benefits of fast visual recovery and little discomfort.

If you opt for LASIK to treat your myopia or hyperopia, it makes a world of sense to have your astigmatism dealt with at the same time, before the cap is put back in place. Except in cases of extreme astigmatism, however, having Astigmatic LASIK as a touch-up procedure, or by itself, is not worth the risks, given that there are effective, less-invasive, alternatives.

UPDATE   The day before this book went to press, the FDA Ophthalmic Devices Panel recommended approval of the VISX Star laser for the treatment of astigmatism. The FDA panel based its recommendation on data gathered from hundreds of patient cases at five clinical trial sites in the U.S. as well as from controlled studies in Canada and the United Kingdom. Mark Logan, CEO of VISX said, "The VISX laser for the treatment of astigmatism will give consumers a safe alternative to AK, an invasive surgical technique. With well over 50% of the nearsighted population having some degree of astigmatism, I think it is safe to assume that final FDA approval will lead to greater consumer satisfaction and an increase in the overall number of procedures performed in the U.S."

AK PATIENTS GIVE THEIR REPORT

Some of the patients whose PRK cases are reported in other chapters had APRK at the same time. On the following pages are the reports of two patients who were treated successfully with AK. One had AK during PRK. The other had AK more than a year after PRK.

FAITH IN HIS OWN PR

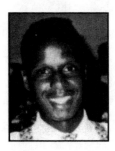

Name
Byron Tucker, 30

Occupation
Public relations executive,
California

Pre-Op Vision
-3.0 with
3.0 astigmatism

-3.75 with
1.75 astigmatism

Procedures
PRK/AK

Post-Op Vision
20/20, 20/30

Surgeon
Robert Maloney, MD

Byron Tucker came to PRK through his job: He handled the announcement of the FDA's approval of PRK for the Jules Stein Eye Institute at UCLA, which was a trial site. At the time we spoke, Mr. Tucker's first eye was four months post-op and his second eye had been treated just two weeks prior to our conversation.

"I already knew about PRK, because I had written the materials for the announcement. Then I went to the Bahamas and it really struck me that there was so much I couldn't do on the spur of the moment because I was afraid I'd lose my contacts in the water. If I wanted to go scuba diving or water skiing, I'd have to go all the way back to my room and get my glasses.

"Basketball was another problem because sweat was always getting in my eyes and messing up the contact lenses.

"Other than this, I was satisfied with contacts: I put them in and took them out every day for 15 years without a problem except for sports and the fact that I lost at least 4-5 pairs of lenses a year during college.

"But PRK has made a tremendous improvement to my life, and not just in sports. Even during the period between eyes when I had to wear one contact lens, I noticed a big change. It took so much less time in the morning to get ready for work. My bathroom cabinets are much neater now without all the little bottles of cleaner. I save all that money on lens solutions.

"After both eyes I was able to see 20/30 within two days. My first eye is 20/20 now. With my second eye I'm already at 20/30 and it has only been two weeks.

A Good Way to Wreck an Evening   "I had a little bit of trouble with recovery after the first eye. After the procedure my mom came over to cook for me and I went to taste something right from the pan. I don't know if it was steam or pepper, but something got in my eye and so I took off the bandage lens. Only someone who has done this knows what it feels like.

"Dr. Maloney said I could come in for a new lens, but I was in so much pain, I didn't want to go through a drive all the way back to L.A. in rush-hour traffic. I thought I could tough it out. So I just suffered from about 3 p.m. until 9:30 the next morning. I don't know if the AK incisions made this worse than it would have been with PRK alone, but it was brutal. I didn't want anyone to talk to me or even look at me!

"When I went in the next morning, Dr. Maloney put in a new lens and some anesthetic and the pain just disappeared. But for about two weeks that eye was extremely sensitive to light. I had to wear two pairs of sunglasses to drive and I had problems seeing the computer at work.

A Different Story "The second eye was a piece of cake. While I was focusing on the light during the procedure, it got clearer and clearer. I sat up and could see immediately. There was no pain at all except, strangely, I had a tingling sensation on the fourth day. I didn't even mention it to the doctor, though—it was nothing to cry about. Yesterday when I was in line to renew my driver's license, I noticed I could read the 20/30 line in the vision test from about double the distance.

"What advice do I have for someone who's thinking about it? Get the procedure done late in the day so you can just go to sleep. Shop ahead of time, don't cook, and whatever you do, don't take out the bandage lens!"

AR - RESTED OFFICER

Name
Joyce Puckett, 44

Occupation
Police dispatcher,
reserve officer,
California

Pre-Op Vision
-5.0 with
2.0 astigmatism

Procedure
PRK/AK

Post-Op Vision
20/30, 20/25

Surgeon
Robert Maloney, MD

Joyce Puckett was part of the FDA Phase III clinical trials for PRK. Her first eye was treated in late '94 and the second eye treated a year later. As discussed in Chapter 11, doctors in the FDA trials were not allowed to use a bandage contact lens or anti-inflammatory drops to prevent pain. The only way they could treat post-op swelling, which can cause severe pain, was with an eye patch and pain medications.

"I had been interested in PRK ever since I first heard about it. One day my brother told me he knew of someone who was part of a study at UCLA. I made the call the same day and it turned out I was one of the very last candidates they accepted into the FDA trials.

"I was legally blind without glasses, but I felt handicapped *with* them! Glasses kept me from becoming a police officer, which is what I always wanted to do. I went into the technical reserves but because of my vision, I couldn't receive training in firearms, driving, or use of force.

"I wore contacts for about 12 years—I was very young and very *vain*, so I was willing to put up with the hassle, but when it got to the point that I was working two jobs, my eyes just got very tired. So I switched to glasses for about a year. When I went back for new contacts, I couldn't seem to get a pair that were comfortable, and I just didn't have the motivation to keep trying. It was too much trouble.

Lazy Days   "I had my first eye done very early in the morning and the doctor gave me Valium beforehand and Demerol to take after. I went home with the eye patch on, went to bed and slept all day and night. I pretty much babied myself. My boyfriend, my mom and my sister all came to wait on me hand and foot— and I took advantage of it! I didn't do anything for four days except sleep and eat.

"I had very little discomfort except the first day. When they took the patch off the next day I could see much, much better than I ever had before. By the third day I was fully recovered. I was seeing pretty well out of that eye but I was constantly testing it and I knew it wasn't quite perfect. It took about three months to get to 20/20.

"Then in January of '95 we had the L.A. earthquake and I was on special duty for months, so I had to put off getting my second eye done. I wore a pair of glasses with no prescription over the eye that had been treated. Finally I was able to schedule the second eye.

Staying Conscious "Dr. Maloney's office called me one day shortly after I made the appointment and said they had an earlier opening—did I want my second eye done two weeks sooner? My family was out of town and I was taking care of my sister's dogs, but I thought 'Hey, what the heck.' My boyfriend took me in, brought me home, and went back to work. That first day I slept.

"The next morning, after my eye was unpatched, I noticed my sister's dog was acting strange. I was afraid to drive, but I didn't want to chance anything happening to her dog, so I stopped taking pain pills and made a vet appointment for a few hours later. Then I put on two pairs of sunglasses, put the dog in the truck and drove six miles to the vet. When I got home I realized I had done it without a problem. So I didn't take any more pain medicine and just went back to work. Now I realize that it was the pain medication that kept me in bed so long after the first eye!

"Quite honestly, you really don't need all that strong medication." She's right, and today most patients take a non-aspirin pain reliever, such as Tylenol, or nothing.

"Six months later, Dr. Maloney performed an AK to treat astigmatism in my first eye. Then he put in a bandage lens, and I was out driving a few hours later. It was just super. For a couple of days my eye felt a little dry, but there was no pain at all.

"My message to other people is do it! PRK has changed my life. It has given me more confidence and I can do more now. When I was a kid I always felt ugly because of my glasses. Now I feel just like anyone else."

17

Monovision: Having Your Cake and Seeing It Too

*I*f you are nearsighted and 35 or older, or farsighted and need lenses to see both near *and* far, this chapter will help you understand an important option you should discuss with your doctor *before* you have your vision treated.

Presbyopia, inability to focus up close, eventually affects nearly everyone, so doctors are trying to solve it. All the procedures described in Chapters 14, 15 and 18 can be used to compensate for presbyopia. They include:

- For the nearsighted: PRK, RK, implantable contact lenses, intrastromal cornea ring segments and LASIK.
- For the farsighted: HPRK, HH, H-LASIK, implantable contact lenses and clear lens extraction, all discussed in the next chapter.

What's so Bad About Reading Glasses?

If you're a fairly inactive person who stays in one place and spends most of your time reading or doing near-vision tasks, having to wear reading glasses probably isn't a bother. You just put them on and forget about them.

QUICK REVIEW   Presbyopia is the age-related inability to bring close-in or small objects into focus. Loss of focusing ability begins at birth but usually doesn't make itself felt until sometime after the age of 40. A very few lucky people never lose the ability to read fine print while others (especially the farsighted) have difficulties much earlier.

If you're like me, however, it's not quite that easy. You spend your day visually jumping from the computer to the phone book to the freeway, and physically jumping from house to yard, office to restaurant and car to plane. Wherever you go, your glasses are supposed to follow. But do they? If you're becoming presbyopic and wear contacts, consider how many times you have needed reading glasses and didn't have them handy for:

- Setting your alarm clock
- Reading a menu
- Dialing the phone
- Seeing a map or directions at night in the car
- Figuring out which of your prescription bottles contains which medicine
- Seeing your flight or seat information on an airline ticket
- Removing a splinter from your hand or foot
- Reading the cooking directions on a food package
- Figuring out what channel a program you wanted to watch was on.
- Reading a magazine in a waiting room
- Reading dosage instructions on medications and pesticides
- Sewing a button back on
- Reading a theater program
- Changing the connections on your computer, video or stereo system
- Adjusting the thermostat or sprinkler timer
- Reading the nutrition information on packages in the grocery store
- Doing any close-in task upstairs when your glasses are downstairs, or *vice versa*.

You get the drift, I'm sure. There are times when being unable to see up close is more than an irksome inconvenience. During my brief life as a presbyope I fantasized about launching a national initiative to ban light blue print on over-the-counter medicine bottles and force disposable reading glasses to be packaged with everything that had print less than a half-inch high.

I'm serious (sort of). My worst experience was the day my oven caught on fire and I couldn't read the directions on the fire extinguisher. Luckily a box of baking soda solved the problem before the fire cured my presbyopia once and for all!

About 20% of the population never has to confront the issue of glasses until they reach fortysomething. Then their arms just seem to get shorter with every passing year.

"You read it. I don't have my glasses."

—Sean Connery to Nicholas Cage in *The Rock*

For the rest of us, myopes and hyperopes alike, presbyopia adds insult to disability: If we wear contacts, we either need to go back for a monovision fit or we have to add reading glasses. If we wear glasses, then we're talking about bifocals, trifocals or progressive lenses.

When Will You Need Reading Glasses?

As Chapter 5 explained in some depth, losing the ability to focus on small printed words on a page is natural and usually begins to be noticeable around the age of 40-45.

In order to read, someone with no refractive error (0.0) either needs natural focusing power of two diopters, which she probably has if she's under 40, or she will need to make up the difference with magnifying glasses. The older she gets, the stronger the glasses will need to be.

On the other hand, someone with -2.0 myopia is naturally focused at about 20"—fine for reading, but legally blind without glasses for distance. When he begins to lose focusing ability, he can simply remove his distance glasses and read just fine. If he wears contacts, that's harder to do.

Farsighted people tend to need reading glasses sooner than anyone because their eyes have to focus for reading even when they are young.

Who'll Be the Last to Go?

Some people need reading glasses sooner than others. You'll keep your focusing ability longer if you:

- Avoid reading through a "distance" prescription: Many optometrists believe that this can overtax the focusing muscles because it forces the eye muscles to pull images into focus that otherwise could be seen without focusing. The stronger the distance prescription, the more focusing ability you need in order to read. If your nearsightedness is increasing with every new pair of glasses and you are reading with your distance glasses on, these doctors believe you might be creating permanent strain on your focusing muscles (see Chapter 5).

- Don't wear reading glasses if you don't have to. Doctors tell patients that the longer they can stand to go without help reading, the longer they'll be able to read without help.
- Don't have refractive surgery. As other chapters have pointed out, having your vision corrected doesn't *cause* presbyopia but it does create the effect of reading through a distance prescription, which puts extra demand on your focusing ability. If this ability is starting to weaken before you have surgery, you *might* need reading glasses after it unless you go for monovision or end up with a multifocal cornea (see below).
- Don't inherit the wrong genes. There are people who can read just fine without glasses all their lives. Pick two of them for your parents and you might never need reading glasses!

THE MONOVISION OPTION

Monovision is a way to compensate for near-vision problems without reading glasses. Not everyone is a candidate for this, but some contact lens wearers have had monovision prescriptions for decades, sidestepping the need for bifocals and trifocals by wearing only one contact lens, or by wearing one with a "distance" prescription and the other with a "reading" prescription. The same effect can be achieved with PRK for some patients if it is planned for as part of the treatment.

Two-Eyed Vision *vs* Monovision

When our two eyes work together harmoniously, we have "stereoscopic" vision—an important element of depth perception. Each eye records an image from two slightly different angles, the brain puts them together for us, and that's how we can tell if one object is in front of another or if one is moving faster than the other.

USE IT OR LOSE IT   This slogan applies to the eye's focusing power as much as it does to your quadriceps. The longer you can go without reading glasses, the longer you'll be able to read without them. At some point the inconvenience of reading glasses gets balanced against the pain of eyestrain and most people succumb to bifocals, trifocals, dime-store readers and half-glasses. Monovision is a way around the entire problem.

Now, let's say you have a contact in one eye and see 20/20 with it, and you put a contact in your other eye which only lets it see 20/30. Ideally, your brain will adjust rapidly to the difference in acuity and automatically use the 20/20 eye for distance vision and the other eye for seeing up close. That's *monovision* —using one eye for distance and the other eye for near—and it's an option you should consider, along with its effect on depth perception, before you have PRK or another vision-correction procedure.

Some people are naturally mono-sighted and don't understand what the fuss is all about. You'll hear some of them bragging at parties that they are 55 and don't need reading glasses. Dr. Steinert says most of these people have at least one slightly nearsighted eye with some mild astigmatism which increases their depth of focus.

Those of us who rely on glasses or contacts typically don't experience monovision unless a doctor suggests it to us, because doctors usually attempt to correct both eyes to 20/20—or as close to it as possible.

Patients who wear contacts are natural candidates for monovision, however: the doctor simply prescribes a full correction lens for the distance eye and a slightly lower-correction lens for the reading eye. If the patient is lucky enough to have natural 20/20 vision in one or both eyes, the doctor can prescribe a 20/25 contact only for one eye.

The same effect can be achieved with PRK and other techniques. Sometimes it works, and sometimes the patient keeps right on improving in the "reading" eye to 20/20 or better. Even then, the patient might be able read.

It is very difficult to achieve comfortable monovision with glasses: the lenses in the glasses are too far out in front of the cornea, and this tends to exaggerate the difference between the powers of the lenses.

The Secret to Enjoying Monovision
Three factors affect whether you will be able to tolerate monovision:
1) Visual balance: The difference in vision between the two eyes should be very small. The larger the difference, the more "out of balance" you will feel. An ideal monovision correction would be 20/20 in one eye and 20/25 or 20/30 in the other.
2) Eye dominance: Monovision seems to work best in people who have no strong dominance in one eye or the other. If one eye is dominant, it usually is corrected for distance and the non-dominant eye is left, or made, slightly nearsighted for reading.

WHAT IT TAKES TO SEE 3-D

We don't need vision in both eyes to be aware of depth—just as we see depth in photographs and art. But true stereoscopic vision is like watching a 3-D movie: light from an object enters each eye slightly differently, producing slightly different images—a more complete picture, in other words.

Two-dimensional depth perception works best when the objects or environments are familiar, because we know the sizes of objects in reality. That's why we can look at images in a photo or on a television or movie screen and perceive them as having three dimensions: our mind fills in the missing information from our experience. Our experience also guides us in the real world: When something appears to be small that we know in reality is very large—like a tanker ship—our brain tells us it's far away, even if it is alone on the horizon and we have nothing else to compare it to. By knowing the sizes of objects and how they look from different angles, we can rapidly calculate where they are in relation to each other and ourselves.

This is what two-eyed vision gives us: the ability to gauge where objects are in relation to each other and us. If you were to cover one eye, chances are you could get along pretty well once you adjusted for a few minutes. You might bump into some walls, but your experience with the way objects really are would help you judge *where* they are. Driving or operating equipment would be harder because the brain has to make detailed calculations very rapidly. With only half the input, the conclusions you would make might leave your car looking a little worse for wear, to say the least.

---

3) Individual adaptation: There is no way of knowing ahead of time who will be happy with monovision and who won't. In addition, lifestyle factors, such as the need for good depth perception on the job, could influence whether monovision is right for you. But you can try out monovision before you have PRK (see below).

Understanding Eye Dominance

Most of us have a dominant hand and a dominant foot. You can test for foot dominance just by dropping a ball in front of you and kicking it. Chances are you'll kick it with your dominant foot.

Most of us also have a rotational dominance—we are more comfortable spinning in one direction than the other. You can see this in action in any skating rink: People in North America, at least, prefer to—or learn to—rotate to the left, so when the guy up in the booth calls out "Reverse direction," arms start windmilling and former hotshots suddenly look very awkward. It just so happens, and perhaps not coincidentally, that our rotational preference is the same as the direction water swirls when it goes down the drain north of the equator. I'd like to know whether skating rinks south of the equator require people to skate in circles to the right.

We chew with one side of our mouths more than the other, and we tend to sleep on one side more comfortably. With all these distinct preferences, then, it isn't surprising that most of us also have a dominant eye.

Do You Have a Dominant Eye?

You can test yourself to find out if you have a dominant eye:

1) Make a "telescope" out of your hands by putting one partially closed fist on top of the other, then hold it up about 20 inches out in front of your eyes.

2) Now look through it and aim it at some small object across the room. Center the object through it with both eyes open.

3) When you have the object perfectly centered, close your left eye without moving your hands. Is the object still centered in your telescope or did it appear to jump to one side? If you can see the object through the telescope with your right eye, most likely you are right-eye dominant.

Try it with the right eye closed. Now start over with other objects; if you have a dominant eye, the object will always be centered when you are looking at it with that eye open.

If neither eye is dominant, you might find the object jumping no matter which eye you close, or the object might appear centered with either eye. Having no strong eye dominance makes adjusting to monovision easier.

As a final test, pick up a normal camera (not a video camera) and look through the viewfinder. Which eye did you use? That's probably your dominant eye. I was amazed to see how difficult it was to look through a viewfinder with my nondominant eye. Try it.

WHICH EYE DO YOU PREFER?   Dr. Roger Steinert told me that our dominant eye usually is on the same side as our dominant hand, but this is not an accurate test of eye dominance. "If doctors rely on handedness alone to determine eye dominance, many patients will end up unhappy with monovision," he cautioned.

Why Eye Dominance Can Matter
The dominant eye is the one we use to do most of our vision work, and this usually isn't a problem. In some people, one eye is so dominant that a cataract or some other vision problem can develop in the nondominant eye and go unnoticed until that eye is almost blind—just one more reason to get your eyes checked every year!

When one eye is so dominant that the other one, which is perfectly capable of seeing, stops working altogether, the result is a childhood condition called "lazy eye" or *amblyopia* which ultimately can result in blindness in the nondominant eye if it isn't quickly diagnosed and treated (usually by patching the dominant eye).

With monovision, the dominant eye usually is corrected for distance—because that's the one most people seem to prefer—and the other eye is undercorrected for reading, which requires less depth of focus.

When the Nondominant Eye Is Better for Distance Vision
In some cases it is better to correct the nondominant eye for distance:
- When the dominant eye is 20/30 or 20/25 and the nondominant eye is much more nearsighted or farsighted, it might be possible to treat only the nondominant eye. If the patient isn't comfortable with this after a few weeks, the dominant eye can be fully corrected.
- If your job requires you to look in one direction for near or distant viewing, that should be taken into consideration. For example, a data-entry clerk who places material to be typed on the right side of his desk might want the right eye treated for near vision.
- If most of your time is spent doing close-in work, you might prefer your dominant eye for near vision.

Other Considerations
In addition to lifestyle and eye dominance questions, your doctor will consider your individual vision. A high degree of astigmatism, for example, might caution against a monovision correction.

Monovision for the Farsighted
It works the same way. The only difference is that one eye is *over*corrected—made a little nearsighted—rather than undercorrected. The other eye is corrected to as close to 20/20 as possible.

THE FDA LOOKS AT MONOVISION In 1994 the FDA decided monovision contact lenses were safe and effective. Their approval included a warning that monovision "might not be optimal" for:

1) Visually demanding situations such as operating dangerous machinery or performing other hazardous activities; and
2) Driving (especially at night). If patients cannot pass drivers' license vision tests with monovision correction, they should not drive with this correction or they should add glasses when they drive.[1]

WHO CAN LIVE WITH MONOVISION?

Doctors have told me that the best candidates for monovision tend to be between the ages of 40 and 55. After about age 55 the "reading eye" needs to be so much weaker than the "distance" eye that the imbalance can cause visual discomfort and loss of stereopsis—depth perception.

If you're not yet 40, you might not understand what the fuss is all about. Before he had PRK, Dr. Steinert had to teach himself what lack of focusing ability meant by using a contact lens which made him slightly farsighted. "Then I could appreciate what it's like not to be able to read." As a result, Dr. Steinert planned his PRK treatment to include monovision and doesn't expect this to create problems in his work. "When I perform microsurgery, where perfect 3-D vision is necessary, I can adjust the microscope to compensate for the undercorrected eye." Dr. Steinert's wife, on the other hand, is a dentist who specializes in root canal therapy and doesn't use a microscope. "When I did her PRK last year, she insisted on full distance correction in both eyes."

Dr. Lin said that about 80% of his patients who request a monovision correction with PRK are happy with it. The rest ask to be retreated so that both eyes have the same vision. "If a patient has tried monovision with contacts and liked it, chances are she'll like it with PRK."

Try Before You Buy

If you can tolerate contact lenses, you can easily find out whether you might like monovision by asking your eye doctor to fit you with some inexpensive monovision contacts or to give you a weaker lens for your nondominant eye. Then test the effects, first in the doctor's office and then in a familiar environment.

Some people react instantly even to the tiniest imbalance in their vision: they get headaches, nausea, lose their balance and feel basically "out of whack." Unless you fall into this group, give yourself a couple of weeks to adjust—it can take that long. Try to wear the lenses all day, except when you drive, because switching from monovision to single vision is an even bigger challenge for the brain. During this adjustment period don't drive with the monovision lens: Swap with a perfect distance lens or ask your doctor to prescribe compensating glasses for driving. Once you're used to monovision, you probably won't need them.

If you still experience eyestrain or poor depth perception, but are motivated to try a little harder, ask your optometrist to reverse the prescriptions—making your nondominant eye the "distance" eye. Sometimes this works. If it doesn't, give it up: The rewards won't be worth the discomfort—especially as you lose all your ability to focus.

Is the Contacts Test 100% Accurate?

Dr. Mihai Pop advises patients who are interested in monovision to do a small trial with contacts before deciding, but he warns them that this test isn't a perfect predictor of how they'll feel with monovision after PRK. "Monovision with contacts can be easier than permanent monovision," he said, "because you can remove the contacts and let the eye rest. Monovision twenty-four hours a day can create fatigue. The greater the difference between the two eyes, the greater this effect."

What Are the Chances Monovision Will Work for You?

A recent one-year study of patients fitted with monovision contact lenses found that 53% were successfully wearing the contacts at the end of the year. Of these, 63% were able to see 20/25 or better in *both* eyes *despite* the fact that one eye was undercorrected. 82% passed reading vision tests with flying colors.[2]

Nearly 60% of the patients had reduced contrast sensitivity in their near vision, but only about 20% had a loss of contrast sensitivity in their distance vision. 14 patients gave up on monovision because of poor distance vision, 14 gave up because of poor near vision, and four gave up because of "ghosted" images.

The Trade-offs: What Do You *Really* Want to See?

Monovision requires compromise: you give up a little distance acuity in order to gain the ability to read without glasses. For 25-year-olds, this compromise isn't worth the price—they would be giving up 20 years of great distance vision when they still have the focusing powers to read. For a 45-year-old, the compromise makes more sense.

Dr. Richard Lindstrom tells his patients, "If you're 20, go for 20/20. If you're 40, you should take into consideration the near demands and consider leaving one eye a little nearsighted."

But if you have a job or hobby that requires great depth perception (such as skeetshooting), or fantastic contrast sensitivity (such as trout fishing), you should think twice about trying for permanent monovision.

Dr. Lindstrom says that monovision patients are more prone to night-induced myopia (see Chapter 11) because they don't have full distance acuity to start with. This can be solved by wearing weak distance glasses for driving at night.

What if You Change Your Mind Later?
Happily, patients who try monovision with PRK and find they don't like it can be retreated with little discomfort and usually great success. Such a small amount has to be "dusted" off the cornea, that the healing period is very fast. There should be few side effects and even fewer complications. Most doctors offer retreatments at no charge if they are done within the first year. Be forewarned, however, that "taking just a little off" can result in taking too much off—overcorrection. The decision to retreat has to take this risk into consideration.

Going the other direction—having your eyes corrected perfectly for distance and then later (when you're older) having one eye treated for monovision—is becoming more of a viable option every year (see below).

Ultimately, I believe, safe, effective procedures will eliminate the need for anyone to wear glasses or contacts at any age, for any reason.

Multifocal Corneas: An Accident by Design
The nature of the PRK procedure—which removes more tissue in the center of the treatment zone (flattening it) and less around the edges (steepening it)—can have the effect of creating a bifocal cornea.

When this effect coincides with the right pupil size and the right placement of the steeper/flatter sections, the patient can read and see into the distance with the same eye *without* using any, or very little, focusing ability.

This happens in about 25-30% of PRK cases, according to Dr. Mihai Pop. RK can have the same effect, by causing the periphery of the cornea to be steeper than the center.

Giorgio Dorin of Sunrise Technologies believes that the holmium laser treatments (see Chapter 18) can be used predictably and safely to create multifocal corneas either on mildly farsighted eyes or on those with no refractive error.

"After treatment with the holmium, the cornea is steeper in the 3- to 6-millimeter zone than it is in the very center. The patient potentially can read with the outer edges and see into the distance with the center," Mr. Dorin said.

ON THE HORIZON: NEW CURES FOR PRESBYOPIA

In addition to PRK and the newer holmium laser treatments, doctors in seven countries are experimenting with an incisional cure for presbyopia. In this procedure, called anterior ciliary sclerotomy, short incisions are cut into the white part (sclera) of the eye just outside the boundary between the cornea/ iris and the sclera. Researchers believe that the incisions help relax the sclera, which tightens up during the aging process, and provide more room for the eye's focusing components. Clinical trials will determine whether the effects of this surgery are predictable, effective and safe.

IT WORKED FOR ME

I think I have a multifocal cornea in one eye, because I can read perfectly without glasses until I'm in low-light conditions—probably because then my pupil dilates beyond the section that the eye uses to see close up, and my near vision blurs.

I'm grateful for the near vision I now have, however, because I've experienced what it's like to be unable to read without glasses: I was losing focusing ability by the diopter in the months before I had PRK.

First, I had to take my distance glasses off to read: All day long, it was on-off, on-off. Then I began to have trouble focusing on the computer screen, so I tried monovision with contacts and had instant success. Unfortunately, I couldn't wear the contacts! Progressive bifocals are what drove me to PRK.

I requested monovision with my PRK and it was attempted. But to undercorrect my left eye, my doctor had to leave a little astigmatism behind, because to remove it would have made the eye too close to 20/20. As a result, I have some double vision in that eye—which causes blurring only in my near vision when I close the other eye. My distance vision in the undercorrected eye is 20/25.

For the first few months after PRK I was disappointed because I still couldn't read without glasses, but as my right eye began to heal fully, I found my reading vision improving every week. At six months the eye was 20/20 and I could read without glasses. It wasn't until I began talking with doctors for this book that I learned about the multi-focal effects of PRK.

Not a Cure for Eyestrain   But reading printed material is only half the battle for someone who works at a computer; writing this book taught me that. The first day after I spent 18 hours at the computer, my eyes began to burn, tear and ache. The second day I began feeling nauseated and thought I was getting the flu. A friend suggested it might be eyestrain (a novel concept, since I was writing a book on vision!) so I wondered if it was my residual astigmatism causing the problem.

I ran out to one of those one-hour glasses stores and had them put some lenses that would correct only my astigmatism in an old pair of frames. This made the situation much worse. In fact, my computer table looked crooked and I started getting headaches. The optician said that it would take time to adjust, but I didn't want to wear the glasses for anything but working at my computer. Finally I tossed the new $60 lenses onto my glasses "bonepile" where they will make their way to the Lion's collection box.

By that time I was certain my eyes were at the center of the problem and I was desperate: Two months to deadline and I couldn't stand to write more than 15 minutes at a time! By trial and error I worked out an eight-step solution that I still use whenever I have to work long hours at the computer. Perhaps it will work for you.

As I write this it has been six weeks and I dont have much eyestrain— even though I've worked 72-hour stretches twice a week since my first bout with the problem. I remove the reading glasses whenever I turn away from the computer, because I don't want to become dependent on them. I plan to have the residual astigmatism in my nondominant eye corrected and keep my fingers crossed that the multifocal cornea in my right eye will be enough to allow me to read.

EIGHT-STEP PROGRAM FOR AVOIDING COMPUTER EYESTRAIN

1) Wear a pair of the weakest possible reading glasses *only* when using the computer.

2) Bump up the size of the type on the screen to 14 points. You can bump it back down again before you save or print the file.

3) If you have a window, minimize glare on the screen by angling the office blinds closed in the daytime.

4) Turn off any lights that shine directly down on the monitor.

5) Raise the monitor up on so your eyes are more in direct line with it.

6) Rest your eyes every half hour by covering them with your hands and looking into the darkness.

7) Raise your blinds and look out the window whenever you talk on the phone or stop to read, or at least try to gaze into the far distance to allow your focusing muscles to relax.

8) Take tasks that you can do away from your desk outdoors if at all possible so you can get some natural light every now and then. I did all m y editing while walking on the local bike trail (yes, it is possible to read, write and walk at the same time).

New Treatments
for Farsightedness

A permanent cure for farsightedness has been slower coming than ones for nearsightedness, but it hasn't been for lack of effort. Doctors have used every method described in this book—and others— in an attempt to solve the vexing problem of making the human eye optically longer or making its focusing powers stronger.

Believe me, the medical community is motivated to help, because there are many more farsighted folk in the population than there are nearsighted. According to one report, about 60% of the U.S. citizenry has more than one diopter of farsightedness.[1]

It's easier to take material away from the cornea than to add more to it. As a result, solutions for hyperopia have focused on steepening the curvature of the eye rather than lengthening the distance between the tear film and the retina. A steeper cornea bends light at more of an angle, which can bring light waves to a sharper focus on the retina.

Some methods for achieving this have worked better than others, but none have been entirely satisfactory. More often than not, the treatment either undercorrects, causes an overcorrection to nearsightedness, or the effects regress over time.

QUICK REVIEW   Farsightedness, or hyperopia, is caused by an eye that effectively is too short or too flat. As described in Chapter 5, light waves enter the eye but aren't bent at enough of an angle, so they never come to focus on the retina. This can cause blurring of both near and far objects.

Happily, lasers have put the medical world right on the brink of solving this problem. Even better, many of the cures are non-invasive and relatively risk-free. So even while the fine points of treatments are being worked out, patients who enroll in trials for the non-incisional procedures stand a good chance of improving their vision and probably won't end up worse off than they are today.

WHAT'S BEEN AVAILABLE UNTIL NOW?

Outside clinical trials or experimental treatments in Canada and other countries, there really have been only two alternatives for solving hyperopia. Both involve incisions and risk.

Hyperopic ALK

Hyperopic ALK uses a combination suction/cutting tool called the "microkeratome" to cut a cap off the front of the cornea. Doctors make a deeper cut for hyperopic treatments than with ALK for nearsightedness—about 60% of the total thickness of the cornea—but they don't have to cut anything out of the underlying cornea: They simply lift up the cap and put it back down.

The procedure works by weakening the center of the cornea so that the pressure inside the eye causes it to bulge out, effectively steepening the curve

Dr. Richard Lindstrom believes that ALK for moderate degrees of hyperopia (+1.0 - +4.0) can be effectivE, but a major problem with ALK for hyperopia is that doctors can't control the degree of steepening. "ALK for hyperopia, even when it is done by the best surgeons in the world, is extremely unpredictable," said Dr. James Salz. "I've seen patients after hyperopic ALK who started out at +3.0 and ended up at -9.0." In other words, they started out moderately farsighted and ended up extremely nearsighted.

"Patients are putting themselves at risk of long-term instability," Dr. Salz continued. "The eye bulges in the center and becomes nearsighted because it becomes more curved. That might be OK in the short term, but the long-term results show that the eyes continue to bulge. That's why many of the surgeons who started doing ALK for hyperopia have stopped."

In addition, because microkeratomes are not 100% accurate, caps can be cut too deep, resulting in myopia or irregular astigmatism. An article published by the American Academy of Ophthalmology in May 1996 said that Dr. Luis Ruiz of Bogota, the world's leading expert in surgical cures for hyperopia, had "performed more than 200 cornea transplants to correct [the problems caused by ALK] in his patients." [2]

Hyperopic ALK is subject to the same risks as ALK for nearsightedness and LASIK—(see Chapter 15).

Hyperopic Incisions

Efforts have been made to use cuts into the cornea to correct hyperopia, usually in a hexagonal pattern around the periphery. The trouble with this approach is its unpredictability coupled with the known risks of incisional surgery.

According to Dr. Vance Thompson, incisional procedures to steepen the cornea have "horrible results. They just don't work."

LASER TREATMENTS FOR HYPEROPIA

Just as for nearsightedness, the future that doctors are working on now involves either laser treatments or incisional treatments, or a combination of both.

Hyperopic PRK (HPRK)

Hyperopic PRK is performed with the excimer laser—so all the benefits of its precision apply (see Chapter 6).

How HPRK Works

The two laser manufacturers approved for PRK use different approaches to achieving the same result: a cornea that is steeper in the center and flatter toward the sides. Both methods are identical to PRK for nearsightedness from the patient's point of view, so all the information in Part II is relevant to patients considering HPRK.

The Erodable-Mask Method

With this method, a disk of polymer plastic is attached to the lens of the laser beam. When the laser is pulsed, the energy in the center of the beam is absorbed by the plastic, but the outer perimeter of the beam is absorbed by the cornea (Figure 18.1). This has the effect of creating a gradually deepening channel about 6.5 millimeters from the center of the cornea. Another pass of the laser transitions the treatment zone out to 9.5 millimeters.

STILL IN TRIALS IN THE USA   Hyperopic PRK is rapidly working its way through FDA trials in the U.S. In Canada, doctors have been refining the procedure over the last two years. Both U.S. laser manufacturers sell HPRK systems to all countries outside the U.S.

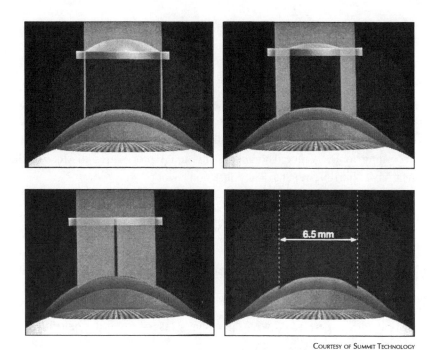

FIGURE 18.1   As this 4-stage animation demonstrates, the erodable mask technique allows most of the laser energy to be absorbed in the 6.5-millimeter zone with a transition from the inner and outer edges of the treatment zone.

The Scanning Method of HPRK

With this method, an off-centered beam is projected through a slit in the laser's aperture and rotated in a revolving pattern.

As the beam scans around the periphery of the cornea, it creates an ablation which is gradually transitioned toward the pupil and toward the outer edges of the cornea. This has the effect of steepening the center of the cornea, which then allows the tear film to refract light at a steeper angle (Figure 18.2).

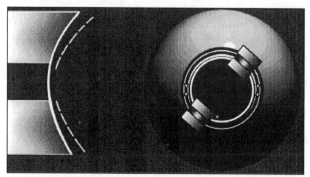

FIGURE 18.2   The scanning method rotates the beam in a circular pattern.

How Well Does HPRK Work?

A very encouraging study of HPRK on 15 eyes ranging from +2.0 to +7.5 demonstrated that at the end of a year 80% had achieved 20/40 or better and twelve were within one diopter of perfect refraction. There was no loss of best-corrected acuity.[3]

Summit presents one-year data on five patients who were an average of +4.0 prior to HPRK. The first month after surgery patients were a little nearsighted (-1.0) but over 3-6 months they regressed towards 0.0 and their vision held "relatively stable" through the end of their first year.

In October of 1995, Dr. Bruce Jackson together with two other doctors performed the first 25 hyperopic procedures on normal sighted eyes using the VISX Star excimer laser. "Patients were between +1.0 and +4.0. At the end of six months, 80% had 20/25 vision or better and 2 had 20/40 or better. Initially the eyes were slightly overcorrected to allow for regression during the first four months," Dr. Jackson said. "All the patients in the study want their second eyes treated."

Dr. Donald Johnson has used four different lasers for HPRK to treat patients from +1.0 to +7.5. "I have been quite happy with the results we've obtained using a narrow scanning laser beam and two passes. This creates a very smooth transition between the treatment zone and the untreated portions of the cornea," Dr. Johnson said. "The intrastromal lasers [see below] might even be a better way to go, because we won't have to remove the epithelium."

At the time I spoke with him, Dr. Mihai Pop had performed about 100 HPRKs in patients with farsightedness up to +6.0. "We don't have long-term follow-up data on these patients yet. We know we've been able to get them very safely to 20/20 or close, but we don't know if the effects will regress over time."

Dr. Michael Gordon said, "International results on HPRK are excellent. I think it's going to prove to be a very worthwhile procedure."

Recovery after HPRK

Dr. Lindstrom said that in his early trials of HPRK, "many patients achieved 20/40 results on the first day with no pain."

Epithelial healing after hyperopic PRK takes a little longer than myopic PRK, according to Dr. Jackson. "About 50% of the patients were healed by Day Three and the other half by Day Four." Bandage lenses were not used with these patients, however, so that could have affected results. Nearsighted patients treated with the bandage lens usually are healed within the first two days. Also, in HPRK a 33% wider treatment zone is used, so more epithelium is removed and has to grow back.

"Downtime is getting shorter for all the laser procedures," Dr. Jackson added. "Visual recovery is getting faster, patients are much more comfortable. There's no reason we won't see this trend continue."

Side Effects and Complications

Most of the side effects and complications that occur with PRK for nearsightedness (see chapter 11) also can occur with HPRK, but because most of the tissue removal during HPRK occurs outside the central visual area, there is less of a risk that haze will interfere with vision.

The primary difficulty with HPRK could be the same that has plagued other attempts to cure hyperopia: regression of effect. The cornea likes to heal itself, and to the extent it rebuilds, the steepened area gradually flattens out and the effect of the treatment diminishes. Dr. Lindstrom believes that HPRK will not be out of clinical trials until late 1998—so we have a while to wait before we will know if the effects of HPRK treatments are long lasting.

In Dr. Jackson's study there was only slight regression within the first six months. All but one of the patients developed trace haze, and there were other side effects similar to those following PRK.

Who Can Benefit from HPRK?

At this time the range of effective treatment isn't known, but, as described above, doctors are using HPRK to treat fairly high levels of hyperopia. HPRK is also used to treat overcorrection after PRK as well as other refractive vision-correction procedures for nearsightedness.

The same physical conditions which would prohibit or delay PRK (see Chapter 3) most likely would affect your candidacy for HPRK.

The Cost

HPRK costs the same as PRK: about $1,500-2,000 per eye.

Hyperopic Holmium (HH): "Honey, I Shrank the Cornea"

For many years researchers have experimented with ways to steepen the cornea by shrinking it. More than 100 years ago a doctor reported that applying a heated probe to the periphery of his patient's corneas would cause changes in the shape of the corneas (be happy you weren't farsighted back then!) This technique was updated during the 1970s when the famous Russian doctor who invented RK, Dr. Svyatoslav Fyodorov, used heated wire needles to accomplish the same result.

Dr. Roger Steinert explained that these treatments did work, short term, because they caused the collagen fibers that make up most of the cornea to contract, or shrink. "The first laser approach for hyperopia used an infrared laser but the results were not permanent," he said. Most often the corneas healed and, *voilá,* the patients were back to wearing glasses.

Now we have another high-tech tool for corneal shrinkage: the Holmium laser for hyperopia—HH. Unlike the earlier needles, wires or lasers, which got the cornea too hot, the Holmium heats the water inside the cornea just enough, it is said, to shrink a tiny amount of tissue without stimulating an aggressive healing response.

How HH Works

In a nearsighted patient, the eye either is too long or the cornea is too steep in the center. Hyperopic patients have corneas that are too short or are too flat in the center.

The Holmium laser, which works through the same slit-lamp microscope doctors use to test your vision—simultaneously shoots pulses of eight tiny beams of infrared light in two octagonal patterns around the edges of the

---

HO-*HUH?* The holmium:yttrium-aluminum-garnet laser (Ho:YAG for short) was developed in the late 1980s. It produces pulses of an infrared (thermal) beam. In HH, moisture in the cornea absorbs the energy in the laser pulses, which heat up and cause the cornea to shrink. By contrast, the excimer laser beam is cool, which is perfect for removing excess from the front surface of the cornea because it doesn't affect the part that remains.

---

pupil. When the beams reach the cornea, any fluid present heats up to about 158°F (~70°C). All the laser energy is totally absorbed in 400 microns of corneal tissue (as opposed to an excimer pulse, which is absorbed in 0.25 microns of tissue). The heated fluid causes collagen fibers to contract, and this creates a tiny crater. (Figure 18.3)

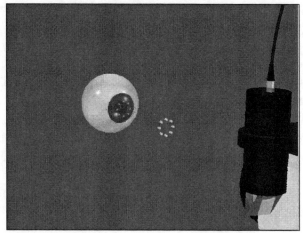

COURTESY OF SUNRISE TECHNOLOGIES

FIGURE 18.3 Like tiny water-seeking missiles, holmium beams simultaneously leave the laser and land at points around the edges of the pupil. This frame from a computer animation shows the second ring in mid-flight. The first ring of beams has already arrived at the cornea.

The shrinkage caused by the laser has the effect of pulling in the periphery of the cornea which causes the center to bulge, or steepen. The amount of correction targeted determines the number of pulses, the number of beams and rings, and the diameters of the circles around the pupil. (Figure 18.4)

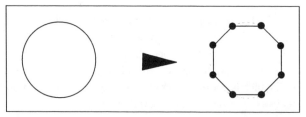

GRAPHIC BY JOSEPH SCHMALENBACH

FIGURE 18.4 This graphic illustrates the "belt-tightening" effect of shrinking points around the periphery of the cornea. When the eight spots around the periphery of the cornea are "burned," they shrink, causing the circle to pull in.

Subsequent HH treatments could help maintain near-vision capabilities. "As patients get older and their focusing powers diminish, we can retreat them to maintain their ability to read and see into the distance," Mr. Dorin said.

Others who could benefit from subsequent HH are patients who are overcorrected by PRK, LASIK or other vision-correction surgeries for nearsightedness.

The same physical conditions which would prohibit or delay PRK or HPRK (see Chapter 3) most likely also would affect your candidacy for HH.

How Well Does It Work?

Like patients treated with HPRK, patients start out slightly nearsighted after HH, according to material produced by Sunrise showing the results of 15 cases. Patients were slightly nearsighted on average, had about -1.25 vision right after the procedure, dropped back to about -0.5 at three months, and tended to stabilize there for the next 18 months.

A published report of FDA Phase I (10 patients) and Phase II (16 patients) trials for HH stated that 79% of the Phase II patients were within +1.0 to -1.0 at six months. 75% had an improvement in their near vision. Irregular astigmatism caused 43% to lose one line, and 7% to lose two lines of best-corrected acuity. The researchers concluded that accurately centering the treatment on the eye is crucial and that it was still unknown whether regression would undo the positive effects of the treatment.[4]

In a study of 15 patients with hyperopia of up to +3.0 who were treated with HH and followed for two years, 73% achieved a correction of about 1.1 diopters from two weeks after surgery through the first

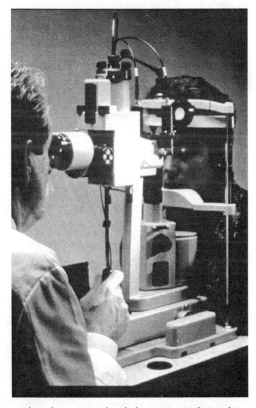

A patient (at right) is being treated with the Sunrise Holmium laser.

two years. The rest of the patients did not experience much correction at all. A small amount of astigmatism (0.18 diopter) was created by the procedure.[5]

Doctors in Canada are beginning to use the holmium in small numbers of cases. Dr. Donald Johnson said, "The holmium might be a solution for up to +1.5 to +1.75 diopters of hyperopia, but above that we're looking at HPRK."

HH Side Effects and Complications

The biggest concern with HH is the same as with all previous cornea-shrinking techniques: Will the effect be permanent? Dr. Salz said, "It's very hard to steepen the cornea and make it stay that way. I don't think the holmium treatments will be proven predictable or stable for more than a couple of diopters of farsightedness in older patients."

In addition, there are risks of induced irregular astigmatism (if the treatment is off-centered or one side of the cornea heals differently than another), short- or long-term nearsightedness, and undercorrection. Any discomfort should be minor and temporary and the risk of infection should be the same as with HPRK—minimal.

A study of four eyes treated in various ways with HH found that after a year, eyes treated with two rings of eight pulsed beams achieved about 1.5 diopters of correction. Most of the regression occurred in the first three months. Corneal topographies of these and five more eyes showed that very mild (about 0.33 diopters) astigmatism resulted in all but one of the eyes.[6]

The Cost

The Holmium laser for HH costs about 75% less than an excimer for PRK. It also requires less space and ancillary equipment and fewer supplies. Surgeon skill and follow-up requirements are not as high. As a result, HH treatments should be far less expensive than HPRK, but no prices were available at press time.

When Will HH be Available?

It will be at least 1998 before laser treatments for HH show up outside of clinical trials in the U.S. Doctors in Canada are performing the treatments on a very limited basis.

INCISIONAL CURES FOR HYPEROPIA

Two incisional approaches to hyperopia which have been used in the last ten years were discussed at the top of this chapter. The ones discussed below currently are being tested in clinical trials.

H-LASIK

Hyperopic LASIK (H-LASIK) combines the incision of ALK with the laser treatment of HPRK. A flap is cut from the front of the cornea and then then HPRK is performed. The flap is carefully replaced and it seals without requiring stitches.

LASIK was discussed in detail in Chapter 15, so we won't go through all that again except to say that the only difference between LASIK for nearsightedness and LASIK for hyperopia is the way the laser beam is used to remove tissue from the cornea. If you are considering H-LASIK, I hope you will read that section.

During H-LASIK the beam removes more tissue from the periphery of the treatment zone than from the center, just as during HPRK.

All the other aspects of LASIK and HLASIK are the same, as are the potential side effects and complications. And, as with other treatments for hyperopia, the long-term stability of the correction achieved with H-LASIK has not been proven.

At this time there are no long-term trial results to indicate whether H-LASIK is safe, predictable or effective. Most of the doctors I spoke to said that it will be a few years before it is known if the procedure is as reliable as standard PRK is for myopia.

Who Can Benefit?

During LASIK all the treatment is done under a flap, so the epithelium is hardly disturbed. For treating nearsightedness this provides the benefits of faster visual recovery and less haze. For hyperopic treatments, the benefits could be even greater because less of a healing response is stimulated. This might make it possible to treat even high levels of hyperopia without much regression of effect.

As with any surgery, the potential gains have to be measured against the risks. While flap surgery is risky, the only other option in wide use today for the very farsighted is even more invasive—cutting into the eye and replacing the lens (see below). For mild-to-moderate hyperopia (below +4.0 or +5.0) HPRK or HH might prove to be a safer way to go.

What the Doctors Say About H-LASIK

Dr. Jeffrey Robin is using H-LASIK to treat both hyperopia and presbyopia. "The flap gives us a smooth, blended surface between the center and the sides of the cornea."

By mid-1996, Dr. Howard Gimbel had performed about 150 HPRKs and H-LASIKs. "I prefer H-LASIK for treating natural hyperopia but I sometimes use HPRK to treat patients who are overcorrected after they had RK and PRK for myopia. The 9-millimeter treatment zone seems to be giving us quite stable and consistent results."

Dr. David Lin said, "I'm waiting for long-term results before I start using LASIK for hyperopia. It's being done and preliminary results are quite promising. HPRK seems to be prone to significant regression, so doing it under a LASIK flap might be the way to go."

Dr. Richard Lindstrom added, "Hyperopic PRK and hyperopic LASIK are working well all over the world, but we're still a few years away from having good, reliable data on the results. Right now, for natural [not surgery-induced] hyperopia in the range of +1 to +4, I'm still using ALK."

REVERSIBLE, ADJUSTABLE
TREATMENTS FOR HYPEROPIA

Two treatments currently being studied have appeal for treating hyperopia because they are very precise or are reversible/adjustable. Dr. James Salz, who is investigating both techniques said, "These are the only realistic treatments on the horizon for very high hyperopia (over +4.0) and both are extremely promising."

Clear Lens Extraction (CLE)

Think of this as cataract surgery without the cataracts—which cause a clouding of the naturally clear lens of the eye or of the membrane which holds it.

During CLE, the natural lens is removed and an artificial one is put in its place. The membrane that held the natural lens now holds the artificial one. As with lenses for cataract surgery, the prescription of the artificial lens is precise, so the patient's vision can end up very close to the target. "When I do CLE on a patient's first eye, I intentionally overcorrect it to -1.0 or -2.0 to allow for a little regression and so the patient can read," Dr. Salz said. "Then I watch how the patient responds after a few months and use this information to try to get him as close to 20/20 as possible in the second eye."

Dr. Salz currently is investigating CLE for high hyperopia in an Institutional Review Board study at Beverly Hills Wilshire Surgery Center. "The lenses are the same ones we use for cataract surgery, so they don't have to go through FDA trials," Dr. Salz said. "However, we are doing a controlled study to identify any unexpected complications unique to farsighted patients." Dr. Salz primarily is including patients over age 40 in his study so that reading vision can be taken into consideration at the same time hyperopia is corrected.

Who Can Benefit from CLE?
While Dr. Salz believes that CLE is *not* a viable option for high myopes, he thinks it will prove to be the best option for farsightedness over +5. "Unlike high myopes, who tend to have large eyes and a greater chance of retinal detachment, high hyperopes tend to have smaller eyes and the risk of detachment is much lower.

How Well Does CLE Work?
"We've obtained wonderful results with CLE for high hyperopia," Dr. Salz continued. "Patients sit up right after the surgery and see 20/40."

A 1994 study of CLE reported results on six extremely hyperopic eyes followed an average of 20 months. 100% achieved 20/40 or better. There were no retinal problems observed during the follow-up period, but there were instances of clouding of the membrane that held the new lenses.[7]

Another 1994 study reported that CLE was performed on 5 eyes that were between +7 and +10 and followed for 18 months. All eyes had 20/30 or better vision, with the average being 20/25.[8]

Side Effects and Complications
The risks of CLE are the same as for any intraocular (open-eye) surgery: damage to the eye and post-op infection. "We are cutting open the eye—so it's very delicate and requires extensive expertise," Dr. Salz said. "The worst risk is severe infection, which can happen in one out of every 2000 cases, and can cause total loss of the eye."

"When patients have more than 4 diopters of farsightedness, however, they are extremely visually handicapped," Dr. Salz continued. "For them, the risks of intraocular surgery are outweighed by what the surgery can offer them." Having said that, Dr. Salz is quick to add, "Patients should go only to surgeons highly experienced in lens-replacement procedures."

The Cost of CLE

In 1996 Dr. Salz said that at his center the cost of CLE was $2500 per eye, including follow-up care.

Implantable Contact Lens (ICL)

This approach along with its benefits and potential risks is described at the end of Chapter 14 and is available only through clinical trials. It involves inserting a microscopic contact into the cornea through a slit in the side. For high hyperopes ICL might turn out to be the ultimate solution.

"Even if the ICLs end up causing cataracts, they might be the best first step for high hyperopes," Dr. Salz said, "because the only alternative would be Clear Lens Extraction—which is the equivalent of cataract surgery. By doing an ICL we can postpone or even eliminate the need for this more-invasive procedure."

IT'S NOT THE MOON, BUT IT WORKS!

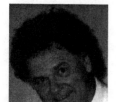

Name
Johnny T. Deen MD, 57

Occupation
Ophthalmologist,
Thomaston, Georgia

Pre-Op Vision
+1.75 (hyperopia)
+1.75 (reading glasses
strength

Procedure
HH

Post-Op Vision
20/20 distance
Needs +2.0 contacts
for reading

Dr. Deen had been wearing bifocals for 15 years when he attended a holmium laser conference in March of 1994. He was so convinced by what he saw, that he had one eye treated before lunch and the other eye after—the first ophthalmic surgeon to have the treatment. His eye was treated in 16 spots with the holmium laser in two concentric rings.

"Before I was treated I couldn't see the TV without contacts. My eyes felt a little scratchy after the procedure, but I attended that evening's cocktail party and dinner with no problem. When I woke up the next morning my eyes were a little sensitive to light and still scratchy. The next day it was like nothing had even been done.

"I had perfect vision at the start. I was seeing 20/15 on day one. Five days after I had the treatment my vision was 20/15 for distance and perfect for near. I had a multifocal cornea with no astigmatism."

I talked with Dr. Deen a little over two years after his HH treatment. His unaided vision was still good for distance, but he needed help to read because his vision required a 3.5 diopter correction (1.75 +1.75) and he only ended up with a 1.5 diopter correction. The multifocal cornea effect HH gave him meant that he can wear contact lenses for reading and still see into the distance.

"Today I wear a +2.0 disposable contact in each eye—I sleep with them, read with them, drive with them, do surgery with them. I'm seeing up a storm. When I pull the contact out, my vision is slightly clearer for the distance. But the benefit is, with the contacts I've got good vision in both eyes for far and near, not just in one like you get with monovision. I've got the eyes of a 20-year-old just by wearing these cheap, throw-away contact lenses.

"I don't think the holmium is going to help all people totally get rid of their glasses and contacts. It's not going to correct both distance and near vision for most people. I have a patient who's a retired orthodontist who thinks I hung the moon for him because I took him to Brussels and gave him the holmium treatment. His vision was like mine going in. It's been 18 months and he still has 20/15 for distance and perfect reading. He regressed during the first 4-6 months but now he's stable. I think he'll stay there.

"But I think that's the exception. For me, what I have now is just fine. It works."

Note: HH is not yet approved by the FDA and Dr. Deen does not provide HH treatments in the U.S. or Europe.

Therapeutic Laser Treatments (PTK)

The first time an excimer laser was approved for eye surgery was in March of 1994 when the FDA approved PTK. It was an easier decision for the FDA panel to make than approving PRK. Unlike PRK, which is performed on healthy eyes to treat problems that can be solved without any surgery at all, PTK is performed on diseased and injured eyes, and all the alternative treatments involve much more risk.

In other words, for the right patients, PTK is a procedure from heaven.

Who Needs PTK?

According to Dr. Vance Thompson, a national medical monitor for Summit Technology's FDA clinical trials, PTK replaces corneal transplants and other procedures such as ALK which require more surgical expertise, involve more risk to the patient, and are more invasive and costly.

Patients who once had no alternative to corneal transplants now can try PTK first.

"Because doing a cornea transplant is a very big deal and the visual results are not always the best, some people sit in never-never land—with vision not quite bad enough to justify a corneal transplant, but not good enough to make

---

WHAT IS PTK? PTK is short for *phototherapeutic keratectomy:* the use of laser *light* to *treat* conditions of the *cornea* by *removing* tiny amounts of tissue.

---

them happy. Now they have a viable, effective option. Just a few drops of topical anesthesia, a couple of minutes in the chair—they don't even change clothes," he said. "Discomfort lasts a day or two and then they're back in action."

If you have one of the conditions on the PTK Hit List (see sidebar), you probably know it. If it's interfering with your vision and your doctor isn't trained in PTK, you might save your sight and the pain of a cornea transplant by consulting with a doctor who can tell you whether PTK is right for you (see Chapter 7 for a list of some experts in PTK).

How PTK Works

PTK's precision is one of the reasons it is such an advancement over other techniques. By using the excimer laser to dust off only $\frac{1}{4}$ micron of cornea tissue per pulse, PTK can delicately remove only the portion of the cornea that is affected, without disturbing healthy tissue. This is especially important in treating conditions which are naturally progressive or likely to recur.

"The excimer laser is the most precise tool for removing layers of tissue in the history of corneal surgery," Dr. Thompson said.

PTK HIT LIST   Studies indicate that PTK can effectively treat a wide variety of corneal irregularities and pathologies including:

- Adenoviral subepithelial opacity
- Corneal plaques
- Dystrophies (Reis Bucklers', Lattice, Avelino, Granular and others)
- Irregular astigmatism
- Keratopathies
- Leukomas
- Nodes caused by keratoconus
- Pterygia (primary and recurrent)
- Recurrent corneal erosion
- Salzmann's nodules
- Scars from trauma to the eye
- Scars from infections and diseases
- Scars from viruses (herpes simplex and zoster)
- Scars from eye surgeries (RK, PRK, ALK)
- Shield ulcers
- Superficial opacities

The PTK Procedure

First, the depth of the scar and amount of irregularity is determined using techniques such as slit-lamp examination, videokeratography (corneal mapping), and ultrasound.

When it has been determined that enough healthy cornea remains under the irregularity to make treatment worthwhile, PTK can be scheduled.

The PTK procedure is almost identical to PRK (see Chapter 9) except that instead of a gradually widening beam, the PTK beam is set to open and remain at the full treatment width. This helps minimize any change in the refractive powers of the cornea. (Figure 19.1)

When the patient also has myopia, hyperopia or astigmatism, PRK can be used to treat the eye after his vision has completely stabilized—usually in 4-6 months.

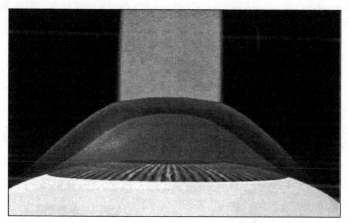

COURTESY OF SUMMIT TECHNOLOGY

The diameter of the laser beam remains constant throughout a PTK procedure to reduce the chance of making the eye more near- or farsighted.

How Well Does PTK Work?

With PRK, the goal is the same for all patients: 20/20 or close to it. With PTK, the goals are individual and are determined by the nature of the patient's problem.

For some patients, achieving temporary improvement in vision is a world of help. For some, removing scars and irregularities that cause constant discomfort makes PTK worth the trip. And PTK can help others get to the point where procedures such as PRK or cataract surgery can help them achieve good vision.

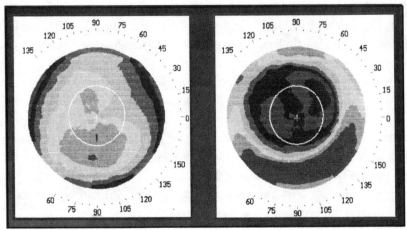

These photos show a scarred cornea before and after PTK. In the photo on the left, a white haze indicates a scar. After PRK the central visual area (circled) has no remaining haze.

Research indicates that most patients who are candidates for PTK are helped by it:

- In a long-term study of 166 eyes, 84% achieved the improvement goal set before surgery for their vision.[1]
- In 11 eyes with Reis Bucklers' dystrophy (including two that had already had a cornea transplant), the recurrent dystrophy was stopped. Visual acuity improved in all the eyes. The researchers concluded, "PTK is now the procedure of choice once surgery is required in Reis Bucklers' dystrophy."[2]
- Out of 28 eyes with a variety of cornea problems that were treated with PTK, best-corrected acuity improved in 20 eyes and worsened in five. Only two patients did not experience enough improvement to avoid cornea transplants.[3]
- Another study investigated the results of PTK on four different types of cases: dystrophies, corneal erosion, pterygia, and scars caused by infections or trauma. Of the 39 eyes followed an average of nine months, nine gained two or more lines of best-corrected acuity, one eye lost two lines because of increased astigmatism and half of the eyes achieved all the goals established prior to surgery.[4]

The Rewards *vs* the Risks

"PTK lets competent eye surgeons achieve quality results in cases that used to require an extremely skilled surgeon," Dr. Thompson said. Other advantages of PTK over the alternatives are that it is:

- Noninvasive (no incisions are made), so there's far less risk of infection.
- More precise, so there's less risk of harm to healthy tissue.
- More predictable, because of the precision.
- Computer controlled, so there's little risk of human error.
- Done under local anesthetic, so the risks of general anesthesia are eliminated.

PTK also has practical benefits. It:

- Reduces time off work to just a couple of days if any, compared to weeks after corneal transplants.
- Requires far fewer follow-up visits than a corneal transplant.
- Costs about a tenth of a corneal transplant.

Side Effects and Complications

When a patient looks at the risks of PTK he has a different point of view than someone considering PRK. Since his vision is compromised already (and likely worsening), the potential gain quite often outweighs virtually any degree of risk. The decision then centers on whether it is likely PTK can solve his problem.

All the side effects that occur with PRK (see Chapter 11) also can occur after PTK, including glare, haze, and halos.

PTK also can cause the same complications as PRK, including overcorrection (more common) and undercorrection (less common), loss of best-corrected acuity, and induced astigmatism.[5] "We might get rid of the scar or dystrophy, but the patient's vision without glasses might end up worse," said Dr. Thompson. "If this happens, we can address it with PRK or the patient can wear glasses or contacts."

In addition, PTK might not fully treat the condition or the condition might recur and require retreatment.[6]

A risk in patients with previous herpes simplex or zoster is that the wound healing stimulated by PTK can cause a recurrence of the virus. Doctors take steps to minimize this risk. "We wait for the virus to be quiet for at least a year before performing PTK," Dr. Thompson said, "and we put these patients on anti-viral medications before and after the procedure."

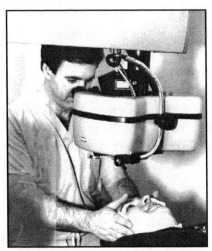

COURTESY OF ST. LUKE'S REGIONAL MEDICAL CENTER, IOWA

Dr. Vance Thompson uses the laser's microscope to align the laser beam with the patient's eye just prior to beginning the PTK procedure.

The Alternatives to PTK

If there is sufficient healthy cornea, the alternative to PTK is Lamellar Keratoplasty (LK) or Automated Lamellar Keratoplasty (ALK) (described in chapter 15). Essentially, these procedures use a surgical knife or special device called a *microkeratome* to slice off the diseased or irregular part of the cornea. "This is a technically difficult procedure to perform," said Dr. Thompson, who has performed many, "and involves significantly higher risks than PTK."

When there isn't enough healthy cornea left for PTK to work successfully, the only alternative is a cornea transplant, which is done under local anesthesia, requires much more time off work, and at least a dozen follow-up visits the first year (compared to five or six with PTK).

During a cornea transplant the entire cornea is removed and replaced by a cornea from a human donor. "It's a big surgery," Dr. Thompson said, "and if you can avoid it, you do. The patient has to undergo more anesthesia and you have to open up the eye. The risks are greater, though serious complications are relatively rare.

"Then there's the *forever*-risk of rejection," Dr. Thompson added.

By contrast, using the laser to remove cornea pathologies lets the patient go home with her own cornea. "Everybody is happier when that can happen," Dr. Thompson said.

PTK-LASIK?

As described in detail in Chapter 15, LASIK is a technique for treating the interior of the cornea with PRK without disturbing the surface much. According to Dr. Thompson, researchers are looking at whether PTK could be done the same way in cases in which the front of the cornea is normal and the disease or damage is deep or at the back of the cornea. Doctors would simply lift up a flap, zap the cornea with the PTK beam, and then set the flap back down. All the benefits and risks of LASIK would apply to PTK-LASIK, but again, those risks have to measured against the risks of the alternatives, or of doing nothing.

Where to Go for PTK

Any doctor who performs PRK theoretically can use his laser for PTK, but that doesn't mean he should. Diagnosing and treating nonrefractive conditions of the cornea should be left to cornea specialists. The tips for finding the right doctor in Chapter 7 apply equally to PTK: You need an experienced ophthalmic surgeon with a subspecialty in corneal diseases who has performed and followed many PTK cases. The resource list contains the names of a few. Another good source would be referrals from your nearest university medical center.

The Cost of PRK

PTK is much less expensive than its alternatives. At this writing, PTK prices range from $1250-1950 per eye, according to Dr. Thompson. "I charge $1750 per eye regardless of the type or severity of the problem."

Who Pays?

Unlike PRK, which is considered cosmetic by insurance companies, PTK should be covered by your health insurance, even if you don't have vision coverage. Consult with your doctor prior to billing the insurance company, because many companies haven't yet updated their procedure codes to include PTK. The doctor might have to bill the procedure under a "lamellar keratoplasty" code or otherwise spend a great deal of time on the phone explaining the procedure to an insurance company representative.

"Medicare doesn't yet recognize PTK," Dr. Thompson said, "but eventually this will change because PTK is so much more cost effective than any of the alternatives. Until then, we bill PTK to Medicare under the lamellar keratoplasty code."

"OH, MAN! IT WAS SO MUCH BETTER!"

Name
Larry Wiebelhaus, 40

Occupation
Truck driver, Iowa

Pre-Op Vision
20/40 best-corrected
acuity
Recurrent lattice
dystrophy

Procedure
PTK both eyes

Post-Op Vision
20/20 best-corrected
acuity

Surgeon
Vance Thompson, MD

In 1992 Larry Wiebelhaus was one of the first patients in the FDA trials for PTK to have the procedure. He had a rare form of cornea disease called *recurrent lattice dystrophy* which he inherited from his mother's side of the family. Of the five kids in his family, three of them have the disease, and all three have had cornea transplants in both eyes.

"Lattice dystrophy seems to affect people with dark brown eyes and it works from the inside out. When it hits the cornea, that's where it does its damage. I've had it all my life. It's kind of like a cataract—it makes everything look like you're seeing through a frosted window. When I was younger my eyes would get really sore. It would lay me up days at a time.

"Glasses can only help so much. My best-corrected vision was 20/40, so I couldn't drive at night. I drive a semi truck between Sioux City and Sioux Falls—that's 100 miles—and I had to do the route in the daytime.

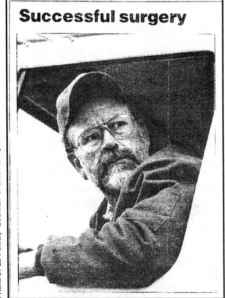

Successful surgery

PHOTO BY ED PORTER, COURTESY OF SIOUX CITY JOURNAL

"In 1981 my condition had progressed to the point that I really couldn't see, so I had a cornea transplant in one eye and then five years later had one in the other eye. You're talking 20-plus stitches and not being able to see for days. You can't lift anything heavy because you don't want to increase your eye pressure and break the stitches. You wear an eye patch at night to keep from scratching because the stitches itch so much that you could scratch the new cornea right off. In fact, one morning I woke up with my eye patch off. Luckily, the cornea was still on.

"After each transplant I had to take eight weeks off work and there were so many trips to the doctor because they could only take two or three stitches out at a time. Once the corneas started to heal, I started rejecting them, which caused redness, soreness and blurry vision. The solution was shots right in my eye. Unbelievably painful! But they saved the corneas because my doctor caught the problem early enough.

"In 1986 the dystrophy started to come back in one eye, so I signed up for the PTK trials in 1992—anything to avoid more transplants! The laser surgery was nothing. There's no comparison. It's so simple, you see better immediately, and there was no downtime at all. I had the bandage lens and there was no pain, no eye patch, just a little discomfort. My vision got a little cloudy soon after the procedure and took about three days to clear up. Then I just had to put drops in my eye three times a day for awhile.

"By 1995 my other eye was getting bad, so I had PTK on it just a few months ago. And it was just as easy—in fact I drove myself home afterward.

"I have the best vision I've ever had in my life now—20/20. I still wear glasses because I have astigmatism, which I could have fixed with PRK if I wanted to. But let me tell you, that's the least of my worries.

"I suppose if you never had eye surgery you might think PTK was a big deal, but it was like nothing for me after what I had been through. The best part is that I know I can get it done again any time I need it and I'll never have to have another cornea transplant!"

KEEPING IT IN THE FAMILY   Back in the late 1950s Mr. Wiebelhaus' mother had one of the very early cornea transplants performed by the legendary eye surgeon, Dr. Max Fine of San Francisco. "It was really tough back then because they had no way to treat rejection. She was laid up for three months—couldn't bathe or get anything near her eyes."

Twenty-five years later, when Mr. Wiebelhaus consulted a surgeon in Texas for his first transplant, the surgeon recognized the Wiebelhaus name, went through some old files and discovered that he had assisted Dr. Fine in treating Mr. Wiebelhaus' mom. "It was so strange because I picked this doctor out of the phone book." When Mr. Wiebelhaus had his second transplant a few years later, it turned out that the *new* doctor had been trained by his *first* doctor who had been trained by his *mom's* doctor. Now, his sister is following in his footsteps and has had PTK in both eyes with the same success.

On The Horizon: Water-Jet Keratectomy?

As described at the end of Chapter 15, new water-jet instruments, called "hydrokeratomes" are currently in FDA clinical trials. These instruments have the potential to eliminate some of the risks of corneal transplants in cases where transplants are unavoidable as well as offer another alternative for treating corneal scars, ulcers and other irregularities. The simplicity of the instruments undoubtedly will result in a lower cost than PTK.

OTHER LASERS FOR VISION PROBLEMS

The excimer laser isn't the only laser used to treat eye conditions. Unlike PRK and PTK, which are performed on the surface of the cornea, there are lasers that can be used to operate on the eye's interior (see chart). The laser beam enters the eye through the pupil or a tear duct, so no incision is necessary. The procedures usually are quick and painless and the patient can resume normal activities shortly after.

If you have one of the conditions listed in Table 11.1, you might save your sight by finding a highly trained ophthalmologist experienced in using the type of laser appropriate for your condition. For help locating the right doctor, see the list in Chapter 7 (most of these doctors either perform these procedures or can refer you to a specialist in them) or call your local medical association and ask for names of several surgeons who specialize in diseases of the eye or cornea and who use lasers. Remember, just because new treatments are available doesn't mean that every doctor has the right equipment or the right training to perform them. It might take a little research and a few consultations to find the right doctor, but the time spent could be well worth it.

LASER CURES FOR EYE DISEASES

Table 11.1

Condition	Symptom/Cause	Laser Treatment
Scars, dystrophies, ulcers, plaques, nodules, opacities, leukomas, irregular astigmatism, pterygias, keratopathies, erosions	These cause a clouding, disturbance or irregularity of the cornea which impairs sight.	Excimer PTK is used to remove damaged tissue.
Cataract	A clouding of the normally clear lens of the eye or the membrane which supports the lens.	Nd:YAG* laser is used to vaporize the cloudiness.
Glaucoma	A blockage of the tear canal results in build-up of fluid pressure inside the eye.	If medications don't reduce the pressure, an Nd:YAG laser beam is used to open the canals so the eye can drain.
Macular Degeneration	In the most severe form, blood vessels start to grow and leak blood under the macula at the back of the retina. This can cause blindness very quickly by destroying the macular cells.	When caught early enough, an Argon laser is used to seal the blood vessels and prevent leakage.
Ocular Histoplasmosis	A fungus which grows in the Southeast and Midwest parts of the U.S. and causes a form of macular degeneration.	Argon laser as above.
Diabetic Retinopathy	A complication of diabetes in which blood vessels in the retina leak and cause scarring and loss of vision.	The Argon laser can stop blindness caused by diabetes by sealing off blood vessels in the retina.

*Nd:YAG is laser-talk for "Neodymium:yttrium-aluminum garnet."

For the Next Edition...

The world of vision correction is changing so rapidly, I will be starting the next edition as this one goes to press. I would love to hear from you if you had an unusual vision problem that was solved by laser vision correction, or if you feel your experience would be helpful to future patients. If you are willing to be interviewed, please include your full name and telephone number, including the best times to reach you, with your letter.

Doctors, and manufacturers, I'd like to hear from you, too, if you have new information that can help future readers, or data on clinical trials. Please indicate who I can contact to arrange an interview if appropriate.

You can reach me via the Internet:
laserviz@aol.com

or via my publisher:
UC Books
Attn: Franette Armstrong, *Beyond Glasses!*
43 Danville Square, Box 1036
Danville, California 94526

References

CHAPTER 2

1. Temme, LA, Still, DL, Fatcheric AJ, Jet Pilot, Helicopter Pilot, and College Student:A Comparison of Central Vision *Journal of Aviation, Space, and Environmental Medicine*, 1995; 4:297-302.

CHAPTER 3

1. Schallhorn SC, Blanton CL, Kaupp SE, *et al.*, Preliminary Results of Photorefractive Keratectomy In Active-Duty United States Navy Personnel, *Ophthalmology*, 1996; 1:5-21.

2. Singh D, Photorefractive Keratectomy in Pediatric Patients, *Journal of Cataract and Refractive Surgery*, 1995; 11:630-632.

3. Kelly P, Naval Medical Center Involved in an FDA Test of Excimer Laser, *Drydock*, August 27, 1993.

CHAPTER 5

1. National Health and Nutrition Examination Survey, 1972 as reported in Stein H, Cheskes A, Stein R, The Excimer, Fundamentals and Clinical Use, *Slack Inc.*, Thorofare, New Jersey, 1995;21.

2. Stein H, Cheskes A, Stein R, The Excimer, Fundamentals and Clinical Use, *Slack Inc.* Thorofare, New Jersey, 1995;21.

3. See note 2.

4. Wildsoet C, Wallman J, Choroidal and Scleral Mechanisms of Compensation for Spectacle Lenses in Chicks, *Vision Research*, 1995; 5:1175-1194.

5. Weale R, Why Does the Human Visual System Age in the Way It Does? *Experimental Eye Research*:1:1995

6. Steinert R, Refractive Surgery Q&A, *Outlook Newsletter of the American Academy of Ophthalmology Refractive Surgery Interest Group*, Fall, 1995.

CHAPTER 6

Personal communications with Drs. Stephen Trokel, Marguerite McDonald, Francis L'Esperance, Roger Steinert, Charles Munnerlyn, Ph.D and Mr. Terrance Clapham. March-May, 1996.

Tulleken CA, Verdaasdonk RM, First Clinical Experience with Excimer-Assisted High-Flow Bypass Surgery of the Brain, *Acta. Neurochir. (Wien)*, 1995; 134:66-70.

CHAPTER 7

1. Dougherty PJ, Wellish KL, Maloney RK, Excimer Laser Ablation Rate and Corneal Hydration, *American Journal of Ophthalmology*, 1994; 8:169-175.

2. Thornton SP, JCRS Study & Discussion Questions:*Journal of Cataract and Refractive Surgery*, 1996; January-February.

CHAPTER 8

1. Schallhorn SC, Blanton CL, Kaupp SE, *et al.*, Preliminary Results of Photorefractive Keratectomy In Active-Duty United States Navy Personnel,*Ophthalmology*, 1996; 1:5-21.

CHAPTER 9

1. Gimbel HV, DeBroff BM, Beldavs RA, *et al.*, Comparison of Laser and Manual Removal of Corneal Epithelium for Photorefractive Keratectomy, *Journal of Refractive Surgery*, 1195; 1-2:36-41.

CHAPTER 10

Niizuma T, Ito S, Hayashi M, *et al.*, Cooling the Cornea to Prevent Side Effects of Photorefractive Keratectomy,*Journal of Refractive and Corneal Surgery*, 1994; 3-4:S262-266.

Ho SS, Coel MN, Kagawa R, Richardson AB, The Effects on Ice on Blood Flow and Bone Metabolism in Knees, *American Journal of Sports Medicine*, 1994; 7-8:537-540.

CHAPTER 11

1. Summit Technology, Inc. *Purchaser's and Users Requirements*, Rev. A, 1995; 11:3.

2. VISX, Incorporated, *Summary of VISX Clinical Studies:Photorefractive Keratectomy (PRK) with the VISX Excimer Laser System*, WP96-01, 1996.

3. Wang W, Zheng W, Pang G, *et al.*, Excimer laser photorefractive keratectomy for myopia in China. A report of 750 eyes with a 6-month follow-up, *Chinese Medical Journal*, 1995; 8:601-605.

4. Talley AR, Hardten DR, Sher NA, Results one year after using the 193-nm excimer laser for photorefractive keratectomy in mild to moderate myopia, *American Journal of Ophthalmology*, 1994; 9:304-311.

5. "Summit Clinical Trial Results" as summarized in the *Summit Patient Information Booklet* 10/23/1995. and *20/20 Laser Centers Summary Business Plan*, 2/23/96, p3-4.

6. Segal M, Not a Cure-All:Eye Surgery Helps Some See Better, F*DA Consumer*, July/August 1995, revised November, 1995.

7. See note 5.

8. Mathers WD, Daley TE, Tear Flow and Evaporation in Patients with the without Dry Eye, *Ophthalmology*, 1996; 4:664-669.

9. O'Brart DP, Lohmann CP, Fitzke FW, Disturbances in Night Vision after Excimer Laser Photorefractive Keratectomy, *Eye*, 1994; 8:46-51.

10. See note 5.

11. See note 1.

12. See note 6.

13. Kim JH, Sah WJ, Hahn TW, Lee YC, Some Problems after Photorefractive Keratectomy, *Journal of Refractive and Corneal Surgery,* 1994; 3-4:S226-S230.

14. See note 2.

15. Schallhorn SC, Blanton C. Kaupp SE, *et al.,* Preliminary Results of Photorefractive Keratectomy In Active-Duty United States Navy Personnel:*Ophthalmology,* 1996; 1:5-21.

16. See note 4.

17. Liu JC, McDonald MB, Varnell R, Myopic Excimer Laser Photorefractive Keratectomy:An Analysis of Clinical Correlations, Journal *of Refractive and Corneal Surgery,* 1990; 9-10:321-328.

18. Spigelman AV, Albert WC, Cozean CH, Treatment of Myopic Astigmatism with the 193 nm Excimer Laser Utilizing Aperture Elements, *Journal of Cataract and Refractive Surgery,* Vol 20 Supplement, 1994; 258.

19. See note 15.

20. See note 2.

21. Snibson GR, McCarty CA, Aldred GF, Retreatment after excimer laser photorefractive keratectomy. The Melbourne Excimer Laser Group, American Journal of Ophthalmology, 1996; 3:250-257.

22. See note 15.

23. Loewenstein A, Lipshitz I, Lazar M, Scraping of Epithelium for Treatment of Undercorrection and Haze after Photorefractive Keratectomy. *Journal of Refractive and Corneal Surgery,* 1994; 3-4:S274-S276.

24. Matta CS, Piebenga LW, Deitz MR, Tauber J, Excimer retreatment for myopic photorefractive keratectomy failurs. Six-to 18-Month Follow-up, *Ophthalmology,* 1996; 3:444-451.

25. Meyer JC, Stulting RD, Thompson KP, Durrie DS, Late Onset of Corneal Scar after Excimer Laser Photorefractive Keratectomy. *American Journal of Ophthalmology,* 1996; 5:529-539.

26. See note 15.

27. Goggin M, Foley-Nolan A, Algawi K, O'Keefe M, Regression after Photorefractive Keratectomy for Myopia.*Journal of Cataract and Refractive Surgery,* 1996; 3:194-196.

28. See note 15.

29. Schipper I, Businger U, Pfarrer R, Fitting Contact Lenses after Excimer Laser Photorefractive Keratectomy for Myopia, Contact Lens Association of Ophthalmologists Journal, 1995; 10:281-284.

30. See note 1.

31. See note 1.

32. See note 15.

33. Maguen E, Salz JJ, Nesburn AB, *et al.,* Results of Excimer Laser Photorefractive Keratectomy for the Correction of Myopia, *Ophthalmology,* 1994, 9:1548-1557.

34. See note 18.

35. See note 4.

36. Terrell J, Bechara SJ, Nesburn A, The Effect of Globe Fixation on Ablation Zone Centration in Photorefractive Keratectomy, *American Journal of Ophthalmology,* 1995; 5:612-619.

Additional Sources for Chapter 11

Busin M, Meller D, Corneal Epithelial Dots Following Excimer Laser Photorefractive Keratectomy, *Journal of Refractive and Corneal Surgery,* 1994:5-6:357-359.

Carones F, Brancato R, Venturi E, *et al.,* The Corneal Endothelium after Myopic Excimer Laser Photorefractive Keratectomy, *Archives of Ophthalmology,* 1994; 7:920-924.

David T, Rieck P, Corneal Wound Healing Modulation Using Basic Fibroblast Growth Factor after Excimer Laser Photorefractive Keratectomy, *Cornea,* 1995, 5-227-234.

Donnenfeld ED, Selkin BA, Perry HD, *et al.,* Controlled Evaluation of a Bandage Contact Lens and a Topical Nonsteroidal Anti-Inflammatory Drug in Treating Traumatic Corneal Abrasions, *Ophthalmology,* 1995; 6:979-984.

Epstein D, Fagerholm P, *et al.,* Twenty-Four -Month Follow-Up of Excimer Laser Photorefractive Keratectomy for Myopia:Refractive and Visual Acuity Results, *Ophthalmology,* 1994; 8:1558-64.

Ferrari M, Use of Topical Nonsteroidal Anti-inflammatory Drugs after Photorefractive Keratectomy *Journal of Refractive and Corneal Surgery,* 1994; 3-4:S287-S289.

Lin DT, Corneal Topographic Analysis after Excimer Photorefractive Keratectomy, *Ophthalmology,* 1994, 8:1432-1439.

McDonald MB, Frantz JM, Klyce SD, Central Photorefractive Keratectomy for Myopia:The Blind Eye Study, *Archives of Ophthalmology,* 1990, 6:799-808.

McDonald MB, Frantz JM, Klyce SD, One-Year Refractive Results of Central Photorefractive Keratectomy for Myopia in the Nonhuman Primate Cornea, *Archives of Ophthalmology,* 1990, 1:40-47.

Palmer RM, McDonald MB, A Corneal Lens Shield System for the Promotion of Postoperative Corneal Epithelial Healing, *Journal of Refractive Surgery,* 1995; 3:125-126.

Seiler T, McDonnell PJ, Major Review:Excimer Laser Photorefractive Keratectomy, *Survey of Ophthalmology,* 1995; September/October.

CHAPTER 12

1. Persico J, Who Wants PRK? *Review of Ophthalmology,* October, 1995.

CHAPTER 13

1. Segal M, Not a Cure-all, Eye Surgery Helps Some See Better, *FDA Consumer,* July-August 1995, Updated October, 1995.

2. Office of Device Evaluation Division of Ophthalmic Devices, Draft Clinical Guidance for the Preparation and Contents of an Investigational Device Exemption (IDE) Applications for Excimer Laser Devices Used in Ophthalmic Surgery for Myopic Photorefractive Keratectomy (PRK), *Federal Drug Administration,* June 8, 1990.

3. Summary Minutes of the Ophthalmic Devices Panel Meeting, *Federal Drug Administration,* April 1, 1996.

CHAPTER 14

1. Segal M, Not a Cure-All:Eye Surgery Helps Some See Better, F*DA Consumer,* July-August, 1995.

2. Waring GO, Lynn MJ, McDonnell PJ, Results of the Prospective Evaluation of the Radial Keratotomy (PERK) Study 10 Years After Surgery, *Archives of Ophthalmology,* 1994; 10:1298-1308.

3. Lindstrom RL, Minimally Invasive Radial Keratotomy:Mini-RK, J*ournal of Cataract and Refractive Surgery,*1995; 1:27-34.

4. See note 1.

5. Epstein RL, Laurence EP, Effect of Topical Diclofenac Solution on Discomfort after Radial Keratotomy, *Journal of Cataract and Refractive Surgery*, 1994; 6:378-380.

6. Thornton SP, RK Offers Immediate Visual Improvement with Few Complications, *Ocular Surgery News*, 1996:Jan 15.

7. Waring GO, Lynn MJ, Fielding B, et al., Results of the Prospective Evaluation of Radial Keratotomy (PERK) Study 4 Years after Surgery for Myopia, *Journal of the American Medical Association*, 1990; 2:1083-1091.

8. See note 6.

9. Parmley V, Ng J, Gee B, Penetrating Keratoplasty after Radial Keratotomy. A Report of Six Patients. Ophthalmology, 1995; 6:947-950.

10. Durrie DS, Schumer DJ, Cavanaugh TB, Photorefractive Keratectormy for Residual Myopia after Previous Radial Keratotomy*Journal of Cataract and Refractive Surgery*, 1994; 3-4:S235-S238.

11. Nordan LT, Binder PS, Kassar BS, Heitzmann J, Photorefractive Keratectomy to Treat Myopia and Astigmatism after Radial Keratotomy and Penetrating Keratoplasty, *Journal of Cataract and Refractive Surgery*, 1995; 5:268-273.

12. Maloney RK, Chan WK, Steinert R et al., A Multicenter Trial of Photorefractive Keratectomy for Residual Myopia Following Previous Ocular Surgery, *Ophthalmology*, 1995; 107:1042-1053.

13. Waisberg Y, Bilateral High Hyperopia after Radial Keratotomy, *Journal of Cataract and Refractive Surgery*, 1993; 1:88-89.

14. McDonnell PJ, Nizam A, Lynn MJ, Morning-to-Evening Change in Refraction, Corneal Curvature, and Visual Acuity 11 Years after Radial Keratotomy in the Prospective Evaluation of Radial Keratotomy Study, *Ophthalmology*,1996; 2:233:239.

15. See note 2.

16. See note 7.

17. Mader TH, White LJ, Refractive Changes at Extreme Altitude after Radial Keratotomy, *American Journal of Ophthalmology*, 1995; 6:733-737.

18. Ng JD, White LJ, Parmley VC, et al., Effects of Simulated High Altitude on Patients Who Have Had Radial Keratotomy, *Ophthalmology*, 1996; 3:452-457.

19. McDonnell PJ, Excimer Laser Corneal Surgery:New Strategies and Old Enemies, *Investigative Ophthalmology and Visual Science*, 1995; 1:4-8.

20. Gussler JR, Miller D, Jaffe M, Alfonso EC, Infection After Radial Keratotomy, *American Journal of Ophthalmology*, 1995; 6:798-799.

21. Casebeer JC, Shapiro DR, Phillips S, Severe Ocular Trauma without Corneal Rupture after RK, *Journal of Cataract and Refractive Surgery*, 1994; 1-2:31-33.

22. Pinheiro MN, Bryant MR, Tayyanipour R, et al., Corneal Integrity after Refractive Surgery, *Ophthalmology*, 1995, 2:297-301.

23. Campos M, Lee M, McDonnell PJ, Ocular Integrity after Refractive Surgery:Effects of Photorefractive Keratectomy, Phototherapeutic Keratectomy, and Radial Keratotomy, *Ophthalmic Surgery*, 1992; 9:598-602.

24. Lee BL, Manche EE, Glasgow BJ, Rupture of Radial and Arcuate Keratotomy Scars by Blunt Trauma 91 months after Incisional Keratotomy, *American Journal of Ophthalmology*, 1995; 7:108-110.

25. Salz JJ, Traumatic Corneal Abrasions Following Photorefractive Keratectomy, *Journal of Cataract and Refractive Surgery*, 1994; 1-2:36-37.

26. See note 22.

27. Burnstein Y, Klapper D, Hersh PS, Experimental Globe Rupture after Excimer Laser Photorefractive Keratectomy, *Archives of Ophthalmology*, 1995; 8:1056-1059.

28. Moreira H, Kolahdouz-Isfahani AH, Englanoff JS, *et al.*, Retrospective Comparison of Simultaneous and Non-Simultaneous Bilateral Radial Keratotomy, *Journal of Refractive and Corneal Surgery*, 1994; 10:545-549.

29. Szerenyi K, McDonnell JM, Smith RE, Keratitis as a Complication of Bilateral Simultaneous Radial Keratotomy, *American Journal of Ophthalmology*, 1994; 4:462-467.

30. Hong, JC, Salz JJ, Retrospective Comparison of Photorefractive Keratectomy and Radial Keratotomy, *Journal of Refractive Surgery*, 1995; 11/12-477-484.

31. American Academy of Ophthalmology, Radial Keratotomy for Myopia, *Ophthalmology*, 1993; 7:1103-1115.

32. Salz JJ, Foldable IOL Corrects High Myopia, Moderate Myopia, *Outlook Newsletter of the American Academy of Ophthalmology Refractive Surgery Interest Group*, Fall, 1995.

Additional Sources for Chapter 14

Alio J, Ismail M, Management of Radial Keratotomy Overcorrections by Corneal Sutures, *Journal of Cataract and Refractive Surgery*, 1993; 9:595-599.

Friedberg ML, Imperia PS, Elander R, et al., Results of Radial and Astigmatic Keratotomy by Beginning Refractive Surgeons, *Ophthalmology*, 1993; 5:746-751.

Jester JV, Villasensor RA, Schanzlin DJ, *et al.*, Variations in Corneal Wound Healing after Radial Keratotomy:Possible Insights into Mechanisms of Clinical Complications and Refractive Effects, *Cornea*, 1192; 5:191-199.

MacRae S, Cox W, Bedrossian R, Rich LF, The Treatment of Persistent Wound Leak after Radial Keratotomy, *Refractive Corneal Surgery*, 1993; 1-2:62-64.

Mader TH, Blanton CL, Gilbert BN, *et al.*, Refractive changes during 72-hour Exposure to High Altitude after Refractive Surgery, 1996; *Ophthalmology*, 8:1188-1195.

Olson RJ, Biddulph MC, Hyperopia, Anisometropia, and Irregular Astigmatism in a Patient Following Revisional Radial Keratotomy, *Ophthalmic Surgery*, 1992; 11:782-783.

Simon G, Ren Q, Biomechanical Behavior of the Cornea and its Response to Radial Keratotomy, *Journal of Cataract and Refractive Surgery*, 1994; 5-6:268-273.

CHAPTER 15

1. Sher NA, Hardten DR, Fundingsland B, et al., 193-nm excimer photorefractive keratectomy in high myopia. *Ophthalmology*, 1994; 9:1575-1582.

2. Snibson GR, McCarty CA, Aldred GF, Retreatment after Excimer Laser Photorefractive Keratectomy. The Melbourne Excimer Laser Group, *American Journal of Ophthalmology*, 1996; 3:250-257.

3. Krueger RR, Talamo JH, McDonald MB, *et al.*, Clinical Analysis of Excimer Laser Photorefractive Keratectomy Using a Multiple Zone Technique for Severe Myopia, *American Journal of Ophthalmology*, 1995; 119:263-274.

4. Pop M, Aras, M, Multizone Photorefractive Keratectomy:Six Month Results, *Journal of Cataract & Refractive Surgery*, 1995; 11:633-643.

5. Stein HA, Cheskes A, Stein RM, The Excimer Fundamentals and Clinical Use, *Slack Incorporated,* Thorofare, New Jersey,1995:84-93.

6. Lyle WA, Jin GJ, Initial Results of Automated Lamellar Keratoplasty for Correction of Myopia:One-Year Follow-up, *Journal of Cataract and Refractive Surgery,,* 1996; 1-2:31-43.

7. FDA Publication No. 96-1227, *Federal Drug Administration.*

8. McDonald MB, Will LASIK Supplant PRK by the Year 2000?, *Outlook Newsletter of the American Academy of Ophthalmology Refractive Surgery Interest Group,* Fall, 1995.

9. Brint, SF, Ostrick, OD, Fisher C, et al., Six-month results of the Multicenter Phase I study of Excimer Laser Myopic Keratomileusis, *Journal of Cataract & Refractive Surgery,* 1994; 11:610-615.

10. Kremer I, Blumenthal M, Myopic Keratomileusis In Situ Combined With Visx 20/20 Photorefractive Keratectomy. *Journal of Cataract & Refractive Surgery,* 1995; 9:508-511.

11. Salah T, Waring GO, el Maghraby A, Excimer Laser In Situ Keratomileusis Under a Corneal Flap for Myopia of 2 to 20 Diopters, American Journal of Ophthalmology, 1996; 2:143-155.

12. Guell JL, Muller A, Laser In Situ Keratomileusis (LASIK) for Myopia from -7 to -18 Diopters, Journal of Refractive Surgery, 1996; 2:222-228.

13. Helmy SA, Salah A, Badawy TT , Sidky AN, Photorefractive Keratectomy and Laser In-Situ Keratomileusis for Myopia between 6.00 and 10.00 Diopters, *Journal of Cataract & Refractive Surgery,* 1996; 3:417-421.

14. Hofman RF, Bechara SJ, An Independent Evaluation of Second Generation Suction Microkeratomes. *Refractive & Corneal Surgery,* 1992; 9-10:348-354.

15. Wachtlin J, Schuler A, Hoffmann F, Accuracy of Corneal Lenticules Produced for Lamellar Refractive Corneal Surgery, *Cornea,* 1995; 5:235-242.

16. See note 10.

17. American Academy of Ophthalmology, Automated Lamellar Keratoplasty—Preliminary Procedure Assessment, *Ophthalmology,* 1996; 5:852-861.

18. See note 6.

19. See note 9.

20. Frueh BE, Bohnke M, Endothelial Cell Morphology after Phototherapeutic Keratectomy, *German Journal of Ophthalmology,* 1995; 3:86-90.

21. See note 9.

22. See note 10.

23. See note 9.

24. See note 13.

25. Lyle WA, Jin GJ, Clear Lens Extraction for The Correction of High Refractive Error, *Journal of Cataract & Refractive Surgery,* 1994; 5:273-276.

26. Knorr HL, Jonas JB, Retinal Detachments by Squash Ball Accidents, *American Journal of Ophthalmology,* 1996; 8:260-261.

Additional Sources for Chapter 15

Pallikaris IG, Papatzanaki ME, Siganos DS, Tsilimbaris MK, A Corneal Flap Technique for Laser In Situ Keratomileusis. Human Studies, *Archives of Ophthalmology,* 1991; 12:1699-1702.

Stonecipher KG, Parmley VC, Rowsey JJ, *et al.*, Refractive Corneal Surgery with The Draeger Rotary Microkeratome in Human Cadaver Eyes. *Journal of Cataract & Refractive Surgery*, 1994; 1-2:49-55.

CHAPTER 16

1. Mortensen J, Ohrstrom A, Excimer Laser Photorefractive Keratectomy for Treatment of Keratoconus, *Journal of Refractive and Corneal Surgery*, 1994; 5-6:368-372.

2. Wilson SE, Klyce SD, Screening for Corneal Topographic Abnormalities before Refractive Surgery, Ophthalmology, 1994; 1:147-152.

3. Snibson GR, Carson CA, Aldred GF, Taylor HR, One-Year Evaluation of Excimer Laser Photorefractive Keratectomy for Myopia and Myopic Astigmatism, Melbourne Excimer Laser Group, *Archives of Ophthalmology*, 1995; 8:994-1000.

4. Spegelman AV, Albert WC, Cozean CH, *et al.*, Treatment of Myopic Astigmatism with the 193 nm Excimer Laser Utilizing Aperture Elements, *Journal of Refractive and Corneal Surgery*, 1994; 3:258-261.

5. Pender PM, Photorefractive Keratectomy for Myopic Astigmatism:Phase IIA of the Federal Drug Administration Study (12 to 18 Months Follow-up). Excimer Laser Study Group, J*ournal of Refractive and Corneal Surgery*, 1994; 1:13-17.

6. Price FW, Grene RB, Marks RG, Gonzales JS, ARC-T Study Group, Astigmatism Reduction Clinical Trial:a Multicenter Prospective Evaluation of the Predictability of Arcuate Keratotomy, *Archives of Ophthalmology*, 1995; 3:277-282.

7. Hvding G, Corneal Astigmatism. The Effect of Transverse corneal incisions, Acta Ophthalmol Scandinavia, 1995; 2:25-28.

8. Lipshitz I, Loewenstein A, Astigmatic Keratotomy followed by Photorefractive Keratectomy in the Treatment of Compound Myopic Astigmatism, *Journal of R*10b]994:3-4:S282-S284.

9. Pulaski JP, Transverse Incisions for Mixed and Myopic Idiopathic Astigmatism, J*ournal of Refractive and Corneal Surgery*, 1996; 4:307-312.

10. Alio JL, Ismail MM, Management of Astigmatic Keratotomy Overcorrections by Corneal Sutures, *Journal of Refractive and Corneal Surgery*, 1995; 5:348-350.

11. Chavez S, Chayet A, Celikkol L, Analysis of Astigmatic Keratotomy with a 5.0-mm Optical Clear Zone, *American Journal of Ophthalmology*, 1996; 1:65-76.

12. Martin RG, Wedge Resection in the Cone after Failed Refractive Surgery in a Patient with Keratoconus, *Journal of Refractive and Corneal Surgery*, 1995; 5:348-350.

Additional Sources for Chapter 16

Friedberg ML, Imperia PS, Elander R, Results of Radial and Astigmatic Keratotomy by Beginning Refractive Surgeons, Ophthalmology, 1993; 5:746-751.

CHAPTER 17

1. Department of Health and Human Services, Procedures for Adding the Monovison Fitting Technique to the Labeling of Class III Single Vision Contact Lenses for Managing Presbyopia, *Food and Drug Administration*, March 8, 1994.

2. Bierly JR, Furgason, TG, *et al* ., *Contact Lens Association of Opthalmologists Journal, 1995*; 4:96-98.

CHAPTER 18

1. Kraff CR, Excimer Correction of Hyperopia:A Look at the Clinical Challenges, O*utlook Newsletter of the Refractive Surgery Interest Group*, Fall, 1995.

2. American Academy of Ophthalmology, Automated Lamellar Keratoplasty—Preliminary Procedure Assessment, *Ophthalmology,* 1996; 5:852-861.

3. Dausch D, Klein R, Schroder E, Excimer Laser Photorefractive Keratectomy for Hyperopia. *Refractive Corneal Surgery,* 1993; 1-2:20-28.

4. Durrie DS, Schumer DJ, Cavanaugh TB, *Journal of Refractive and Corneal Surgery,* 1994; 3-4:S277-S280.

5. Koch DD, Abarca A, Villarreal R, *et al.* Hyperopia Correction by Noncontact Holmium:YAG Laser Thermal Keratoplasy, Clinical Study with Two-Year Follow-up, *Ophthalmology,* 1996; 5:731-740.

6. Kohnen T, Husain SE, Koch DD, Corneal Topographic Changes after Noncontact Holmium:YAG Laser Thermal Keratoplasty to Correct Hyperopia, *Journal of Refractive and Corneal Surgery,* 1996; 5:427-435.

7. Lyle WA, Jin GJ, Clear Lens Extraction For The Correction of High Refractive Error, *Journal of Refractive and Corneal Surgery,* 1994; 5:273-276.

8. Siganos DS, Siganos CS, Pallikaris IG, Clear Lens Extraction and Intraocular Lens Implantation in Normally Sighted Hyperopic Eyes, *Journal of Refractive and Corneal Surgery,* 1994; 3-4:117-121.

Additional Sources for Chapter 18

Jackson WB, Mintsioulis G, Agapitos PJ, Casson E, Excimer Laser Photorefractive Keratectomy for Low Hyperopia: An Assessment of Safety and Efficacy, *University of Ottawa Eye Institute, Ottawa General Hospital,* (Ottawa, Ontario).

Vrabec MP, Durrie DS, Hunkeler JD, Arcuate Keratotomy for The Correction of Spherical Hyperopia in Human Cadaver Eyes. *Refractive Corneal Surgery,* 1993; 102:2388-391.

CHAPTER 19

1. Fagerholm P, Fitzsimmons TD, Orndahl M, Ohman L, Tengroth B, Phototherapeutic Keratectomy:Long-term Results in 166 Eyes, *Refractive Corneal Surgery,* 1993; 3-4:S76 -S81.

2. Rogers C, Cohen P, Lawless M, Phototherapeutic Keratectomy for Reis Bucklers' Corneal Dystrophy, *Australia/New Zealand Journal of Ophthalmology,* 1993; 11:247-250.

3. Hersh PS, Burnstein Y, Carr J, *et al.,* Excimer Laser Phototherapeutic Keratectomy. Surgical Strategies and Clinical Outcomes, *Ophthalmology,* 1996; 8:1210-1222.

4. Tuunanen TH, Tervo TM, Excimer Laser Phototherapeutic Keratectomy for Corneal Diseases:A Follow-up Study, *Contact Lens Association of Opthalmologists Journal,* 1995;1:67-72.

5. See note 1.

6. Binder PS, Anderson JA, Rock ME, Vrabec MP, Human Excimer Laser Keratectomy. Clinical and histopathologic Correlations, *Ophthalmology,* 1994; 6:979-989.

Additional Sources for Chapter 19

Anastas CN, McGhee CN, Webber SK, Bryce IG, Corneal Tattooing Revisited:Excimer Laser in the Treatment of Unsightly Leucomata, *Australia New Zealand Journal of Ophthalmology,* 1995:8:227-230.

Chan WK, Hunt, KE, Glasgow BJ, Mondino BJ, Corneal Scarring after Photorefractive Keratectomy in a Penetrating Keratoplasty, *American Journal of Ophthalmology,* 1996; 5:570-571.

Lazzaro DR, Haight DH, Belmont SC, *et al.,* Excimer Laser Keratectomy for Astigmatism Occurring after Penetrating Keratoplasty, *Ophthalmology,* 1996; 3:458-464.

Index

Is Someone You Care About Considering Vision Correction?

Here's how to order more copies of Beyond Glasses!
Shipping is Free!

1. YOUR NAME

Name_____

Company_____

Street/box:_____

City_____

State/Province_____Zip/Postal Code_____

Day Telephone: Very important! (_____) _____ - _____

2. SHIP TO ADDRESS (if different from above)

Name_____

Company_____

Street/box:_____

City_____

State/Province_____Zip/Postal Code_____

3. GIFT? Please tell us what message you would like included:

_____

_____

4. HOW MANY?

_____ copies of *Beyond Glasses!*

5. CALCULATE YOUR TOTAL

Number of copies _____ X $19.95 ($28.95 Canada)=_____

$1.65 sales tax *per copy* (CA residents only):   =_____

Your Total: $_____

6. MAIL CHECK AND ORDER FORM TO:

UC Books
43 Danville Square, Box 1036
Danville, California 94526

Please allow 7-10 days for delivery.

Is Someone You Care About Considering Vision Correction?

Here's how to order more copies of Beyond Glasses!
Shipping is Free!

---

1. YOUR NAME

Name_____

Company_____

Street/box:_____

City_____

State/Province_____Zip/Postal Code_____

Day Telephone: Very important! (_____) _____ - _____

2. SHIP TO ADDRESS (if different from above)

Name_____

Company_____

Street/box:_____

City_____

State/Province_____Zip/Postal Code_____

3. GIFT? Please tell us what message you would like included:

_____

_____

4. HOW MANY?

_____ copies of *Beyond Glasses!*

5. CALCULATE YOUR TOTAL

Number of copies _____ X $19.95 ($28.95 Canada)=_____

$1.65 sales tax *per copy* (CA residents only):   =_____

Your Total: $_____

6. MAIL CHECK AND ORDER FORM TO:

UC Books
43 Danville Square, Box 1036
Danville, California 94526

Please allow 7-10 days for delivery.

About the Author

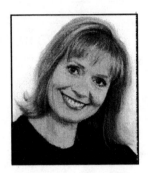

*F*ranette Armstrong has translated the benefits of technology to consumers since the earliest microcomputers and is the president of a marketing communications agency serving some of the nation's largest corporations. She and her husband live in the San Francisco Bay Area where, thanks to laser vision correction, she enjoys good natural vision for the first time in her life.

"I wrote *Beyond Glasses!* to help others understand how they can safely take advantage of the new treatments," the author explained. "Laser vision correction is a modern miracle, there's no doubt about it, but every procedure isn't right for every person. Since the FDA approved PRK, some doctors have begun to promote related procedures that are quite risky compared to standard PRK, haven't been adequately studied, and haven't yet been approved. I knew nothing about any of this when I had my own vision corrected, and I was lucky. With this book, people won't have to rely on luck to see what they've been missing."

Ms. Armstrong has written several books in the fields of business and education as well as numerous articles, scripts and business publications.